Topographic Mapping of Brain Electrical Activity

Participants in "Progress in Topographic Mapping of Neurophysiologic Data," October 16–17, 1984, Boston, Massachusetts.

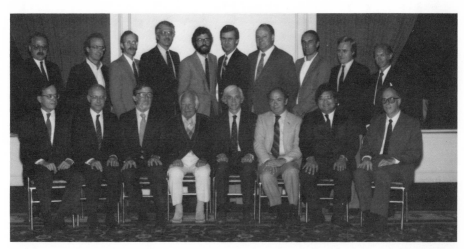

FROM LEFT TO RIGHT: *Front Row:* J.E. Desmedt, D. Lehmann, D.O. Walter, R.G. Bickford, F.H. Duffy, M.S. Buchsbaum, J.M. Morihisa, H. Petsche. *Back Row:* A.F. Schatzberg, P. Etevenon, R. Coppola, R.N. Harner, G. Sandini, D.G. Childers, P.H. Bartels, G. Pfurt-scheller, P. Rappelsberger, A. Persson.

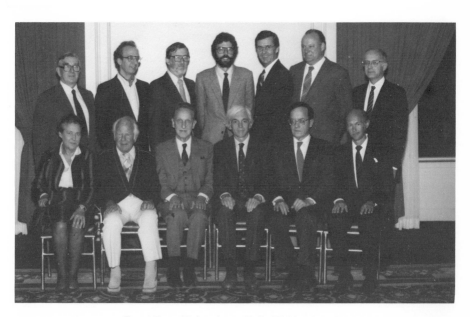

FROM LEFT TO RIGHT: *Front Row:* N. Lesèvre, R.G. Bickford, A. Rémond, F.H. Duffy, J.E. Desmedt, A. Persson. *Back Row:* D. Fender, P. Etevenon, D.O. Walter, G. Sandini, D.G. Childers, P.H. Bartels, D. Lehmann.

Topographic Mapping of Brain Electrical Activity

Edited by
Frank H. Duffy, M.D.

Associate Professor of Neurology, Harvard Medical School,
and Director of Developmental Neurophysiology,
The Children's Hospital, Boston, Massachusetts

With 45 contributing authors

Butterworths

Boston London Durban Singapore Sydney Toronto Wellington

*Every effort has been made to ensure that the drug dosage schedules
within this text are accurate and conform to standards accepted at
time of publication. However, as treatment recommendations vary in
light of continuing research and clinical experience, the reader is
advised to verify drug dosage schedules herein with information
found on product information sheets. This is especially true in cases
of new or infrequently used drugs.*

Library of Congress Cataloging in Publication Data
Main entry under title:

Topographic mapping of brain electrical activity.

    Includes index.
    1. Electroencephalography.   2. Evoked potentials
(Electrophysiology) I. Duffy, Frank H.
RC386.6.E43T67   1986   616.8'047547   85-15156
ISBN 0-409-90008-7

Butterworth Publishers
80 Montvale Avenue
Stoneham, MA   02180

10 9 8 7 6 5 4 3 2 1

Printed in the United States of America

To N. David Culver,
in appreciation

Contents

Contributing Authors

Barry Allen, Ph.D.
Vice-President Research and
Development, Allen
Microcomputer Services, Inc.,
San Diego, California

Ron Ball, M.S.
Senior Programmer, Department of
Psychiatry, University of California,
Irvine, Irvine, California

Hubert G. Bartels, M.S.E.
Senior Programmer, Optical
Sciences Center, University of
Arizona, Tucson, Arizona

Peter H. Bartels, Ph.D.
Professor of Optical Sciences and of
Pathology, University of Arizona
School of Medicine, Tucson,
Arizona

I. Bertoldi
Neurological Testing Service,
Centre Hospitalier et Universitaire
de Rouen, Rouen, France

Reginald G. Bickford, M.D.,
F.R.C.P.
Professor Emeritus of
Neurosciences, University of
California, San Diego, School of
Medicine, La Jolla, California

Monte S. Buchsbaum, M.D.
Professor of Psychiatry, University
of California, Irvine, College of
Medicine, Irvine, California

Keith H. Chiappa, M.D.
Assistant Professor of Neurology,
Harvard Medical School, Boston,
Massachusetts

Donald G. Childers, Ph.D.
Professor of Electrical Engineering,
University of Florida, Gainesville,
Florida

Richard Coppola, D.Sc.
Senior Scientist, Laboratory of
Psychology and Psychopathology,
National Institute of Mental Health,
Bethesda, Maryland

John E. Desmedt, M.D.
Professor and Director, Brain
Research Unit, University of
Brussels, Brussels, Belgium

J. Y. Doris
Neurological Testing Service,
Centre Hospitalier et Universitaire
de Rouen, Rouen, France

E. Dreano
Neurological Testing Service,
Centre Hospitalier et Universitaire
de Rouen, Rouen, France

Frank H. Duffy, M.D.
Associate Professor of Neurology,
Harvard Medical School, Boston,
Massachusetts

Glen R. Elliott, M.D.
Research Physician, Department of
Psychiatry and Behavioral Sciences,
Stanford University School of
Medicine, Stanford, California

Pierre Etevenon, D.Sc.
Director of Research (Université
René Descartes, Paris V),
Quantitative EEG Laboratory,
Centre Hospitalier Ste.-Anne and
INSERM, Paris, France

Richard N. Harner, M.D.
Professor and Vice Chairman,
Department of Neurology, Medical
College of Pennsylvania,
Philadelphia, Pennsylvania

Erin Hazlett
Staff Research Associate,
Department of Psychiatry,
University of California, Irvine,
Irvine, California

Bo Hjorth, Dr.Med.Sc.
Research Engineer, Research and
Development Laboratory, Siemens-
Elema AB, Solna, Sweden

Steven Johnson, M.D.
Resident Physician, Department of
Psychiatry, University of California,
Irvine Medical Center, Long Beach
Veterans Administration Medical
Center, Orange, California

Dietrich Lehmann, M.D.
Professor of Neurology and Clinical
Neurophysiology, University
Hospitals, Zurich, Switzerland

Jan E. Lerbinger, B.A.
Research Assistant,
Psychopharmacological Program,
McLean Hospital, Belmont,
Massachusetts

Nicole Lesèvre, Ph.D.
Director, CNRS Experimental
Electrophysiology and
Neurophysiology Research Group,
Hôpital de la Salpêtrière, Paris,
France

Barbara Marcel, M.S.
Clinical and Research Fellow,
McLean Hospital, Belmont,
Massachusetts

Robert W. McCarley, M.D.
Professor of Psychiatry, Harvard
Medical School, Boston,
Laboratory of Neurophysiology,
Massachusetts Mental Health
Center, Boston, Massachusetts, The
Brockton V.A. Center

John M. Morihisa, M.D.
Psychiatrist-in-Chief, VAMC,
Washington, D.C., Professor of
Psychiatry, Georgetown University,
School of Medicine, Washington,
D.C.

Ken Nagata, M.D.
Division of Neurology, Research
Institute for Brain and Blood
Vessels–Akita, Akita, Japan

Anders Persson, M.D.
Assistant Professor of Clinical
Neurophysiology, Karolinska
Institutet, Stockholm, Sweden

Hellmuth Petsche, Dr.med.
University Professor and Director,
Institute of Neurophysiology,
University of Vienna, Vienna,
Austria

Gert Pfurtscheller, Ph.D.
Professor, Department of
Computing, Institute of Biomedical
Engineering, Technical University
of Graz, Graz, Austria

Helmut Pockberger
Institute of Neurophysiology,
University of Vienna, Vienna,
Austria

Peter Rappelsberger
Institute of Neurophysiology,
University of Vienna, Vienna,
Austria

Antoine Rémond, M.D.
Director of Research, Laboratory of
Electrophysiology and Applied
Neurophysiology, Hôpital de la
Salpêtrière, Paris, France

Paolo Romano, M.D.
Research Associate, Department of
Communication, Computer, and
Systems Sciences, University of
Genoa, Genoa, Italy

D. Samson-Dollfus
Director, Neurological Testing
Service, Centre Hospitalier et
Universitaire de Rouen, Rouen,
France

Giulio Sandini, Ph.D.
Associate Professor, Department of
Communication, Computer, and
Systems Science, University of
Genoa, Genoa, Italy

Alan F. Schatzberg, M.D.
Interim Psychiatrist-in-Chief,
McLean Hospital, Belmont,
Massachusetts

Harold W. Shipton, C.Eng.
Professor of Biomedical
Engineering, Washington
University, St. Louis, Missouri

Fumio Shishido, M.D.
Senior Researcher, Department of
Radiology and Nuclear Medicine,
Research Institute for Brain and
Blood Vessels–Akita, Akita, Japan

Nancy Sicotte
Research Associate, Department of
Psychiatry, University of California,
Irvine, Irvine, California

Wolfgang Skrandies, Ph.D.
Department of Experimental
Ophthalmology, Max Planck
Institute for Physiological and
Clinical Research, Bad Nauheim,
Federal Republic of Germany

Koichi Tagawa, M.D.
Director, Division of Neurology,
Research Institute for Brain and
Blood Vessels–Akita, Akita, Japan

Michael W. Torello, Ph.D.
Assistant Professor of Psychiatry,
Department of Psychiatry, The
Ohio State University College of
Medicine, Columbus, Ohio

Z. Tsouria
Instructor in Psychiatry, National
Institute of Medicine, Oran, Algeria

H. Richard Tyler, M.D.
Division of Neurology, Brigham
and Women's Hospital, Boston,
Massachusetts

Kazuo Uemura, M.D.
Director, Division of Radiology and
Nuclear Medicine, Research
Institute for Brain and Blood
Vessels–Akita, Akita, Japan

Preface

Topographic mapping has been used for many years in a number of disciplines, including electroencephalography. Recent technological advances, primarily computerization, have spurred renewed research into applications of the technique. The intent of this book is to clarify the current state of this emerging technology, to assess its potential for substantive contributions to brain research, to delineate necessary areas of further research, and to envision resultant clinical applications.

The impetus for this volume was an international symposium, "Progress in Topographic Mapping of Neurophysiological Data," held in Boston under the auspices of The Children's Hospital, Harvard Medical School. Drawing on the interchange of ideas and opinions presented at the conference, participants were asked to prepare a chapter delineating their recent research activities or areas of concern, or to provide critical commentary. The research and discourse of 46 neuroscientists, researchers, and physicians are presented here. These authors, representing research laboratories in many parts of Europe, Japan, and the United States, include both the pioneers and the current experts in this exciting field.

Reflecting the growing interest in the use of topographic mapping to interpret and amplify data on neuroelectrical activity of the brain, the symposium sought to present a diversity of opinion through both favorable and critical commentary. We believe the reader will find that the different chapters present a stimulating range of viewpoints. The spectrum of topics includes summaries of the genesis and development of topographic mapping in medical research, technical aspects of method and analytic paradigms, and clinical applications directed to a range of disorders.

The authors approached both the symposium and their chapter contributions with a high level of enthusiasm and a commitment to substantive dialogue and general excellence. I wish to express my sincere appreciation to all these respected scientists. I would also like to thank Children's Hospital, Inc., of Harvard Medical School and Braintech, Inc., for graciously sponsoring the symposium. I am grateful also to David and Gloria McAnulty for their efforts in organizing the symposium and in the editing of this volume.

Topographic mapping—brain electrical activity mapping—is becoming established as a tool used in the diagnosis and treatment of neurological dysfunction, yet its form has not yet crystalized. Nonetheless, its move to the clinic has begun. I hope this first book wholly devoted to the topic will expand awareness of the potentials and applications of this promising technology.

F. H. Duffy

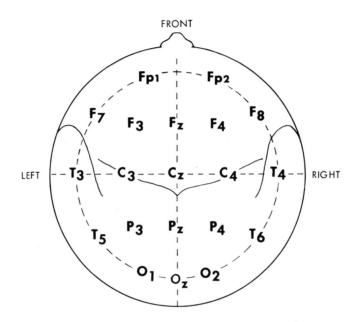

International 10–20 System of Electrode Placement: The figure provides the alphanumeric designations of electrode placement on the scalp for electroencephalographic (EEG) recordings. These standard locations are frequently referenced by our contributing authors in this book.

Color Imaging of Scalp Somatosensory Evoked Potential Fields

John E. Desmedt

Progress in the clinical application of averaged sensory evoked potentials involves a better understanding of the neural generators of the components of recorded profiles, both in health and in disease. However, interpretations based on single or even a few averaged traces may be biased by the selection of electrode sites or montages; some waveform features may be given undue significance, and the true significance of others may be overlooked.

The current data base can be extended by detailed spatial delineation of evoked potential fields. This chapter presents some features of the scalp distribution of human somatosensory evoked potentials (SEP). The use of many channels raises problems of data management unless an accurately computerized display of the embedded spatiotemporal information can be created through novel imaging resources [1–6]. Here the time history of SEP fields was visualized by animation effects through series of frozen maps at approximately 1 msec intervals.

METHODS

The imaging of SEP fields was implemented through appropriate software on a PDP 11–34 Digital Equipment computer. For bit-mapped imaging, 16 electrodes were arranged over both sides of the scalp with earlobe as the common reference. The head, assumed to be spherical, was projected onto a two-dimensional circular outline about the Cz electrode such that the arc length from each electrode to Cz was proportional to its radial distance from center on the two-dimensional circular top view of the head. The system surveyed the entire head. Bit-mapped images were drawn on paper by the microprocessor-based 4695 Tektronix Color Graphics Copier. The maximum width of the graphic field was 256 pixels (picture elements). Each map was created by 1074 pixels.

In map computation the 16 pixels overlying each electrode site were assigned the recorded numerical values of potential. The other pixel values were computed through a four-point linear interpolation algorithm using the 4 nearest electrodes as identified by standard analytic geometry. Potential values were each given a weight that was in inverse linear proportion to the distance from the pixel to each of the four electrodes considered.

Voltage values were then fitted to a scale of discrete levels imaged by different hues. Details are given in Desmedt [7] for recording methods, and in Desmedt and Nguyen [5] and Desmedt and Bourguet [6] for bit-mapped SEP imaging.

RESULTS

This chapter considers recent results about the SEPs elicited by electrical stimulation of fingers or the median nerve at the wrist. With earlobe reference recording, averaged SEPs show no distortion of focal cortical components (Figure 1.1) [8]. These are quite different on either side of the central fissure, and the recording electrodes have been deliberately placed either in front of or behind the central region (where such components tend to be confounded). Early SEP components are labeled as N20 and P27 over the parietal scalp contralateral to the upper limb stimulated, and P22 and N30 over the prerolandic region. The frontal N30 can diffuse with smaller voltage over the ipsilateral parietal region (Figure 1.1B) The earlobe reference recording also displays the P14 far field thought to reflect the medial lemniscus volley (Figure 1.1) [9,10].

Scalp evoked potential fields are displayed as a series of frozen maps at 1-msec intervals for the first 70 msec after the stimulus. To save space, only 15 such maps at selected latencies are shown (Plate 1). Latencies expressed in milliseconds after stimulation are printed below each map. In a given subject, median nerve or fingers I-IV stimulation evokes similar SEP field patterns, but the finger SEPs are delayed by about 3 msec due to extra conduction distance from fingers to wrist.

With the scalp initially at about zero potential (green), the widespread P14 (blue) appears at 11–12 msec in this subject, who has short arms, and hence SEP onset latencies somewhat smaller than the average. The first focal event is negative (black/yellow) over the right (contralateral) parietal scalp at 15 msec and corresponds to the N20 response. One millisecond later, this N20 has increased in voltage (red) while a P22 focus appears over the midfront. The P22 field increases in voltage and area and persists after dissipation of N20 at 20 msec.

The maps evidence a clearly earlier onset of P22 at midfront than over the central region. Hence the P22 onset latency is best measured 3 to 6 cm in front of Cz plane. Mean transit time from N20 next onset to P22 onset is 0.81 msec and P22 never starts before N20 [6].

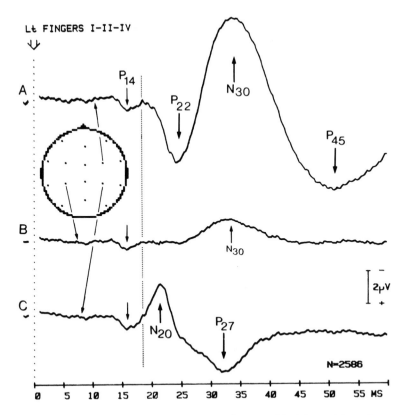

Figure 1.1. SEPs to left fingers I-II-IV, stimulation recorded with right earlobe reference in a normal 23-year-old man. Electrode positions indicated in the figurine (top view of the head). All traces show a P14 far field whose termination is indicated by a vertical dotted line. A: Right (contralateral) prerolandic site with large P22 and N30 followed by a P45. B: Left parietal site with only an attenuated N30 diffusing from frontal regions after the P14. C: Right parietal site with N20 and P27, but no P45 in this example. From Desmedt and Bourguet [6] (with permission from Elsevier Biomedical Press, Amsterdam).

No significant N20-P27 appeared at the ipsilateral parietal scalp [8,11–13]. A large bilateral N30 next develops frontally while a focal P27 (blue) appears at the right parietal region at 22–34 msec. The map at 21 msec is actually hitting two distinct positive foci that probably correspond to P22 and P27, respectively.

DISCUSSION

With current developments in metabolic or anatomical imaging by computerized tomography (CT) or positron emission tomography (PET) scans, xenon blood flow, or magnetic resonance (MR), it is important for electrical brain studies to provide compatible imaging of comprehensive topographic features. Bit-mapped color imaging of evoked potential fields on the volume conductor of head and neck is a highly promising noninvasive method for extracting pertinent information from multichannel electrical recordings of brain potentials.

SEP imaging helps us to reconsider current views of cortical SEP components that were based on descriptions of analog traces. SEP mapping of the scalp convexity proves feasible with a system of 16 channels whereby smooth contours with clear foci can be created (see Plate 1). One important feature of our study has been the avoidance of the central scalp region and use of an electrode system with electrodes about 3.5 cm either in front of or behind the central (Cz) plane: this prevents confounding the precentral with the postcentral neural generators and allows the N20 and P22 sets of SEP components to be clearly delineated [6].

The data substantiate the view that distinct cortical generators are involved in the N20, P27, and P22 SEP components of median nerve stimulation [8,13,14]. The N20 and P27 fields are restricted to the contralateral parietal scalp and do not appear ipsilaterally. The onset of the prerolandic P22 field is about 1 msec after the onset of the N20 field. The P22 offset is not synchronous with that of N20 (see Plate 1).

The prerolandic P22 field is also clearly distinct in timing and scalp location from the parietal P27 field. In other words, P22 reflects activities in prerolandic neuron populations at a time when no P27-related activities have yet appeared, and P27 involves other (parietal) neuron populations at a later time. These results refute the hypothesis that the parietal N20 and prerolandic N22 are mirror images generated concurrently in the depth of the central sulcus by a single dipole generator whose anterior half gives rise to P22 and posterior half to N20. The mapped P27 field that is confined to the contralateral parietal scalp is thought to reflect transactions in somatosensory receiving subareas. Several parietal generators are no doubt involved in both N20 and P27 SEP components.

The mapped N30 field was quite extensive over the precentral region on both sides. N30 and P22 probably do not share identical generators because they can be dissociated in some subjects. For example, N30 decreased in voltage in normal aging while P22 was preserved or actually enhanced [8,13]. The ipsilateral extension of the N30 field did not necessarily reflect the existence of direct ipsilateral projections because no ipsilateral N30 was recorded in the remaining frontal cortex after surgical hemispherectomy [15,16]. The evidence is compatible with generation of N30 in the supplementary motor area (SMA), which is close to the midline (see N30 field, Plate 1) and which receives projections from motor area 4 and parietal areas 1, 2, and 5 [17].

The prerolandic P22 must be generated primarily by motor area 4, which is the direct recipient of thalamocortical projections from ventral posterolateral oralis-ventral lateral candalis VPLo-VLc. However, we do not exclude a contribution to P22 from supplementary motor areas since SEP imaging data disclose extension of the P22 focus over the SMA (see Plate 1). Our emphasis on direct projections to motor cortex does not exclude a corollary role for the known corticocortical connections from parietal area 2 to motor area 4, and from areas 1, 2, and 5 to SMA [17,18]. Further data and discussion of these issues is presented in Desmedt and Bourguet [6].

ACKNOWLEDGMENTS

This research has been supported by the Fonds de la Recherche Scientifique Médicale, Belgium.

REFERENCES

1. Ragot, R.A., and Rémond, A. EEG field mapping. Electroenceph. Clin. Neurophysiol. 1978; 45:417–421.
2. Duffy, F., Burchfiel, J.L., and Lombroso, C.T. Brain electrical activity mapping (BEAM): A method for extending the clinical utility of EEG and evoked potentials data. Ann. Neurol. 1979; 5:309–321.
3. Lehmann, D., and Skrandies, W. Reference-free identification of components of checkerboard-evoked multichannel potential fields. Electroenceph. Clin. Neurophysiol. 1980; 48:609–621.
4. Buchsbaum, M.S., Rigal, F., Coppola, R., et al. A new system for gray-level surface distribution maps of electrical activity. Electroenceph. Clin. Neurophysiol. 1982; 53:237–242.
5. Desmedt, J.E., and Nguyen, T.H. Bit-mapped color imaging of potential fields generated by propagated and segmental subcortical components of somatosensory evoked potentials in man. Electroenceph. Clin. Neurophysiol. 1984; 58:481–497.
6. Desmedt, J.E., and Bourguet, M. Color imaging of scalp topography of parietal and frontal components of somatosensory evoked potentials to stimulation of median or posterior tibial nerve in man. Electroenceph. Clin. Neurophysiol. 1985; 62: 1–17.
7. Desmedt, J.E. Some observations on the methodology of cerebral evoked potentials in man. In J.E. Desmedt, ed., Attention, Voluntary Contraction and Event-Related Cerebral Potentials, Prog. Clin. Neurophysiol. Basel; Karger, 1977; 1: 12–29.
8. Desmedt, J.E., and Cheron, G. Non-cephalic reference recording of early somatosensory potentials to finger stimulation in adult or aging man: Differentiation of widespread N18 and contralateral N20 from the prerolandic P22 and N30 components. Electroenceph. Clin. Neurophysiol. 1981; 52:553–570.
9. Desmedt, J.E., and Cheron, G. Central somatosensory conduction in man: neural generators and interpeak latencies of the far-field components recorded from neck and right or left scalp and earlobes. Electroenceph. Clin. Neurophysiol. 1980; 50: 382–403.

10. Suzuki, I., and Mayanagi, Y. Intracranial recording of short-latency somatosensory evoked potentials in man: Identification of origin of each component. Electroenceph. Clin. Neurophysiol. 1984; 59:286–296.

11. Goff, W.R., Rosner, B.S., and Allison, T. Distribution of somatosensory evoked responses in normal man. Electroenceph. Clin. Neurophysiol. 1962; 14:697–713.

12. Desmedt, J.E. Somatosensory cerebral evoked potentials in man. In A. Rémond, ed., Handbook of Electroencephalography and Clinical Neurophysiology. Amsterdam: Elsevier, 1971; 9:55–82.

13. Desmedt, J.E., and Cheron, G. Somatosensory evoked potentials to finger stimulation in healthy octogenarians and in young adults: Waveforms, scalp topography and transit times of parietal and frontal components. Electroenceph. Clin. Neurophysiol. 1980; 50:404–425.

14. Mauguière, F., Desmedt, J.E., and Courjon, J. Astereognosis and dissociated loss of frontal or parietal components of somatosensory evoked potentials in hemispheric lesions: Detailed correlations with clinical signs and computerized tomography scanning. Brain 1983; 106:271–311.

15. Hazemann, P., Olivier, L., and Dupont, E. Potentiels évoqués somesthésiques recueillis sur le scalp chez 6 hémisphérectomisés. Rev. Neurol. Paris 1969; 121: 246–257.

16. Noel, P., and Desmedt, J.E. Cerebral and farfield somatosensory evoked potentials in neurological disorders. In J.E. Desmedt, ed., Clinical Uses of Cerebral, Brainstem and Spinal Somatosensory Evoked Potentials, Prog. Clin. Neurophysiol. Basel: Karger, 1980; 7:205–230.

17. Jones, E.G., Coulter, J.D., and Hendry, S.H.C. Intracortical connectivity of architectonic fields in the somatic sensory, motor and parietal cortex of monkeys. J. Comp. Neurol. 1978; 181:291–348.

18. Jones, E.G. The nature of the afferent pathways conveying short-latency inputs to the primate motor cortex. In J.E. Desmedt, ed., Motor Control Mechanisms in Health and Disease, New York: Raven Press, 1983; 263–285.

2

Visual Evoked Potential Topography: Methods and Results

Wolfgang Skrandies

Most workers in the fields of electroencephalography and evoked potentials consider topographic analysis to be a method which defines the intracranial sources of scalp-recorded electrical brain activity. It is a physical fact that the potential distribution on the scalp is determined by the instantaneous configuration and location of active intracranial neural populations. But it is important to keep in mind that the reverse is not true: The scalp field configuration does not allow us to predict uniquely the underlying intracranial sources (the "inverse problem"). Computations to localize model dipoles have to rest on certain assumptions regarding conductivity and geometry of intracranial media, as well as the number and arrangement of electrical model dipoles, in order to yield meaningful results [1–3]. Due to the "inverse problem" and the physiological fact that virtually thousands of neural generators are active at any moment in time, the ambitious goal of intracranial generator localization from scalp field data presently appears less attainable and of less practical value than expected.

In this chapter I try to define another goal of topographic analysis. Scalp distributions are being investigated not to identify intracranial sources directly, but to characterize brain electrical events unambiguously in terms of latency and scalp location. Scalp topography provides a basis for testing hypotheses concerning the processing of different aspects of sensory information by the central nervous system. Whether or not the exact intracranial sources of the scalp-recorded brain activity are known, the interpretation of scalp field data, combined with knowledge of the anatomy and physiology of sensory brain systems, allows meaningful conclusions to be drawn. Comparisons of scalp distributions evoked in different experimental conditions give useful information on the identity (or nonidentity) of the neural populations activated in these conditions. Nonidentical scalp fields must be caused by different neural generator mechanisms, whereas identical distributions may or may not be generated by different neural populations. This chapter discusses how scalp-recorded brain activity can be used to gain insight into complex electrical brain mechanisms independent of the inherent shortcomings of the "indirect" recording method which is, in general, the only possible method in humans.

BASIC CONSIDERATIONS

Surface-recorded brain activity reflects the mass response of large neural populations, which spreads instantaneously throughout the brain via volume conduction. Auditory stimuli evoke potential components of very short latency that can be recorded from the intact scalp, and that are believed to reflect the electrical activity at early processing stages of the auditory pathway at the level of the brain stem [4]. In the cat visual system, field potentials generated by the optic nerve and optic tract can be recorded at widespread regions of the brain [5]. The mass activity of the Y-, X-, and W-ganglion cells of the cat retina that is elicited by electrical stimulation of the optic nerve may be discriminated at the optic disc, and the field potentials "stray" from the retina into the vitreous body of the eye and persist even when the electrode is several millimeters in front of the retinal surface [5]. This illustrates that potential components recorded at a given point in the nervous sytem need not be generated at that site. Thus, careful statements about the location of neural generator populations of components of evoked brain activity require a solid experimental and physiological basis.

The problem of the position of the reference electrode is a traditional discussion topic in electroencephalography (EEG) work and has received much attention in the literature. This chapter shows how this issue can be dealt with, and how surface-recorded EEG data can be interpreted unambiguously.

Electrical brain activity is recorded as potential differences between recording points on the human scalp. The position of both the reference and the recording electrode influences the waveform pattern of electrical activity. In general, waveforms are ambiguous in terms of amplitude and phase of electrical events analyzed over time. On the other hand, the characteristics of the underlying electrical fields of the brain (and thus of the scalp fields) are constant and reference-independent at each moment in time, and accordingly, only electrical fields may be interpreted in a meaningful way [6]. A strict topographic analysis can be applied to electrical scalp fields in order to avoid the problem of the reference electrode [7–9].

As illustrated by Lehmann (Chapter 3), mapping the power of different frequency bands of spontaneous EEG activity yields conflicting, reference-dependent results. Confusion also arises when evoked potential waveshapes are analyzed. Visual evoked potentials (VEPs) recorded from nine midline electrodes to a checkerboard reversal stimulus are shown in Figure 2.1. Surprisingly, the occipitally positive component shows different peak latencies in different recording channels (e.g., channel 6 has a peak latency of 99 msec; channel 7: 104 msec; channel 8: 107 msec; channel 9: 114 msec). One might interpret these changes in latency as evoked activity moving from anterior to posterior brain areas. Changing the location of the reference electrode yields an even more complex picture. The same data set recorded against other reference sites is illustrated in Figure 2.2. On the left, the data of Figure 2.1 are referred to the vertex reference, in the center an electrode 2.5 cm posterior to the vertex is used as reference, and on the right an electrode 5 cm posterior to the vertex is used as reference. In addition to the latency differences occurring in different recording channels, there appear to be changes in latency depending on the reference chosen: For example, for electrode 6, we find peak latencies of 101, 102, or 103 msec. It is important to keep in mind that we are looking at identical data (the same set of data recomputed), and that all our statements on peak latencies are correct. There is no reason to prefer one set of waveforms over the other. This dilemma of waveshape variability and ambiguous data interpretation can only be overcome by a reference-independent analysis technique.

In reality, there is no such thing as electrical brain activity wandering over larger distances on the scalp [10], or different component latencies in different recording channels. This becomes clear when the data are treated as an electrical field. In Figure 2.3 the data are displayed as a potential profile at 106 msec latency. This is a simple rearrangement of the data: the amplitude values at 106 msec are measured in each channel and are entered at their respective electrode

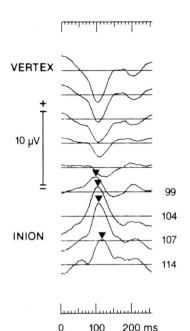

Figure 2.1. Potential wave shapes evoked by a 30-min arc reversing checkerboard pattern presented with 62% contrast as a test field of 8.7-x-11.4-degree arc to the upper hemiretina. Arrowheads and numbers indicate peak latencies. The electrode array starts at the vertex and extends in regular steps to 2 cm below the inion. Data are referred to the average reference.

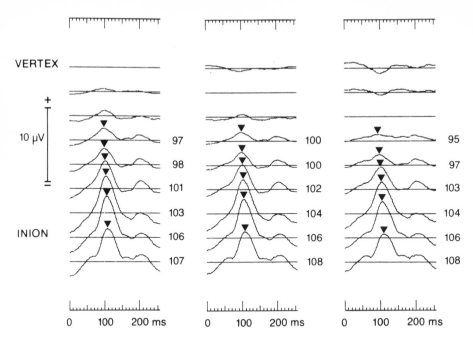

Figure 2.2. Data of Figure 2.1 computed against different reference sites. At the vertex (*left*), 2.5 cm posterior to the vertex (*center*), and 5 cm posterior to the vertex (*right*). Note changes in peak latencies.

positions. The result is a potential profile at this latency. When using a two-dimensional electrode array, equipotential line maps are an adequate topographic display of the electrical brain activity (e.g., Figures 2.7, 2.9, 2.12, or 2.17). The main feature of the profile in Figure 2.3 is an occipital positive peak which is surrounded by steep gradients while over frontal areas a flat distribution results. It is important to note that a change of the reference point does not change the shape of the potential profile. Another reference would simply change the position of the zero potential level and the labeling of the potential values, while potential maxima and minima and gradients remained unaffected.

The information of Figure 2.1 is topographically displayed in Figure 2.4, which shows a series of potential profiles between 4 and 256 msec latency. In contrast to the potential waveshapes, the time axis runs from top to bottom, and the electrode positions from left to right. This display contains the same information as the waveshapes, stressing the topographic aspect of the data.

The latency of an evoked component may reasonably be defined as the occurrence time of maximal activity in the scalp field reflecting the time of synchronous activity of a maximal number of neurons. We have proposed a measure of "field power" that is computed as the mean of all possible potential differences in the field, or a related measure of "potential range" that yields

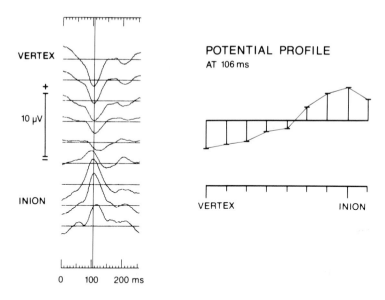

Figure 2.3. Construction of a topographic potential profile at 106-msec latency. Amplitudes measured in each channel are plotted as a function of electrode position. Changing the reference site simply shifts the zero baseline, but leaves the shape of the profile unchanged.

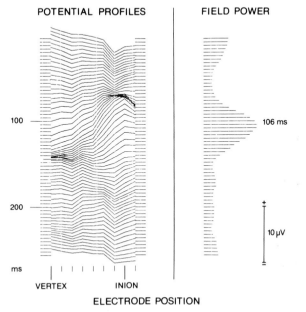

Figure 2.4. Series of potential profiles between 4 and 256 msec (*left*), and global field power (*right*) computed at 4 msec intervals. Same data as Figures 2.1 and 2.2.

similar results [8,9]. These measures quantitatively determine the amount of electrical activity at each time point independent of the reference electrode. Pronounced scalp fields with high peaks and troughs and steep gradients will result in high field power defining the occurrence of a component. On the right side of Figure 2.4 global field power is plotted as a function of time adjacent to the corresponding potential profiles. At early latencies field power is low, and around 100 msec it increases, reaching a maximum at 106 msec. This time defines the latency of the evoked component.

When the potential profiles are plotted at successive time points, topographic changes over time can be analyzed in detail, as illustrated in Figure 2.5. Contrary to what was expected from the potential waveshapes in Figure 2.1, it becomes obvious that there is no change in the scalp location of the occipital component: between 90 and 120 msec the potential maximum remains at the same electrode, and only the potential gradients change.

After determining component latencies, a second step is the analysis of the scalp field features at these component latencies in terms of the location of the potential maxima, minima, and gradients. These derived measures are by definition reference-independent. Different subject populations or different experimental conditions may then be compared statistically. Most important, this analysis strategy defines evoked components independent of a reference point, and thus treats electrical scalp field data unambiguously, thus more meaningfully relating them to intracranial mechanisms.

EVALUATION OF LATENCY AND SCALP LOCATION

A similar analysis strategy is employed in recordings from two-dimensional electrode arrays. In a population of 11 subjects, recordings of visual evoked potentials in 16 channels to a reversing grating stimulus presented to the upper or lower hemiretina were obtained (scalp fields evoked by stimuli of different spatial frequencies are discussed in [11]).

Figure 2.6 shows the grand mean potential waveshapes evoked by upper hemiretina stimuli. Vertical lines indicate times of maximal field power (see also Figure 2.10). In the lower part of the figure, the construction of the potential field at component latency is illustrated. The potential value of each electrode is entered at its respective electrode position, and points of equal potential are connected by lines. A series of potential distribution maps is illustrated in Figure 2.7 in which the data of Figure 2.6 are shown as equipotential line maps between 80 and 132 msec with intervals of 2 msec.

Grand mean potential waveshapes evoked by lower hemiretina stimuli are illustrated in Figure 2.8, and the scalp distribution at component latency shows a posteriorly shifted potential maximum. The whole series of scalp field maps for lower hemiretina stimuli (Figure 2.9) is different from that evoked by

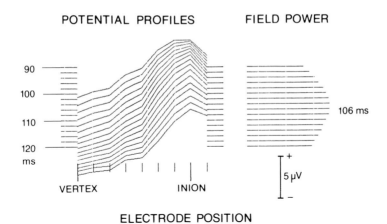

POTENTIAL PROFILES   FIELD POWER

VERTEX   INION

ELECTRODE POSITION

Figure 2.5. Enhanced display of profile series of Figure 2.4 between 90 and 120 msec. Note that there is no change in component location as was suggested in Figure 2.1.

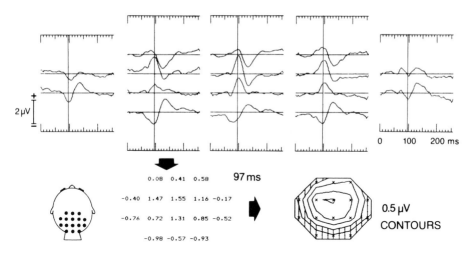

97 ms

0.08 0.41 0.58

-0.40 1.47 1.55 1.16 -0.17

-0.76 0.72 1.31 0.85 -0.52

-0.98 -0.57 -0.93

0.5 µV
CONTOURS

Figure 2.6. Grand mean evoked potential data (waveshapes and map construction) of 11 subjects recorded from 16 electrodes extending in four regular steps from 2 cm below the inion to 7 cm above the inion, and in two steps to 4 cm to the left and right from the mid-line (see inset). Square wave modulated vertical gratings (2.3 cycles per degree, 80% contrast) were presented at a rate of 2 reversals per second as a circular test field of 7-degree arc diameter to the upper hemiretina from a distance of 185 cm.

upper hemiretina stimuli in terms of component location, demonstrating a more posterior location for lower hemiretina evoked components. There are also differences in component latency as determined by global field power shown in Figure 2.10; the maximum for upper hemiretina stimuli occurs at 97

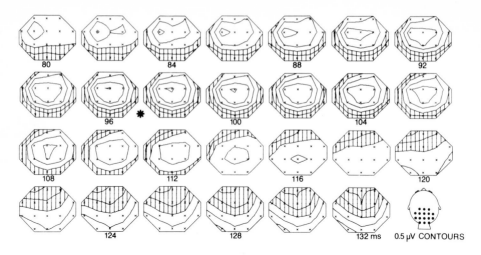

Figure 2.7. Series of grand mean potential field maps evoked by upper hemiretinal stimuli between 80 and 132 msec at 2-msec intervals (hatched areas negative with respect to the average reference). Asterisk indicates time of maximal global field power.

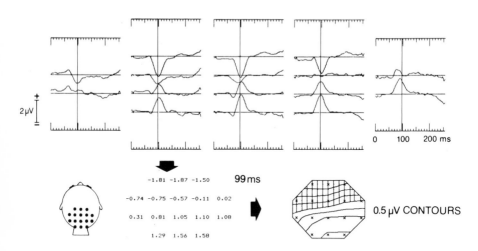

Figure 2.8. Grand mean evoked potential data (waveshapes and map construction) of 11 subjects evoked by lower hemiretina stimulation, same stimulus parameters as in Figure 2.6.

msec, that for the lower hemiretina at 99 msec. These numbers refer to the grand mean data. Paired t-tests on the individual data revealed consistent, and statistically significant differences. The mean latency of the upper hemiretina was 96.4 msec; that of the lower hemiretina, 100.7 msec. This difference was statistically significant ($t = 4.66$; $p < 0.0005$). Component location differences were also tested using the individual data on the location of the occipital positive component in the anterior-posterior direction shown in Figure 2.11; component locations evoked by upper hemiretina stimuli are located more anteriorly than components evoked by lower hemiretina stimuli. The mean location difference was 4.62 cm; this difference was statistically significant ($t = 7.45$; $p < 0.0005$).

A related set of data was obtained in recordings with 45 channels in a population of six healthy subjects (technical details of the recordings can be found in [12]). Figure 2.12 illustrates two map series of scalp potential fields evoked by upper and lower hemiretina stimuli, respectively. Relative global field power curves are also plotted (top left) for the two experimental conditions. Arrowheads in the field power graphs and over maps indicate times of maximal field power which occurred for the upper hemiretina at 113 msec and for the lower hemiretina at 121 msec. Globally, the two map series show a similar pattern of activity taking place at different poststimulus times; an occipital positivity surrounded by steep gradients develops around 100 msec, reaches a maximal pronunciation at component latency, and slowly disappears. This behavior over time is paralleled in the field power curves. There are also differences in the topographic distribution of the occipital component, showing a more anterior scalp location of the positive component for upper than for lower hemiretinal stimuli.

In the subject population, the mean component latency for the upper hemiretina was 99 msec, for the lower 115 msec. Longer component latencies for the lower hemiretina were found in all subjects, and the difference was sta-

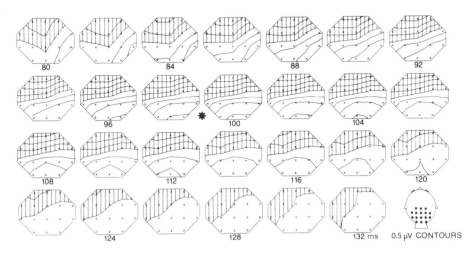

Figure 2.9. Series of grand mean potential field maps evoked by lower hemiretinal stimuli between 80 and 132 msec at 2-msec intervals (hatched areas negative with respect to the average reference). Asterisk indicates time of maximal global field power.

tistically significant. An analysis of the mean scalp locations of the occipital positive components at individual times of maximal field power of the six subjects in the two stimulus conditions showed that components evoked by upper hemiretina stimuli were consistently more anteriorly located than components evoked by lower hemiretina stimuli.

There is supporting evidence that the upper hemiretina is functionally superior, describing regional differences in motor reaction time [14,15], in temporal sensitivity as measured by critical flicker fusion and double flash discrimination [16], and in visual acuity [17], [18], and [19].

These findings have direct implications for the clinical use of visual evoked potentials. The latency of evoked potential components is considered a useful diagnostic measure. The main application of evoked potential recording in the visual modality is the establishment of clinically silent damage to the optic nerve in patients suspected of having multiple sclerosis [20]. Latency pro-

Figure 2.10. Global field power of grand mean data of Figures 2.7 and 2.9. Note that the maximum is reached earlier for upper hemiretina stimuli.

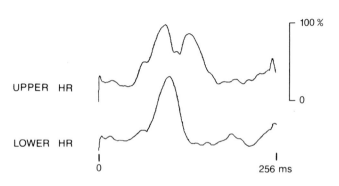

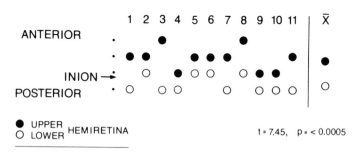

UPPER ● HEMIRETINA
LOWER ○ HEMIRETINA

$t = 7.45$, $p = < 0.0005$

MEAN LATENCIES: UPPER = 96.4,   LOWER = 100.7, $t = 4.66$, $p = < 0.0005$

Figure 2.11. Distribution of potential maxima in the anterior-posterior direction of 11 subjects at individual component latencies for upper and lower hemiretina grating stimuli. The location differences are statistically significant ($t = 7.45$, $p < 0.0005$). Original data of Figures 2.7 and 2.9 were used.

longation of only a few milliseconds may yield a statement of a pathological condition. As shown above, such latency differences may also be caused by the existing physiological differences between the upper and lower retinal systems, and may lead to an incorrect pathological diagnosis. A simple change of fixation toward the lower parts of the stimulus display is followed by prolonged component latencies.

ORIGIN OF VISUAL EVOKED POTENTIAL COMPONENTS

Due to its long latency, the P100 component of the visual evoked potential is presumably of cortical origin, and its scalp distribution after lateralized half-field stimulation supports this assumption [21]. From the anatomical geometry of the cortical representation of the retina, it is expected that small lateralized visual targets activate neurons at the occipital pole of the hemisphere ipsilateral to the hemiretina stimulated, whereas large targets yield an activation at more medial parts of the visual cortex. The data obtained by Skrandies and Lehmann [21] are in agreement with these anatomical expectations.

In this study scalp distribution data were regarded as multidimensional statistical observations, and principal component analysis (PCA) was used to uncover functional components. In contrast to other applications of PCA to evoked potential data [22,23], this spatial PCA treated the electrode positions on the scalp as variables and decomposed the potential field distributions, consisting of 45 amplitude values, into a small number of underlying, statistically independent components. Two component latencies (around 100 and 140 msec) of the scalp distribution data of six subjects evoked by large and small, central and lateralized checkerboard reversal stimuli were identified at times of maximal field power. Scalp distributions evoked by large left and right hemiretinal stimuli of six subjects are illustrated in Figure 2.13. Sixty such field configurations were the basis for the spatial PCA which reduced the 45 amplitude values to three principal components which accounted for 93.4% of the variance. The distribution of the grand mean and of two principal components is shown in Figure 2.14. Component 1 shows anterior-posterior scalp distribution differences with an occipital maximum surrounded by steep gradients, and Component 2 displays lateral differences. The scores on these components define their contribution to the observed potential field in a given experimental condition, and these component scores were analyzed statistically using analyses of variance. Figure 2.14 shows a significant interaction between latency and target size for Component 1: between 100 and 140 msec, a polarity change in the anterior-posterior direction occurred, with higher amplitude values evoked by larger targets. Component 2 displayed a significant interaction between retinal stimulus location, stimulus size, and latency: at 100 msec both small and large left hemiretinal stimuli yielded a positivity over the right hemisphere,

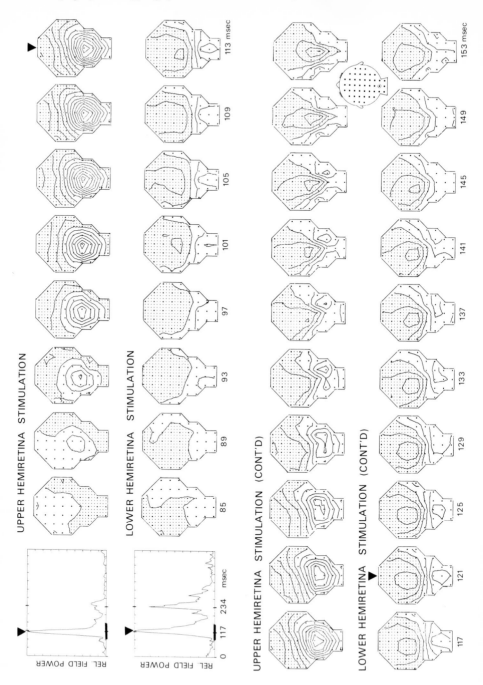

Figure 2.12. (*opposite page*) Global field power curves (*top left*) and series of scalp field maps of potentials evoked by checkerboard reversal stimulation (50-min check size, 15.5-degree arc diameter, 96 % contrast) of the upper or lower hemiretina (the 68-msec epoch during which maps are illustrated is indicated by horizontal bars in the field power plots). Simultaneous recordings in 45 channels as indicated in inset, most anterior electrode at 30% nasion-inion distance, circled electrode at inion. Dotted areas are negative and white areas are positive with respect to the average reference. Equipotential lines in steps of 1.0 µV. Arrowheads in the field power graphs and over maps indicate times of maximal field power. Note the earlier latency time, and the more anterior scalp location of the positive component for upper than lower hemiretinal stimuli. From Lehmann and Skrandies [13] by permission.

whereas right hemiretina stimuli showed a positivity over the left hemisphere. At 140 msec, the negativities are lateralized over the hemisphere contralateral to the stimulated hemiretina. Most interesting, smaller targets are lateralized to a lesser degree than large targets, and central stimuli yield very low scores on this lateralization component, reflecting no lateralization (for a more detailed discussion of these results, see [21]).

Further support for a cortical origin of the P100 component has been found when comparing components evoked by patterns with contrast borders, and by stereoscopic checkerboard patterns that depend on binocular fusion in the visual cortex [24]. Potentials evoked by dynamic random-dot stereograms (RDS) are presumably of cortical origin because in the human visual system the input of the two eyes is separated until the level of the visual cortex. Binocular interactions crucial for stereoscopic depth perception (Julesz's cyclopean retina [25]) are cortical functions. Thus, purely cortical neuronal generator mechanisms can be studied by recording the brain's electrical activity evoked by dynamic RDS stimuli, which operationally skip all stages prior to the activation of cortical binocular disparity neurons. The general morphology of the VEPs is similar for stereoscopic and binocular contrast stimuli: the major feature in both stimulus conditions is an occipital positivity occurring about 120 msec after the stimulus. In our analysis, component latencies were not statistically different in the subject population; however, amplitudes of the RDS evoked components were significantly smaller than those of the binocular contrast VEPs. Figure 2.15 shows the grand mean potential profiles of 15 subjects at their component latencies. Both stimulus conditions evoked a positive, occipital maximum that was located more anteriorly for stereoscopic stimuli. This difference in component location was statistically significant ($t = 3.59$; $p < 0.0025$) in the subject population. The occipital positivity for the stereoscopic stimuli was consistently located further anterior on the scalp (mean 4.25 cm above the inion) than that for the binocular stimulus condition (mean 2.45 cm above the inion).

The finding of much smaller amplitudes for stereoscopically evoked components suggests that fewer neurons are activated synchronously by this stimulus. The difference in scalp field distributions proves that differently located (or oriented) neural generator populations are activated by three-dimensional stimuli. This interpretation is in line with single-unit recordings in the visual cortex of monkeys, where depth sensitive neurons were found [26]. Some authors claimed that area 18 (which lies anterior to primary visual area 17) contains more neurons responding to disparate stimuli [27,28]. In contrast to single-unit studies in which sampling biases may mimic a differential distribution of functional units, evoked components reflect the activity of neural populations, and global functional differences may be investigated. The finding of a more anteriorly located potential peak evoked by stereoscopic stimuli may be interpreted as an indication that more neurons in area 18 than in the primary visual cortex are activated by stereoscopic stimuli. Since potential components evoked by contrast changes have the same latency as the stereoscopic components that are definitely of cortical origin, these results strongly suggest that contrast evoked components with latencies in the order of 100 msec are also of cortical origin.

LEFT HEMIRETINA STIMULI

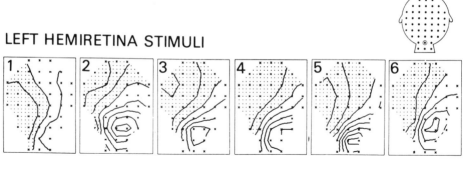

RIGHT HEMIRETINA STIMULI

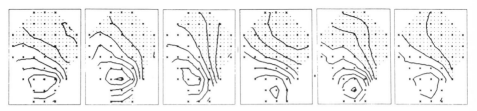

Figure 2.13. Evoked potential maps of six subjects at individual times of maximal field power around 100 msec latency (electrode array, see inset, equipotential lines in steps of 1.0 μV, dotted areas negative, white areas positive with respect to the average reference). *Top.* Fields evoked by 26-degree arc reversal targets on the left hemiretina. *Bottom.* Fields evoked by 26 F-degree arc reversal targets on the right hemiretina. From Skrandies and Lehmann [21], by permission.

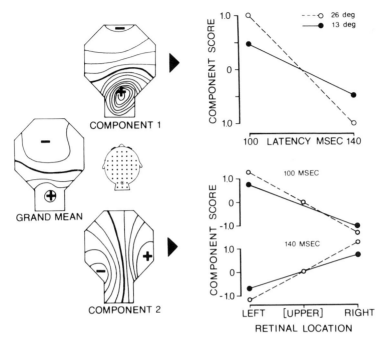

Figure 2.14. Grand mean potential field (mean over subjects and experimental conditions) and configurations of the first two principal components with a score of 1.0 and corresponding component scores. The metric of the components has been restored to μV by multiplying component loadings by their respective standard deviations, equipotential lines in steps of 0.3 μV. Mean scores of Component 1 display a significant interaction between latency and stimulus size. Mean scores of Component 2 show a significant interaction between retinal location, stimulus size, and latency. Note the lesser degree of lateralization for smaller stimuli, and the very low contribution of this component to fields evoked by nonlateralized stimuli (details in Skrandies and Lehmann [21]).

TEMPORAL ACTIVITY PATTERNS

A way to look at activity patterns of longer duration is to plot the most distinct features of the scalp fields (e.g., the locations of the potential maxima and minima) over time. This yields information on the similarity of complete neural activity cycles evoked in different experimental conditions. Figure 2.16 shows that the topographic differences between stereoscopic and contrast stimuli are not restricted to the occurrence times of components but prevail over long durations. These data are the location means over 15 subjects plotted at 5-msec intervals. Significant differences between stereoscopic and contrast evoked activity were established by computing paired *t*-tests (Figure 2.16). These data suggest that the time course of the activation pattern is similar but that the topography is different. Both the potential maxima and minima have different

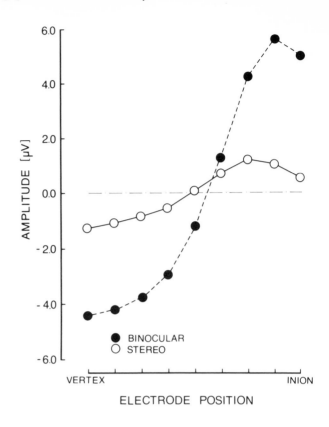

Figure 2.15. Grand mean potential profiles at individual component latencies of 15 subjects recorded from a midline row of nine electrodes equidistantly spaced between the vertex and 5 mm above the inion. Stereoscopic checkerboard reversal stimuli composed of dynamic random-dot patterns (dot size 12-min arc) were shown on two black and white TV monitors to each eye separately every 20 msec using a special visual pattern generator. Conventional binocular checkerboard patterns with the same mean luminance were used for comparison. Note larger amplitudes of components evoked by contrast stimuli and the more anteriorly located potential maximum. From Skrandies and Vomberg [24], by permission.

locations over time, indicating the activity of neural generator populations of different location (or orientation).

SCALP DISTRIBUTIONS AND HIGHER VISUAL INFORMATION PROCESSING

The topography of cognitive evoked components related to attention, expectation, stimulus comparison, and task relevance gives insight into higher visual information processing strategies. Further, the time sequence of processing steps and the involvement of different neural generator structures in various tasks can be investigated. Chapman et al. [22] gave a general description of the basic design of the experiments described in this section. Detailed information is also found in Skrandies [29] and Skrandies et al. [30].

Potential field distributions were constructed from recordings obtained while subjects performed information processing tasks comparing either geometric or alphanumeric stimuli presented randomly and independently in different retinal locations. In the relevant condition (Figure 2.17*A*), times before and shortly after stimulus presentation show field configurations organized around an anterior negative extreme value. However, for irrelevant stimuli (Figure 2.17*B*), at corresponding times, the fields are organized around posi-

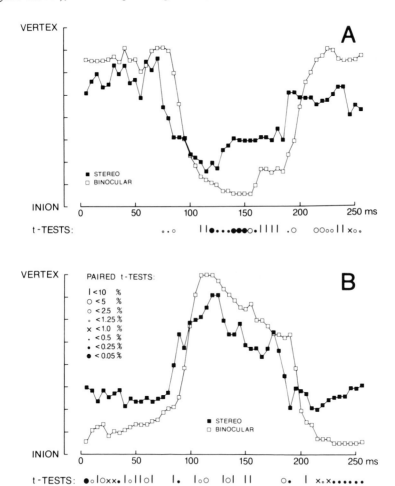

Figure 2.16. Mean distribution in the anterior-posterior direction of potential maxima (*A*) and minima (*B*) of 15 subjects between 5- and 255-msec latency evoked by stereoscopic stimuli or by similar binocular contrast stimuli. Significant differences were established by paired *t*-tests shown below each graph computed on the individual data. Scalp distribution differences persist over longer times indicating activation cycles of different neural populations in the two conditions.

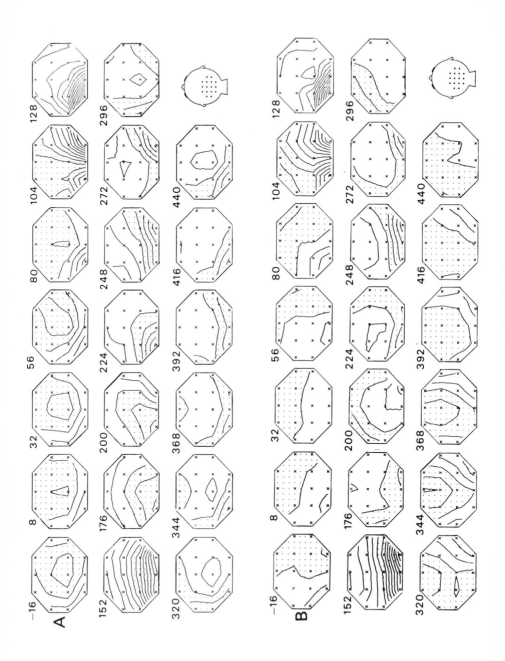

Figure 2.17. (*opposite page*) Map series of scalp distributions evoked by relevant (*A*) and irrelevant (*B*) alphanumeric stimuli which were presented to the left hemiretina. The series range between 16 msec before and 440 msec after the stimulus in intervals of 24 msec. The distributions are similar at 80 msec and 152 msec, and different early (before 80 msec) and late (after 272 msec). Lines are in increments of 1 μV, dotted areas negative with respect to the average reference; electrode array is shown in inset. From Lehmann and Skrandies [13], by permission.

tives. The expected relevant stimuli are preceded by a topographic distribution not unlike that of the contingent negative variation (CNV). In contrast, the irrelevant stimuli evoke fields of opposite polarity. At latencies beyond 300 msec, relevant stimuli evoke scalp fields dominated by a positive parietal peak, whereas in the irrelevant condition this positivity is not seen (compare Figures 2.17*A* and *B*). The late positivities evoked by task relevance are consistent with reports on P300 and Slow Wave components [31,32]. At other times, relevant and irrelevant stimuli yield similar potential fields reflecting more basic physiological processing. For example, at 80 msec, the stimuli presented to the left hemiretina evoke an ipsilateral occipital positivity and a field trough over the right side in both conditions (Figure 2.17). This finding is in line with the correct component lateralization obtained for small visual targets as illustrated above (see Figure 2.14).

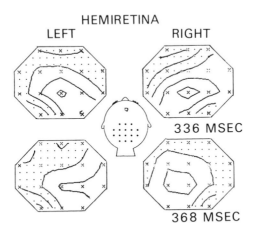

HEMIRETINA
LEFT   RIGHT

336 MSEC

368 MSEC

Figure 2.18. Scalp field distributions evoked by relevant expected stimuli presented to the left or right hemiretina. Both at 336 msec and at 368 msec there are significant differences in the lateralization of the parietal positivity. Lines are in increments of 1 μV, dotted areas are negative with respect to the average reference; electrode array is shown in inset. From Lehmann and Skrandies [13], by permission.

An interesting finding of this study was that the topographic distribution of the P300 component varied with retinal stimulus location. Figure 2.18 illustrates potential fields evoked by task-relevant expected stimuli at 336 and 368 msec latency. Lateralized stimuli produce midline peaks over parietal scalp areas, showing hemispheric differences with a more positive potential distribution over the hemisphere contralateral to the hemiretina stimulated, and with steeper gradients over the ipsilateral hemisphere. These data illustrate that P300 is not exclusively dependent on psychological variables, but it also reflects basic physical stimulus characteristics. Taking into account the strict retinoptic representation of the visual field at cortical visual processing areas, the task-directed activity of visual fixation neurons in the inferior parietal cortex of monkeys [33], and the extensive representation of the visual modality throughout the brain [34], it appears conceivable that higher visual information processing is also influenced by retinal stimulus location.

The preceding topographic analysis strategies are transparent and simple to apply. They yield direct quantitative measures on latencies and scalp locations of evoked components. These reference-independent measures can then be treated statistically and allow comparisons of subject populations or experimental conditions. The application is not restricted to potential fields but can also be used in multivariate statistical data analysis. Both principal component loadings [21] and principal component scores [29,30] were topographically examined. The combination of multivariate statistics and scalp field distribution data proved a powerful tool in the analysis of differences in VEP lateralization [21] and of brain activity evoked by higher information processing tasks [29,30].

As our scalp-recorded data on lateralized visual stimulation and the stereoscopic evoked potential fields demonstrates, the combination of topographic information and detailed knowledge on the physiological processing mechanisms of the visual system is promising. The direct, unambiguous topographic analysis strategies allow meaningful interpretations of neural mass activities in the human nervous system.

REFERENCES

1. Schneider, M.R. A multistage process for computing dipolar sources of EEG discharges from surface information. IEEE Trans. Biomed. Eng. 1972; 19:1–12.
2. Kavanagh, R.N., Darcey, T.M., Lehmann, D., and Fender, D.H. Evaluation of methods for three-dimensional localization of electrical sources in the human brain. IEEE Trans. Biomed. Eng. 1978; 25:421–429.
3. Sidman, R.D., Giambalvo, V., Allison, T., and Bergey, P. A method for localization of sources of human cerebral potentials evoked by sensory stimuli. Sens. Proc. 1978; 2:116–129.

4. Jewett, D.L., Romano, M.N., and Williston, J.S. Human auditory evoked potentials: Possible brain stem components detected on the scalp. Science 1970; 167: 1517–1518.
5. Skrandies, W., Wässle, H., and Peichl, L. Are field potentials an appropriate method for demonstrating connections in the brain? Exp. Neurol. 1978; 60: 509–521.
6. Nunez, P. Electrical Fields of the Brain. New York: Oxford University Press, 1981.
7. Lehmann, D. Human scalp EEG fields: Evoked, alpha, sleep and spike-wave patterns. In H.H. Petsche and M.A.B. Brazier, eds., Synchronization of EEG Activity in Epilepsies, Berlin: Springer, 1972; 307–325.
8. Lehmann, D., and Skrandies, W. Reference-free identification of components of checkerboard-evoked multichannel potential fields. Electroenceph. Clin. Neurophysiol. 1980; 48:609–621.
9. Skrandies, W., and Lehmann, D. Occurrence time and scalp location of components of evoked EEG potential fields. In W.M. Herrmann, ed., Electroencephalography in Drug Research, Stuttgart: Fischer, 1982; 183–192.
10. Lehmann, D. Multichannel topography of human alpha EEG fields. Electroenceph. Clin. Neurophysiol. 1971; 31:439–449.
11. Skrandies, W. Scalp potential fields evoked by grating stimuli: Effects of spatial frequency and orientation. Electroenceph. Clin. Neurophysiol. 1984; 58:325–332.
12. Lehmann, D., and Skrandies, W. Multichannel evoked potential fields show different properties of human upper and lower hemi-retinal systems. Exp. Brain Res. 1979; 35:151–159.
13. Lehmann, D., and Skrandies, W. Spatial analysis of evoked potentials in man: A review. Prog. Neurobiol. 1984; 23:227–250.
14. Hall, G.S., and von Kries, J. Über die Abhängigkeit der Reaktionszeit vom Ort des Reizes. Arch. Anat. Physiol. 1879; suppl.: 1–10.
15. Payne, W.H. Visual reaction times on a circle about the fovea. Science 1965; 155: 481–482.
16. Skrandies, W. Critical flicker fusion and double flash discrimination in different parts of the visual field. Int. J. Neurosci., 1985; 25:225–231.
17. Landolt, E., and Hummelsheim, E. Die Untersuchung der Funktionen des excentrischen Netzhautgebietes. In Graefe-Saemisch Handbuch der gesamten Augenheilkunde, T. Saemisch, ed., Leipzig: Engelmann, 1904; 4:503–583.
18. Low, F.N. The peripheral visual acuity of 100 subjects. Am. J. Physiol. 1943; 140: 83–88.
19. Skrandies, W. Human contrast sensitivity: Regional retinal differences. Human Neurobiol., 1985; 4:95–97.
20. Halliday, A.M., McDonald, W.I., and Mushin, J. The visual evoked response in the diagnosis of multiple sclerosis. Br. Med. J., 1973; 4:661–664.
21. Skrandies, W., and Lehmann, D. Spatial principal components of multichannel maps evoked by lateral visual half-field stimuli. Electroenceph. Clin. Neurophysiol. 1982; 54:662–667.
22. Chapman, R.M., McCrary, J.W., Bragdon, H.R., and Chapman, J.A. Latent components of event-related potentials functionally related to information processing. In J.E. Desmedt, ed., Progress in Clinical Neurophysiology, Basel: Karger, 1979; 6: 80–105.

23. Skrandies, W. Latent components of potentials evoked by visual stimuli in different retinal locations. Int. J. Neurosci. 1981; 14:77–84.
24. Skrandies, W., and Vomberg, H.E. Stereoscopic stimuli activate different cortical neurones in man: Electrophysiological evidence. Int. J. Psychophysiol. 1985; 2: 293–296.
25. Julesz, B. Foundations of Cyclopean Perception. Chicago: University of Chicago Press, 1971.
26. Poggio, G.F., and Fischer, B. Binocular interaction and depth sensitivity in striate and prestriate cortex of behaving rhesus monkey. J. Neurophysiol. 1977; 40: 1392–1405.
27. Hubel, D.H., and Wiesel, T.N. Cells sensitive to binocular depth in area 18 of the macaque monkey cortex. Nature 1970; 225:41–42.
28. von der Heydt, R., Hänni, P., Dürsteler, M., and Peterhans, E. Neuronal responses to stereoscopic stimuli in the alert monkey: A comparison between striate and prestriate cortex. Pflügers Arch. 1981; 391:R34.
29. Skrandies, W. Information processing and evoked potentials: Topography of early and late components. Adv. Biol. Psychiat. 1983; 13:1–12.
30. Skrandies, W., Chapman, R.M., McCrary, J.W., and Chapman, J.A. Distribution of latent components related to information processing. Ann. N.Y. Acad. Sci. 1984; 425:271–277.
31. Sutton, S., Braren M., Zubin, J., and John, E.R. Evoked potential correlates of stimulus uncertainty. Science 1965; 150:1187–1188.
32. Squires, N.C., Squires, K.C., and Hillyard, S.A. Two varieties of long-latency positive waves evoked by unpredictable auditory stimuli in man. Electroenceph. Clin. Neurophysiol. 1975; 38:387–401.
33. Mountcastle, V.B., Lynch, J.C., Georgopoulos, A., Sakata, H., and Acuna, C. Posterior parietal association cortex of the monkey: Command functions for operations within extrapersonal space. J. Neurophysiol. 1975; 38:871–908.
34. Macko, K.A., Kennedy, C., Miyaoka, M., Sokoloff, L., and Mishin, M. Mapping the primate visual system with [2-C^{14}]deoxyglucose. Science 1982; 218:394–397.

3

Spatial Analysis of EEG and Evoked Potential Data

Dietrich Lehmann

Different modes and elements of information processing in the brain are performed by at least partially different neural populations and activity patterns. The activities of these neural populations manifest as the net result in the spatial configuration of the brain's electromagnetic field and its changes over time [1,2], which can be recorded on the scalp even when the active area is deep in the brain [3,4]. However, conventional analysis of the time series of voltages recorded as potential differences between two electrodes cannot be used for unique functional/physiological interpretations of the electrical scalp field data, since these voltage series are ambiguous for a given scalp location (Figure 3.1). Therefore, a first transformation over space in order to obtain unambiguous local values has to precede further analysis. The unambiguous values can then be subjected to reduction, extraction, and analysis over space and time.

MAPPING EEG AND EVOKED POTENTIAL DATA

Mapping is an appropriate strategy to display electroencephalogram (EEG) evoked potential (EP) data, or to display spatial results of the analysis of such data. Mapping in itself, of course, does not constitute data analysis or even reduction. Since maps show the data in a space-oriented form, they ought to display unambiguous local values of the mapped field distribution. The local values are ambiguous if the mapped EEG/EP data are voltages recorded against one real electrode as a reference, since many more voltages than electrode locations are possible. There are as many possible, equally privileged, and meaningful voltages for one location on the scalp at one moment in time as there are additional electrodes on the scalp; i.e., for n electrodes, there are $(n - 1)$ possible voltages, and hence, $n*(n - 1)$ directly measurable, possible time series of voltages or waveshapes (Figure 3.1; for examples of longer data

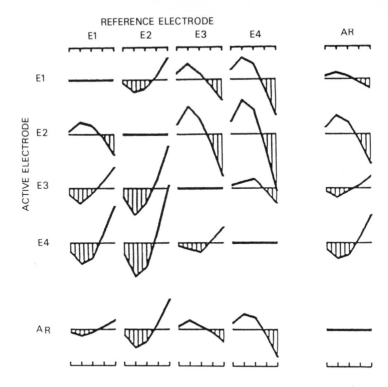

Figure 3.1. All possible wave shapes that are recordable from four electrodes (E1-E4) at five sampling times (horizontal). The five sampling points are indicated by tic marks. The vertical values represent voltage; baseline indicates zero voltage difference between active and reference electrode. Relative positivity of active electrode is shown in white; negativity is striped. there are $n*(n-1) = 12$ directly recordable waveshapes, with an additional $n = 4$ straight lines over time (same electrode as active and as reference) which nevertheless contain crucial information. For instance, the line E4 versus E4 shows that E4 as the active electrode was the most negative point in the sampled scalp field compared with the other electrodes at sampling times 1, 2, and 3. There are nine additional traces of and versus the average reference (AR). One-half of all waveshapes is the polarity-inverted mirror image of the other half. Note also that "latencies" depend on the electrode combination, as for example in E3 versus E4 as opposed to the other combinations.

epochs see Figure 1 in Lehmann and Skrandies [5] and Figure 1 in Lehmann and Skrandies [6]). These $n*(n-1)$ possible time series result in $n*(n-1)/2$ different power spectra [7]. There is no possible proof of electrical inactivity or zero potential for any given location [8,9]. At any rate, since only the distribution of the potential around the brain is of interest, points further away cannot provide useful information.

Obviously, values and descriptors of the brain/scalp field which are not biased by the preselection of a reference must be used for mapping and analysis, if functional/physiological interpretations of the results are planned. Diagnostic classification of results, on the other hand, can be performed with data that are not functionally interpretable, but for which estimates of mean and variance of the target populations are known.

Unambiguous Local Scalp Field Map Values and Descriptors of Scalp Field Maps

The production of unambiguous values or descriptors of a momentary field distribution is a mandatory first step in EEG/EP analysis if there is more than one data channel and if its aim is interpretation (Table 3.1). Unambiguous local values of an instantaneous map are (1) local voltages compared to the average reference (the average reference behaves as "no reference"; this can be said because the mean of the rectified voltages at all electrodes referred to the average reference can be derived from the mean of all rectified, instantaneously possible potential differences within the field without choosing a common reference [5]); or (2) local gradients (the first spatial derivatives); or (3) local current densities (the second spatial derivatives, Laplacian operators), as shown in Figure 3.2 for one map. Unambiguous extracted descriptors or characteristics of an instantaneous map are the locations of maximal and minimal field value and the hilliness or "global power" of the field; a related descriptor is an equivalent dipole fitted into the field [10–12], assuming for the purpose of data reduction the unrealistic existence of only one or two generators.

The recomputation of the local values into voltages compared to the average reference does not change the instantaneous field configurations; it merely removes the spatial dc component (as a spatial high-pass filter), thus reasonably assuming a constant electrical charge on the head over time. However, potential fields, fields of gradients, and fields of current densities of the same data differ in their configurations as they stress different field properties. Reference-independent global or local characteristics can be extracted from any type of field display. These characteristics constitute not only reference-free field descriptors but also meaningful field data reductions. Average reference, gradient, and current density recomputations of evoked and spontaneous activity were long ago introduced into EEG and EP studies [9,13–18], but have as yet received little attention in systematic studies. EEG/EP data typically are reported as time series of potential differences compared to a preselected electrode.

After reference-independent local or global values have been produced at each moment in time, further analytic steps may be selected for the data. Inspection of map sequences (Figures 3.3 through 3.5) show relatively simple field configurations with one or sometimes two peaks and troughs, with field

Table 3.1   Overview of EEG/EP Analysis Steps, and Their Meaningful Sequence

From	Operation	Next Possible
Amplifier/	A. Data: Reference-dependent local values (differences between local potentials); hardware bandpass; ADC.	B/C/
	(OPTION: Digital Filter)	
A/	B. Transformation into reference-free local values (map by map, or via Fourier transformation of predetermined epochs D1/)	C/D/E/F/
	B1. Voltages vs. Average Reference (spatial high pass filter).	
	B2. Gradients (first spatial derivative).	
	B3. Current densities (second spatial derivative).	
A/B/	C. Reduction; extraction of reference-free parameters/field characteristics.	
	C1. Field strength: global field power (maximal value difference "range").	D2/E/F/
	C2. Field configuration: locations of maximal and minimal values. Equivalent dipole fitting.	D3/E/
B/C/E	D. Predetermined epochs or self-adaptive segments.	E/F)
	D1. Predetermined epochs.	
	D2-3-4. Self-definition of segment. Procedures examine time sequences of maps; three ways:	
	D2. Times of maximal field power for component latencies.	
	D3. Field configuration (by locations of maxima/minima) determines component or segment; disregard polarity for spontaneous activity. Autoregression segmentation. Dipole parameters.	
	D4. For evoked fields, peak values issimilarity terminate segment (component).	
B/C/viaD/F/	E. Means/differences over times, subjects, conditions: Global and/or local mean field values, variances. Mean of voltages vs. aver. ref. (from B1/) = 0, local S.D. = power vs. aver. ref. *k.	D(if not from F)/G/

Operations are labeled with letters. Input to each described analysis operation (center column) is indicated in the left column, starting with amplifier output. The right column indicates the next possible operation(s).

Table 3.1   *(continued)*

From	Operation	Next Possible
B/C1/viaD/ (if from A/, B/ after F/)	F. Characteristics of local values of time series of maps: Fourier components. Sine-cosine vector diagrams. Power maps and compromise coherence maps. Frequency-wave number spectra (from C1-global map feature: Frequency spectrum).	E/ (if from A/, B/)
E/	G. Comparisons between times, subjects, conditions, incl. reliability tests. Compare complete fields via global statements; dis-similarity index, extracted characteristics (from E/ via local characteristics). Maps of significant local differences. Spatial PCA.	

lines tending to be concentric around these extreme values. The map sequences give the impression of landscapes with volcanos that erupt and recede here and there; sometimes, while one volcano emerges, another one recedes (Figure 3.4). There are no wave fronts, and over time, the major landmarks tend to be stationary and then change location quickly. Epochs of flat maps alternate with epochs of hilly maps (Figure 3.4). There appears to be little tendency for propagation of major features over larger distances. The latter issue is also a consideration in the interpretation of the multitude of different phase angles that can be measured in data over time (see section, "Spatial Aspects of Frequency Characteristics"), where preselected phase information often is inappropriately used for interpretations.

Avoidance of Biased Display Conventions in Mapping

Although mapping is not analysis, maps of instantaneous scalp field values that are referred to a preselected reference electrode may suggest misleading interpretations of the data. For instance, if the reference electrode was accidentally located at or near the most positive (or most negative) location of all measured locations (not infrequently, the ears are sites of most negative or most positive values [20]), the displayed map will show predominantly negative (or positive) values, as seen in Plate 2. This may suggest to some observers an "event of negative (positive) polarity." Such interpretation could possibly be justified if steeper local gradients existed around the nonreference extreme field value than around the reference, but it is certainly not justified when the reference poten-

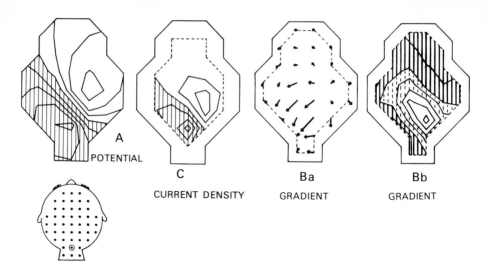

Figure 3.2. Map of an evoked, averaged scalp field at a point in time 72 msec after a visual stimulus. The same data is shown as a map of potential distribution (*A*), as a recomputed map of gradient magnitudes and orientations (*Ba*) and of gradient magnitudes only (*Bb*), and as a recomputed map of current source densities (*C*). Stimulus was the 2/sec checkerboard reversal with 55-min checks in a 16-degree target, shown to the upper hemiretina of the right eye of a normal subject. Activity was simultaneously recorded in 45 channels; for the electrode array, see inset; the most anterior electrode was at 30% nasion-inion distance, with the circled electrode at inion. Head seen from above, nose up. The solid line around each map is the outline of the electrode array. *A*. The field as equipotential contour map. Equipotential lines are linearly interpolated between electrodes in steps of 0.8 μV. Hatched: negative; white; positive relative to average value of all data points (average reference). *Ba*. Same data as in A, recomputed into gradients (first spatial derivative of the potential distribution). Within the electrode array, for each square formed by four electrodes the gradient was computed and entered as an arrow that points in the direction of the resultant gradient. The origin of the arrow is at the center of the four-electrode square. The length shows the relative magnitude of the gradient. *Bb*. Magnitude of local gradients of *Ba* mapped with equigradient lines in steps of 0.2 μV/cm, linearly interpolated between gradient locations of *Ba*. Orientation omitted. Hatched; low gradient; white; high gradient area. *C* Same data as in A, recomputed into current source density (CSD) values (second spatial derivative), using the potential values of the four surrounding electrodes for each CSD computation. Equidensity lines were linearly interpolated in equal steps of arbitrary size (μV/cm^2) between electrode locations. Hatched; positive (sink); white; negative (source). Note the reduction of the result area (broken outlines) compared to recording area (solid outlines) with computation of spatial derivatives; the current density map yields values only at 25 of the 45 electrodes of the potential map A. Note the somewhat different configuration of the potential distribution compared with the current density distribution: The minimum location is identical, but the maximum location is different. Asymmetric field configurations are seen at this latency in many subjects and do not depend on the stimulated eye.

tial value simply happened to be near one of the extreme potential values in the field—wherever the reference was, on the scalp or elsewhere.

Theoretically, these arguments are applicable not only to instantaneous potential fields but also to gradient and current density fields if they are referenced to a particular electrode postulated as zero. It is hoped that the temptation to select a putatively inactive, real electrode location as reference will be small for gradient and current values.

Possibly misleading interpretations of maps are avoided if the average reference is used for data display. The average reference values ensure that there are equal amounts of measured total negativity and positivity in each field map. In particular, the average reference is the only reference that produces negative and positive values in each map, since it is a spatial frequency high-pass filter for each field distribution. For unbiased means and differences between maps, recomputation against the average reference is mandatory in order to avoid privileging of one particular location as a no-change-over-time point in space.

The problem is dramatically illustrated in convolutions of voltage data over time. Maps of band power obtained by Fourier transformations of a given data epoch show very different topographic distributions for different reference electrodes. For n electrodes, $n + 1$ different and correct power maps (including one referred to the average reference) are possible for each frequency (Hz) point in the spectrum (see Figure 3.6). The site of the reference electrode by definition shows a power of zero. All maps are equally correct since there is no possible proof for an "indifferent" real electrode. Only the map of power recomputed against the average reference is privileged and should be used for further functional or physiological considerations.

The necessary interpolation for equipotential or equipower contour lines or areas may be linear or nonlinear between actually measured values. Various strategies have been proposed [21–30]. In our own work we have preferred linear interpolations for map displays [5,6,19,20,31–35]. However, when there are no midline electrodes, nonlinear interpolations might be preferable to avoid undue accidental lateralizations of the displayed data. In any case, further analysis should be done using only those values obtained at the measured locations.

REDUCTION OF MAP SEQUENCES: DETERMINING EPOCHS FOR ANALYSIS

Mapping of the recorded data is a rearrangement of the data into a form which, when chosen appropriately, does not invite biased assessment. Mapping does not reduce the data since there is a map for each data point in time. Maps can be reduced by selecting representative times, or times of particular significance, or by averaging over fixed or adaptively determined

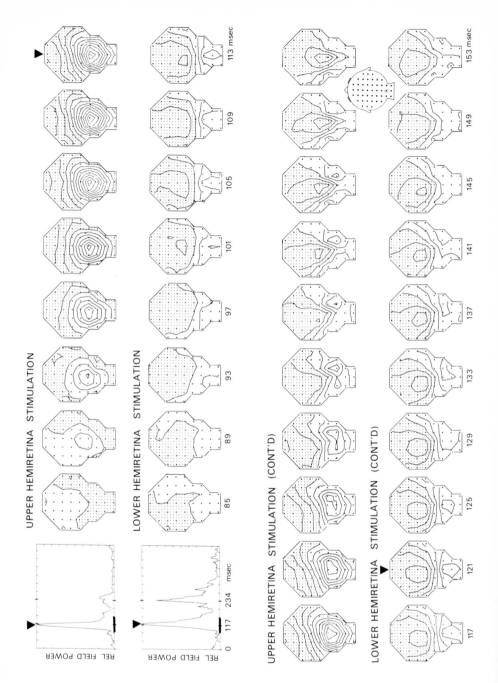

Figure 3.3. Relative global field power curves (*top left*) and equipotential contour field maps (*top right, bottom*) of potentials evoked by 2/sec checkerboard-reversal stimulation (16-degree arc circular target; 50-min arc checks) to the upper and lower hemiretina of the right eye. Recordings were simultaneously obtained from 45 electrodes as indicated in the schematic inset; the most anterior electrode is at 30% nasion-inion distance, circled electrode at inion. Head seen from above, nose up. Dotted area negative, white positive, relative to average of all field values. Equipotential contour lines in given increments of 1.0 µV. Triangles in the field power graphs and over maps indicate the time of maximal global field power (field hilliness or relief), which is 8 msec earlier for upper than for lower hemiretinal responses. The 68-msec epoch during which maps are illustrated is indicated by heavy horizontal bars in the plots of relative field power. Note the difference in location of the evoked positive field maximum between upper (at 113 msec) and lower (at 121 msec) hemiretinal response. From Lehmann and Skrandies [6].

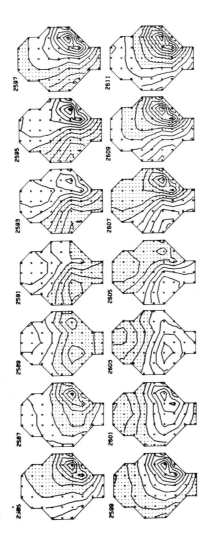

Figure 3.4. Maps of alpha EEG scalp fields recorded with 45 simultaneous channels (digitally filtered 8–12 Hz) during one alpha cycle, at intervals of 7.8 msec between maps (about 100 msec total time; times are coded by map numbers). This figure maps a portion of the data of Figure 3.13 (demarcated by the rectangle) and of Figure 3.5 (the present figure shows maps with high time resolution spanning three of the maps of figure 3.5). Time progresses from left to right, from upper to lower row. The dotted area represents negative, white positive to the average of all measurements. Note relatively high field power (many field lines) in first map, low field power (few field lines) in third map, high power at end of upper row but inverted polarity of the field, low power at middle of lower row, then high power in the last maps, once more with inverted polarity so that the initial configuration and polarity is approximately reestablished. One alpha cycle is completed. Note absence of right-left propagation (two simultaneous minima) of minimal field value in third map, upper row. From Lehmann [19].

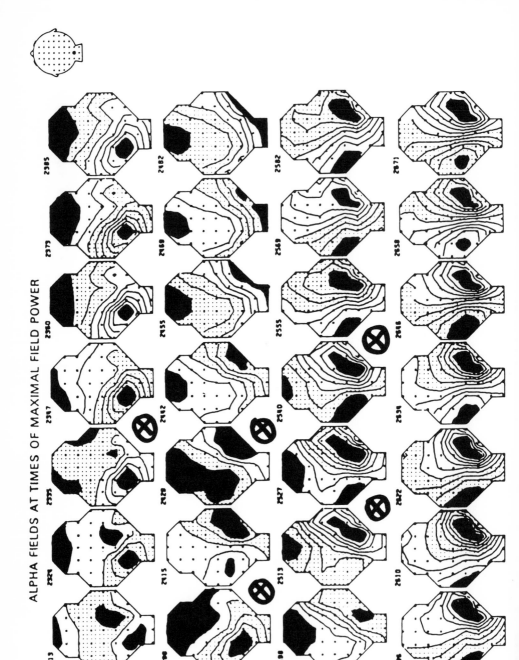

ALPHA FIELDS AT TIMES OF MAXIMAL FIELD POWER

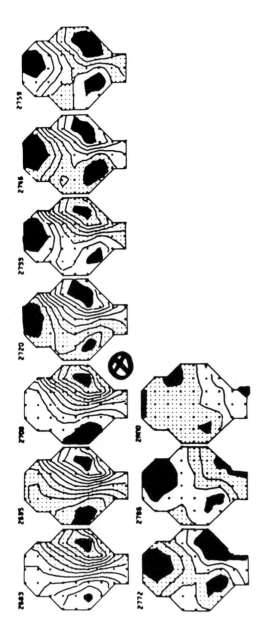

Figure 3.5. Segmentation of a 1.8-sec sequence of alpha EEG scalp field maps (digitally filtered 8–12 Hz activity) into periodically stationary epochs. Scalp potential field distributions were recorded and mapped with 45 simultaneous channels (256 samples/sec/channel; for electrode array, see inset), and equipotential lines in 2 μV increments were linearly computer-interpolated between electrodes. Global power of the scalp fields was computed (see Figure 3.13) and maps for this illustration were selected at times of maximal global field power, which, because of the alpha frequency band, occurred about every 50 msec. Figure 3.4 shows an example of intermediate maps between three of the maps of the present figure. Numbers are computer frames. White, positive; stippled, negative; black, areas of extreme (maximal or minimal) voltage field values. Black (extreme) areas form a configuration in each map, and this configuration stays stable for shorter or longer epochs. The configuration might show three extremes, or a left occipital and an anterior extreme, or a right and a left occipital extreme, etc. Occurrence of an extreme location beyond a neighbor electrode between two successive maps demarcates the end of a stationary segment. Segment terminations are indicated by circled crosses. From Lehmann [7].

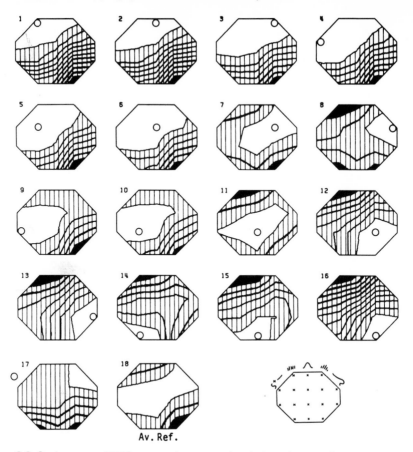

Av. Ref.

Figure 3.6. Scalp maps of EEG power demonstrating their ambiguity. Calculated power at any single recording point depends on the chosen reference. For example, the spatial distributions of EEG power in the 9-Hz frequency band are shown as a function of the reference point (the point arbitrarily set to zero and indicated by a circle) chosen for mapping power. Sixteen scalp electrodes and a left ear electrode were used for simultaneous recordings. Spectra were computed for epochs of 4 sec and averaged over six epochs. Maps 1–16 show power computed against scalp electrodes 1–16, 17 against the left ear, and 18 against the average reference. Equipower contour lines are in arbitrary units, but equal units are used for all maps. The area with lowest power is white, the intermediate is hatched, and the highest power is black in each map. In the schematic, crosses indicate electrodes. The most anterior electrode is at vertex, most posterior at inion, at about equal interelectrode distances. Head seen from above, nose up. There are as many power maps possible as there are electrodes (1–17), and in addition, the power against the average reference can be mapped (18). Although all maps are technically correct, none of them can be identified as indicative of the real source of the mapped power, as there is no possible proof for electrical inactivity in one of the points relative to the others. Only the power distribution computed against the average reference can be interpreted physiologically (see Figure 3.12). The 18 maps cannot be transferred into each other, since phase angles are not included in the power displays. From Lehmann [7].

Figure 3.7. *A*, Dissimilarity of field configuration between successive field distribution maps as a function
of time (see text). *B*, Relative global field power as a
function of time. Bar indicates epoch mapped and analyzed in Figures 3.8 and 3.10. Horizontal, time in msec;
vertical, arbitrary units. From Lehmann and Skrandies
[6].

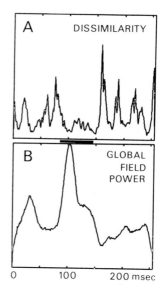

time epochs. A map that consists of many local values can be reduced to
reference-free descriptors of the mapped field distribution.

The Strength Criterion: Field Power Detects
Components and Moments of High Signal-
to-Noise Ratios

Conventionally it is argued in studies of evoked potentials that a time
moment of maximal amplitude of the waveshape indicates a step in information processing. This contention is based on the hypothesis that near-
synchronous activity of a neuronal population (whose particular geometry
might be described) reflects a step in information processing at a specific
latency. Such activity will result in a maximal amplitude of the recorded
scalp potential field. Even though the determination of this time moment
using a few selected, recorded waveshapes is ambiguous, the basic idea can
be applied as an unambiguous strategy to the entire recorded field [5,20]
or to a one-dimensional space slice of the field [35,46]. In principle, this
reference-independent approach determines the greatest potential difference
(maximal field amplitude, or "field voltage range") between any two electrodes for each time moment, eliminating preselection of the reference; the
two extreme values of the instantaneous field (positive and negative) may
occur at any two electrodes.

One can plot this maximal amplitude of the field as a curve over
time. This curve can then be searched for the times of peak amplitude

that identify the occurrence of components defined as times of maximal field strength. (At the determined latencies, the locations of the field maximal and minimal values describe the component topography.) When all measurement points in the field are included in the computation, the general hilliness or flatness of the field is expressed as the mean of all rectified voltages compared to the average reference in the field (mean amplitude/electrode) [20]. This value can be transformed into "global field power" [5], which can also be computed from all possible potential differences within the field, i.e., for n electrodes from the $n*(n-1)$ instantaneously measurable voltages which do not require the selection of a reference. This possibility of transformation also shows that the computed average reference behaves in a way which is different in principal from any other reference. The formula for global field power (for examples over time, see Figures 3.3 and 3.7) produces the root of the mean of the squared potential differences between all possible electrode pairs in the field, and reads as follows:

$$
\text{Global field power} = \left\{ (\tfrac{1}{2n}) \sum_{i=1}^{n} \sum_{j=1}^{n} \left[u(i) - u(j) \right]^2 \right\}^{0.5}
\tag{3.1}
$$

where n about equally distributed electrodes measure the potentials $e(i)$ and $e(j)$; $i,j = 1, \ldots , n$. The observed voltages are $u(i) = e(i) - e$(common reference). Comparisons between curves of this global field power and curves of "field voltage range" over time usually show only minor differences [5]. Spontaneous activity in the alpha range produces field power curves with about 20 field power maxima per second [19,20].

The Field Configuration Criterion: Trajectories of Locations of Maximal and Minimal Values and Field Similarity Determine Stationary Segments

Different configurations of the scalp electrical field must be produced by different neuronal generator populations, whereas similar configurations may or may not be produced by identical populations. Since different types of, or steps in, information handling presumably involve different neural populations, meaningful components of evoked potential data may be identified by the field configuration as criterion, disregarding absolute amplitude which, reflecting strength of the process, does not ensure similarities or differences in nature. In addition, a new step in information processing need not manifest as "stronger" activity. This approach still implies sequential steps of information processing but does not assume the magnitude of the activity to be critical.

We have proposed a global measure of dissimilarity of two field distributions [5] that uses the voltage information and the average reference at all measured points with equal weight in the two fields to be compared. In order to assess the configurations without weighting by absolute field power, we scale the fields to be compared to unity global field power, and then apply the formula that computes the average, across all electrodes locations, of the standard deviations of the local mean values between the two maps (measurements against average reference):

$$
\text{Global dissimilarity} = (1/2n) \sum_{i=1}^{n} \left\{ \left[(u(i,m(1)) - u(i,m(2)) \right]^2 \right\}^{0.5} \qquad (3.2)
$$
(between two maps)

where $u(i)$ is the voltage at electrode i referred to the average reference; i is one of the n electrodes; and $m(1)$ and $m(2)$ are the maps to be compared.

Applying this dissimilarity computation to pairs of successive field distributions over time yields curves that tend to show high values of dissimilarity (which indicate the beginning of a new segment) at times of low global field power, and high similarity at times of high field power (see Figure 3.7). However, when more than one prominent maximum and minimum value exists in the field, field configuration assessment may become a more meaningful determinant of segments than field power.

A related approach to segment an evoked map series into epochs characterized by stationary field configurations is the extraction of reference-independent descriptors of the fields. We have proposed to use a two-statement descriptor based on the locations of the maximal and the minimal field value. For example, the connecting line between the two locations in Figure 3.8 indicates the axis of the net generator process, and its angle can be used for clustering the different segments into meaningful classes. For segmentation, spatial windows are set up around the locations of the two extreme values at the first time point. Then, the locations of the extremes at the next time point are compared against the window; if they have stayed within the windows, the segment continues. If one of them has occurred outside the spatial window, a new segment is started, and the spatial windows around both extremes are redefined. An application is shown in Figure 3.9, where the grand mean locations, over all stimulus conditions and subjects, of the extreme field values along the anterior-posterior and left-right axes are displayed as functions of time. In this 16-

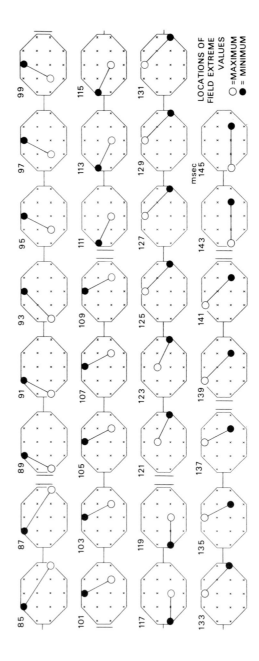

Figure 3.8. Reference-free reduction of evoked scalp fields. Plots are given of locations of field extreme values with only one maximal (circle) and one minimal (dot) value per map, during the marked time of the map sequence analyzed in Figure 3.7. The extrema in each plot are connected by a line, in order to ease visualization of the basic field configurations. This figure illustrates the proposed segmentation procedure. Horizontal lines connect location plots that belong to the same segment. Vertical lines (segment terminations) separate plots where one or both extreme values left their areas defined by the initial location and one neighboring electrode. Figure 3.10 illustrates the dwell times and field orbits of the same data.

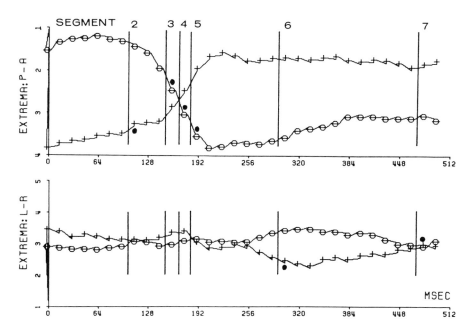

Figure 3.9. Time segmentation of evoked, average map sequence, according to field configuration criteria. Shown are scalp field locations (*vertical*) of maximal (+) and minimal
(−) field values in posterior-anterior (P-A, *upper graph*) and left-right (L-R, *lower graph*)
direction as a function of time. A 16-electrode array was used, with four electrodes (E)
from posterior (E4) to anterior (E1), and at most five electrodes from left (E5) to right (E1).
Data is the grand mean evoked by 8 x 40 = 320 tachistoscopic 30 msec stimuli of 3-de-
gree arc visually structured targets for each of 12 subjects. Every 16 msec, the location of
the maximal and minimal value in the mapped average evoked field was determined, and
averaged over runs and subjects. The grand means were entered in the P-A and L-R
graphs. Starting with data point 1 as base, a segment end (vertical line) was diagnosed
when the location of a new entry exceeded the window of 0.5 electrode distances around
the base entry. The first data point of the new segment was used to reset the window for
all four measures. Dots indicate the entries which started a new segment. Seven segments were identified (vertical lines) during the 512 msec after stimulus onset. Further
statistics can test for each segment the differences of extrema locations between targets. Results from Brandeis and Lehmann, unpublished.

channel recording average, the spatial window was set at 1/2 electrode
distance in both directions from the electrode location.

When mapping the locations of field extreme values over time, one
observes trajectories or orbits, during which the extrema tend to reside at
few electrodes over relatively long times, and at many electrodes at relatively little or no time (Figure 3.10). Similar results are observed with
evoked and with spontaneous activity, in the latter case resulting in near
repetitions of the trajectories over time (Figure 3.11).

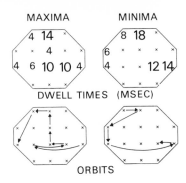

Figure 3.10. Dwell times (msec) and orbits (lines with arrowheads) of the locations of field extreme values (maximal and minimal values) of the evoked potential data shown in Figures 3.7 and 3.8 (85 to 145 msec after stimulus). Numbers indicate dwell time as duration of occurrence of an extreme value at the electrode location; one maximal and minimal value was determined per map; maps at 2-msec intervals. Arrows indicate progression of time. For electrode arrangement see Figure 3.9. Note that many electrode locations showed no extreme field value during the analysis time, and few locations showed many extremes. Note also the jump-like change of locations in space. From Lehmann and Skrandies [6].

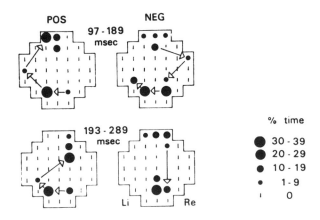

Figure 3.11. Orbits or trajectories of positive and negative extreme values of alpha EEG scalp fields. Upper maps during a first alpha cycle (msec 97–189); lower maps during the subsequent alpha cycle (msec 193–289 of a continuous record). Recordings with 45 channels. Schematic maps portray head seen from above, nose up. Dots and vertical bars show electrode positions. The size of the dots indicates percentage analysis time during which the extreme was observed at the location. Arrows show sequence of observations. Vertical bars represent electrode locations where no extreme value was observed during the two alpha cycles. From Lehmann [32].

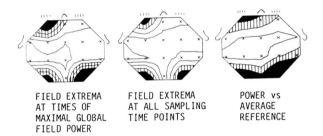

FIELD EXTREMA   FIELD EXTREMA   POWER vs
AT TIMES OF   AT ALL SAMPLING   AVERAGE
MAXIMAL GLOBAL   TIME POINTS   REFERENCE
FIELD POWER

Figure 3.12. Scalp distribution maps of locations of field positive and negative extreme values accumulated at times of maximal global field power (*left*), or at all sampling times (256/second, *center*), and map of alpha band power computed against the average reference, for a 24-sec recording of 16-channel spontaneous EEG (8–12 Hz band) of a healthy subject with eyes closed. From Lehmann, Ozaki, and Pal, unpublished.

For spontaneous activity, mean maps of the extrema locations over time expectedly show spatial distributions that closely resemble the spatial distribution of power computed against the average reference (Figure 3.12), since the average reference is the only reference which, at each moment in time, will assign a negative and a positive value to the two extreme value points in the field. We note in Figure 3.12 that the use of all recording times compared to only the times of maximal global field power for the average of the locations of the extreme field values does not cause a great difference. This is to be expected, since the fields at the times of maximal field power show configurations that are relatively stable over time. The configurations change relatively quickly during short times, typically during times of low field power.

When applied to spontaneous EEG activity the segmentation strategy requires a modification because of the basically periodic nature of spontaneous activity reflected in the concept of "frequencies." When one examines a curve of global field power during alpha EEG, there is a fairly regular (around 20/sec) cycle of maximal and minimal values [19,20] (Figure 3.13). Field configurations at the successive times of maximal global field power typically show similar configuration and inverted polarity (see Figure 3.5). This may continue for several successive occurrences of maximal field power until the configuration changes into a new type of distribution that in turn is repeated over several occurrences of maximal field power (with inverted polarities for successive maps). If one assumes stationary generators of periodically inverting polarity, then a homogeneous segment will be defined by the persistence of the field structure regardless of its polarity. Thus, for the adaptation of the segmentation procedure to spontaneous EEG data, polarity of the field extreme values must be rectified before setting up the space windows—polarity is omitted. In addition, the analysis uses only the data at occurrences of maximal field power in order to avoid the relatively brief epochs of change of field configuration during low field power where intermediate configurations may occur with a low signal-to-noise ratio.

In a segmentation study of spontaneous alpha EEG activity (currently in preparation in collaboration with H. Ozaki and I. Pal) in six subjects (2 minutes analysis time each), 16 electrode positions were used for simultaneous recording; the spatial window around the two initial field extrema locations was defined by the first three direct neighbor electrodes, which became extrema locations at later analysis times. The median duration of the segments was 250 msec; the longest segment lasted for 2.6 seconds. On the average across the six subjects, the most frequent segment class accounted for 20% of the total analysis time, the two most frequent classes for 31%. Figure 3.14 shows an example of successive classes of alpha EEG segments from one subject. The data cover about 5 seconds and illustrate the segment classes as defined by the accumulated locations of the field extreme values over the duration of each segment. The different segments show differing durations, and different classes occur in unsystematic succession. The results suggest that brief epochs of spontaneous EEG of differing durations are stationary in their field configurations, and can thus be hypothesized to reflect functional micro states associated with different types of information treatment [36]; they also suggest that during resting, a relatively large proportion of time is spent in one mode of activity.

It is intriguing to speculate that in the future, segments of specific spatial configuration during map sequences of spontaneous activity could be recognized as identical with segments during evoked potential map sequences, and

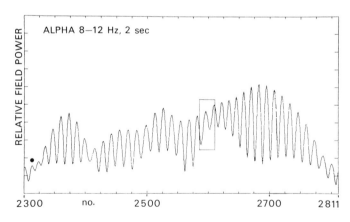

Figure 3.13. Global field power (arbitrary units) (8–12 Hz band) during 2 seconds of alpha activity recorded with 45 channels, using 256 samples per second per channel. Results are for a total of 512 maps. The dot indicates first map shown in the series of Figure 3.5, the rectangle defines the time of the map series of Figure 3.4. Adapted from Lehmann [19].

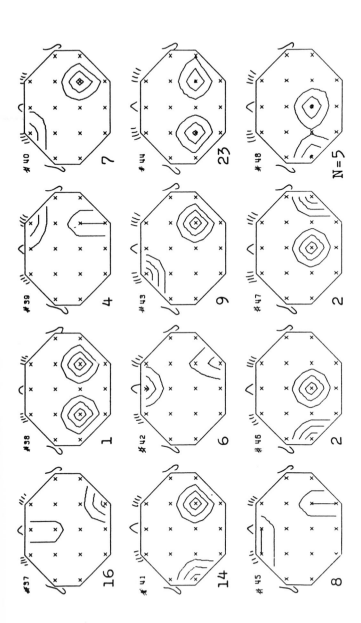

Figure 3.14. Configuration of scalp fields of 12 successive alpha EEG segments; the sample is taken from segmentation of spontaneous 16-channel alpha EEG (8–12 Hz band) of a subject, with closed eyes. Each map shows the occurrence locations of field positive and negative extreme values accumulated during the duration of the segment, and scaled to unity. Head seen from above, nose up. The figure to the left and below each map indicates the number of peak times of global field power (see Figure 3.13) during which the segment lasted (this figure multiplied by 50 is the approximate segment duration in milliseconds). Some classes of segments occurred once, others several times; some were short, others long. The total analysis time covered in this figure is nearly 5 seconds. From Lehmann, Ozaki, and Pal, unpublished.

that this identification might permit the interpretation of parts of spontaneous map sequences as being identical with certain steps of information processing known from studies of event evoked activity.

SPATIAL ASPECTS OF FREQUENCY CHARACTERISTICS: POWER AND PHASE ANGLES OF SPECTRAL ANALYSIS

Fourier analysis produces information on amplitude (power) and phase for voltage series obtained from pairs of scalp locations for each frequency band. The ambiguity of power statements associated with a single electrode location is interrelated with a similar ambiguity of statements about phase angles. This is most evident when the data are displayed in vector diagrams (Figure 3.15) for a given frequency band (one data point of the Fourier series), into which the sine and cosine values of the analysis results for each electrode location are entered. The entries form a figure or constellation not unlike a star map. The circumference of the entries for spontaneous scalp fields is often elliptical, with the largest distances (power) between entries in the anterior-posterior direction of the recorded field. However, even neighboring frequency bands may produce very different constellations of the entries, i.e., different scalp topographies. The constellation of the star map can easily be read as topographic distribution of the power mapped against any of the electrodes as reference. The constellation of the entries to each other is invariant—a newly added reference does not change the relationships, it will merely add another entry. Figure 3.15 illustrates the electrical relation of several popular reference locations to the scalp data during the analyzed epoch. Figure 3.15 also shows that obviously the power or phase results obtained with the same data set compared to a new reference will depend on the choice of reference. The descrepancies between results of power computations against different electrodes as references are particularly evident when all possible maps of power for a given frequency band are displayed (see Figure 3.6) [7].

The interrelation between power and phase becomes evident when one considers the results that would be obtained with the left or right ear as reference in Figure 3.15. Phase angles between the active electrodes (for example, 7 and 15) as well as amplitudes (square root of power; in Figure 3.15, the distances between electrode entries) between the reference and the active electrodes change, depending on the reference choice. In fact, for each point in the Fourier spectrum there are $n*(n-1)*(n-2)/2$ possible phase angles for n electrodes, which illustrates the irrelevance of phase angle information obtained with a real reference when hypothesized traveling of waves across the scalp is considered [32,37,38]. If one imagines a situation where one of the local values remains unchanged by the choice of a new reference, it will have to change relative to other possible references.

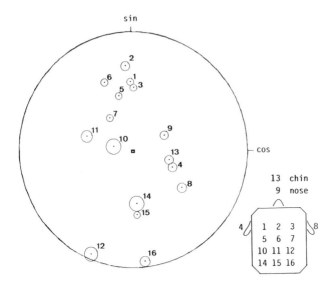

Figure 3.15. Vector diagram shows the mean result of a Fourier analysis of 25 successive EEG epochs of 2 seconds duration during resting. The sine and cosine values of the 10-Hz component of a 16-electrode recording are displayed. For electrode positions, see inset. The sine (vertical) and cosine (horizontal) value determines the position of the electrode in the vector diagram. The circle around each position indicates the standard error of the mean of the results of the 25 averaged epochs. The results were averaged by rotating the 25 diagrams around the average reference (heavy dot at center) into a best fit. This averaging procedure avoids privileging any one electrode as the point of no variance. The amplitude (the distance between two electrode entries) or power (squared distance) of the 10-Hz component between any two electrodes can readily be measured from the graph, as can phase angles ("latencies") between any three of the electrodes. Note that the configuration of the entries, i.e., the geometric relations between the points, is invariant and will not be changed by the introduction of an additional electrode. Note also the different results for left and right ear, and the differences in amplitude and phase angle (i.e., latency) that would result from using, for example, different ears or the nose as reference. Note also the mutual dependence of amplitude and phase. From Ozaki, Pal, and Lehmann, unpublished.

The average reference is the mean of all sine and cosine values within the star map. The average reference is the least deviation compromise between all sine/cosine entries. Power mapped against the average reference is privileged over all other possible power maps against a real electrode as reference (Figure 3.7) [7], because its topographic configuration corresponds to the configuration of the map of the locations of mean occurrence of field maxima and minima values over time (Figure 3.13)[32]; field maxima and minima are reference-independent field descriptors. A line that connects the locations of maximal and minimal potential in each instantaneous map indicates the surface-projected orientation of the net generator process. Accordingly, the line that connects the peaks of the local occurrences of extrema locations over time and (following Figure 3.12) the lines that connect the locations of maximal power versus the average reference indicate the orientations of the net generator processes. The orientation of the line is interpretable, for example, as hemispheric synchrony or counter-phase activity (anterior-posterior orientation in the former case, left-right orientation in the latter). Only the average reference can produce this result for power over time, since all other references may, at some times, be at a location of maximal or minimal potential. In addition, the use of any one of the real electrodes as reference by definition assigns an electrical power of zero to the chosen reference location, a problem which is avoided when the average reference is used.

These considerations lead us to the conclusion that values other than those computed against the average reference cannot yield meaningful interpretations, even though they might be diagnostically useful and efficient. This conclusion likewise applies to the display of spectral analysis as frequency wave number spectra [9,39,40], where once more only average reference data appear worthy of interpretation.

In summary, for the scalp map display of spectral power of time series of voltages, the average reference should be used. The time series of the local values of gradients and of current density carry no ambiguity, and their spectral power can be mapped directly [16,17].

MEAN MAPS AND DIFFERENCE MAPS: COMPARISONS BETWEEN SUBJECTS, TIMES, AND CONDITIONS

For comparisons of data sets with the intention of estimating the statistical probability of chance occurrence of differences, information is necessary about the variance of at least one of two data sets to be compared. Variance information is generated by average or difference computations. For the dissimilarity index, see formula (2).

Mean maps and difference maps of field distributions must be computed with reference-independent values, so that all recording locations carry variance information with equal weight. If a real electrode is chosen as a reference, this reference location in the potential field will show a mean or difference value of zero with a variance of zero—an unjustifiable privilege. Moreover, although the instantaneous configuration (the polarity and the differences between local values) of the mean or difference field is independent from the reference, the magnitude and the polarity of the local values is dependent on it. This dependence may result in misleading conclusionns, such as the statement that a certain area is more negative in field A than in field B. However, a different reference may lead to the opposite interpretation (see Plate 2).

DIFFERENCE SCALP FIELD MAPS (mean of 12 ss),
EVOKED BY "ATTENDED" MINUS "IGNORED" STIMULI
LEFT   VISUAL FIELD STIMULI   RIGHT

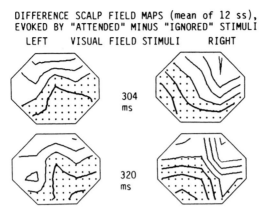

304
ms

320
ms

Figure 3.16. Maps of the differences of mean for 12 subjects of scalp fields evoked by attended and nonattended stimuli, presented to the left or right visual hemifield; difference maps computed at 304 msec and 320 msec latency. Head seen from above, nose up; 16-channel recordings, most anterior electrodes at Cz posterior at inion. Dotted areas show where attended stimuli evoked more negativity; white areas represent the locations where attended stimuli evoked more positivity. All maps were computed as average reference voltages and scaled to unity field power before averaging. From Brandeis and Lehmann, unpublished.

In an application of difference field computations, the mean over subjects of difference fields was computed between the two experimental conditions of requested attention and requested no attention to one of two visual stimuli presented alternately (experiments with D. Brandeis). In some runs the presentation was given to the left visual hemifield, in others to the right. Attended stimuli produced more pronounced negativity than nonattended stimuli at more than 300 msec after stimulus onset occipitally over the hemisphere on the side where the stimulus was entered (Figure 3.16).

In clinical applications it is typically necessary to test possible result aberrations of single cases from normal control group findings. Duffy et al. [41] and Duffy [42] have pointed out that Z-transform significance maps should be used for this purpose. We suggest use of only reference-independent local values for such comparisons, so that unambiguous space-oriented interpretations are possible. In the case of potential maps, these are voltage values referred to average reference values.

Mapping Significances of Difference

Arguments about local ambiguity of referenced values also apply to the mapping of statements of statistical significance of differences of local field values. Such statements are unambiguous only if derived from comparisons of maps whose values are not referred to real electrodes as references (Figure 3.17). Duffy [42] has proposed an extension to mapping significances which identifies the area of interesting differences; optimally, the strategy should be applied to maps of reference-free local values.

Extracted Field Values: Maxima and Minima

The trajectories or orbits of field extreme values (field maxima and minima) in space over time can be treated in prefixed epochs or segmented in time so as to identify stationary epochs. The locations of field extreme values can be determined at selected times (e.g., selected via the field strength criterion). Extrema locations that describe the field configurations in different experimental condditions can be entered into multivariate statistics. Maps of the mean locations of maxima and minima during the analysis time and over subjects can be completed with information on the variance in the anterior-posterior and left-right direction, and they can be tested for significance of difference between groups.

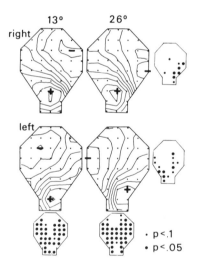

Figure 3.17. Mean equipotential contour line scalp fields for six subjects, evoked by right (*top*) or left (*bottom*) hemiretinal checkerboard reversal stimuli of 13 and 26-degree arc target size. Individual average fields at latencies of maximal, global field power at around 100 msec were scaled for unity amplitude between subjects before mean computation. Head seen from above, nose up; dots indicate the 43 electrode placements. Plus sign indicates positive, minus sign negative extreme mean field value. The small circle-dot arrays to the right and at the bottom give significances of the differences at each electrode site (values of paired *t*-tests) between mean field values evoked by small and large, and right and left hemiretinal targets. Adapted from Lehmann and Skrandies [43].

Examples of Applications

Using the strength criterion for component identification, we studied space and time differences of the mapped potential fields that were evoked by upper and lower hemiretinal checkerboard reversal stimulation. Having established the latency of the component by field power or "voltage range," its location is determined as the potential maximum (minimum) in the field. Since the well-known functional anatomy predicted location differences only in the anterior-posterior dimension, and since this was confirmed in 47-channel field studies (Figure 3.3; see also [35,45], Figure 5 in [19]), we limited the data sampling to one space slice along the scalp midline (see also Chapter 2). The results showed a dominant component around 100 msec latency with a more anterior (around 4 cm) and earlier (about 10%) occipitally positive maximum for upper than for

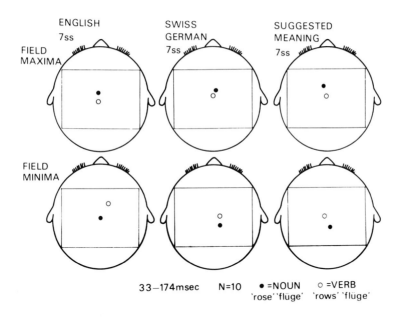

Figure 3.18. Language-evoked scalp fields. The figures provide the locations of field maximal and minimal values over 10 sampling times (between 33 and 174 msec after word onset; the mean of 7 subjects was entered per sampling time) evoked in each of the six stimulus conditions: English noun/verb and Swiss-German noun/verb context meanings of homophone words, and suggested noun/verb context meaning of homophone sounds. Rectangle indicates the outline of the 12-electrode array 4-x-3 which was centered around Cz with interelectrode distances of 5 cm. Head seen from above, nose up. The anterior-posterior differences were significant in all cases with WILCOXON $p < 0.05$; the right-left differences were significant ($p < 0.05$) only for English, minimal field values. Calculated from the data analyzed in Brown and Lehmann [44].

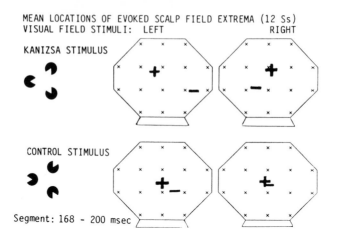

Figure 3.19. Mean locations for 12 subjects of evoked scalp field extreme (positive and negative) values, 168–200 msec after presentation of a KANIZSA figure (*upper graphs*) and a control stimulus (*lower graphs*) to the left or right visual hemifield. The 168–200 msec epoch was identified by the field configuration-based adaptive segmentation procedure (see text) and ANOVA over conditions and segments. The anterior-posterior and left-right distances between the mean extreme locations were significantly larger for KANIZSA than for control stimuli. Simultaneous 16-channel recordings. Head seen from above, nose up. Electrodes between Cz and inion. Note the lateralization of the KANIZSA evoked field minimal values, depending on the input-receiving hemisphere. From Brandeis and Lehmann, unpublished.

lower hemiretinal stimuli [46,47]. This difference of response latency between upper and lower hemiretinal systems deserves attention in clinical applications of pattern evoked visual potentials.

Onset, reversal, and offset mode of the checkerboard stimuli produced systematic differences in locations and latencies of the occipitally positive dominant component around 100 msec [48]. Latencies increased from onset to reversal to offset stimuli, and from upper to lower hemiretinal stimuli. Component location measured as the distance forward from the inion decreased from onset to reversal to offset for upper hemiretinal stimuli, and had an inverted spatial sequence for lower hemiretinal stimuli, in accordance with the projection of the geometrically mirroring cortical visual areas for upper and lower hemiretinal input.

In a similar fashion, maximal field values of binocularly evoked components as compared with monocularly evoked components were more anterior for upper hemiretinal stimuli and more posterior for lower hemiretinal stimuli [47], results which supported the reports of relatively more binocularly excitable elements in higher than lower visual areas.

In a comparison of potential fields evoked by noun and verb meanings of homophone words in different languages we analyzed successive prefixed poststimulus data epochs (Figure 3.18). The evoked maximum field locations for grammatical nouns were significantly more anterior than those for grammatical verbs, and the minimum locations for grammatical nouns were significantly more posterior than the minimum locations for grammatical verbs in two different languages and for two different lexical meanings. These results agreed with results obtained with suggested noun and verb meaning of an unintelligible sound sequence as stimulus [44]. For an application of principal component analysis to field configuration data, see Chapter 2 and Skrandies and Lehmann [49].

Using the adaptive segmentation procedure in a study (in collaboration with D. Brandeis) of potentials evoked by visual figure (subjective KANIZSA contours) and no-figure stimuli of identical visual elements, we determined as the most discriminating time segment, the epoch of 168–200 msec after stimulus onset using an ANOVA procedure. The evoked field extrema locations were averaged over subjects and times during the duration of this segment and for the two conditions. There were significant location differences between conditions (Figure 3.19), with the field minimum residing more laterally over the stimulated hemisphere, and the maximum more anteriorly for figure than for no-figure stimuli. This indicates two at least partially different neural populations which are involved in the processing of the information of the two visual targets, and it indicates also that the processing of the figure information is performed by hemisphere-bound neural populations, depending on which lateral hemifield contained the figure information.

SUMMARY

The overview in Table 3.1 outlines different treatments to which EEG/EP data can be subjected with the aim of obtaining interpretable, unique results. The construction of reference-independent, unique local values is the prerequisite for all subsequent steps for interpretable analysis results of EEG/EP data. In a straightforward treatment, unique local values are obtained by conversion of reference-dependent maps into reference-unbiased maps at each time point; an alternate route is the immediate extraction of reference-free map descriptors. Subsequent treatments may use different approaches. Meaningful, unbiased reduction of the data is the guideline—mapping alone does not reduce the data. Mapping, as well as further treatment, should only be applied to unambiguous data, in order to avoid misleading deductions. Configurations of instantaneous fields invite generator-population (map configuration) oriented segmentation in time. This procedure in turn leads to short stationary epochs in evoked as well as in spontenaous activity, and may thus be a linking method for the two aspects of research on electrical brain fields.

In summary, for functionally or physiologically interpretable results of EEG and EP studies, analysis over space must precede analysis over time. Diagnostic classification can be performed on reference-dependent data analyzed over time, but the results are not amenable to functional or physiological interpretation.

ACKNOWLEDGMENTS

Supported in part by the Swiss National Science Foundation, EMDO Foundation, Hartmann-Mueller Foundation, and Roche Research Foundation. The author thanks D. Brandeis, M. Koukkou, and W. Skrandies for critical comments, I. Pal for computer programs, and J. Müller for photography.

REFERENCES

1. Skrandies, W., Wässel, H., and Peichl, L. Are field potentials an appropriate method for demonstrating connections in the brain? Exp. Neurol. 1978; 60:509–521.
2. Mitzdorf, U., and Singer, W. Excitatory synaptic ensemble properties in the visual cortex of the macaque monkey: A current source density analysis of electrically evoked potentials. J. Comp. Neurol. 1979; 187:71–84.
3. Jewett, D.L., and Williston, J.S. Auditory evoked far fields averaged from the scalp of humans. Brain 1971; 94:681–696.
4. Smith, D.B., Sidman, R.D., Henke, J.S., et al. Scalp and depth recordings of induced deep cerebral potentials. Electroenceph. Clin. Neurophysiol. 1983; 55:145–150.
5. Lehmann, D., and Skrandies, W. Reference-free identification of components of checkerboard-evoked multichannel potential fields. Electroenceph. Clin. Neurophysiol. 1980; 48:609–621.
6. Lehmann, D., and Skrandies, W. Spatial analysis of evoked potentials in man: A review. Prog. Neurobiol. 1984; 23:227–250.
7. Lehmann, D. EEG assessment of brain activity: Spatial aspects, segmentation and imaging. Int. J. Psychophysiol. 1984; 1:267–276.
8. Katznelson, R.D. EEG recording, electrode placement and aspects of generator localization. In P.L. Nunez, Electric Fields of the Brain. New York: Oxford University Press, 1981; 176–213.
9. Nunez, P.L. Electric Fields of the Brain. New York: Oxford University Press, 1981.
10. Kavanagh, R.N., Darcey, T.M., Lehmann, D., and Fender, D.H. Evaluation of methods for three-dimensional localization of electrical sources in the human brain. IEEE Trans. Biomed. Engin. 1978; 25:421–429.
11. Ueno, S., and Fukui, Y. Current dipole model for the electroencephalogram and the magnetoencephalogram, with application to diagnosis of the central nervous

system diseases. Memoirs of the Faculty of Engineering, Kyushu University 1978; 38:207–217.

12. Grandori, F. Dipole localization methods (DLM) and auditory evoked brainstem potentials. Rev. Laryngol. Otol. Rhinol. 1984; 105 (suppl.):171–178.

13. Offner, F.F. The EEG as potential mapping: The value of the average monopolar reference. Electroenceph. Clin. Neurophysiol. 1950; 2:215–216.

14. Rémond, A. Poursuite de la significance en EEG. I. Problème de la référence spatiale. Rev. Neurol. 1960; 102:412–415.

15. Rémond, A. The importance of topographic data in EEG phenomena, and an electrical model to reproduce them. Electroenceph. Clin. Neurophysiol. 1968; suppl. 27:29–49.

16. Hjorth, B. An on-line transformation of EEG scalp potentials into orthogonal source derivations. Electroenceph. Clin. Neurophysiol. 1975; 39:526–530.

17. Hjorth, B. Source derivation simplifies topographical EEG interpretation. Am. J. EEG Technol. 1980; 20:121–132.

18. Persson, A., and Hjorth, B. EEG topogram: An aid in describing EEG to the clinician. Electroenceph. Clin. Neurophysiol. 1983; 56:399–405.

19. Lehmann, D. Spatial analysis of evoked and spontaneous EEG potentials. In N. Yamaguchi and K. Fujisawa, eds., Recent Advances in EEG and EMG Data Processing, Amsterdam: Elsevier, 1981; 117–132.

20. Lehmann, D. Multichannel topography of human alpha EEG fields. Electroenceph. Clin. Neurophysiol. 1971; 31:439–449.

21. Aoyagi, M., Manaka, S., and Sano, K. Study of topographic display of EEG with special reference to spectral encephalography. Clin. Electroenceph. 1979; 21:482–489.

22. Ashida, H., Tatsuno, J., Okamoto, J., and Maru, E. Field mapping of EEG by unbiased polynomial interpolation. Comput. Biomed. Res. 1984; 17:267–276.

23. Buchsbaum, M.S., Rigal, F., Coppola, R. et al. A new system for gray-level surface distribution maps of electrical activity. Electroenceph. Clin. Neurophysiol. 1982; 53:237–242.

24. Duffy, F.H., Burchfiel, J.L., and Lombroso, C.T. Brain electrical activity mapping (BEAM): A method for extending the clinical utility of EEG and evoked potential data. Ann. Neurol. 1979; 5:309–321.

25. Duffy, F.H., Denckla, M.B., Bartels, P.H., and Sandini, G. Dyslexia: Regional differences in brain electrical activity by topographic mapping. Ann. Neurol. 1980; 5:412–420.

26. Nagata, K., Mizukami, M., Araki, G., Kawase, T., and Hirano, M. Topographic electroencephalographic study of cerebral infarction using computed mapping of the EEG. J. Cerebr. Blood Flow Metab. 1982; 2:79–88.

27. Ueno, S., Matsuoka, S., Mizoguchi, T., Nagashima, M., and Cheng, C. Topograhic computer display of abnormal EEG in patients with CNS diseases. Memoirs of the Faculty of Engineering, Kyushu University. 1975; 34:195–209.

28. Ueno, S., and Matsuoka, S. Topographic display of slow wave types of EEG abnomality in patients with brain lesions. Jpn. Med. Electr. Biol. Eng., 1976, 14:118–124.

29. Ueno, S., and Matsuoka, S. Topographic computer display of abnormal EEG activities in patients with brain lesions. Digest of the 11th International Conference on Medical and Biological Engineering, Ottawa, 1976; 218–219.

30. Walter, D.O., Etevenon, P., Pidoux, B., Tortrat, D., and Guillou, S. Computerized topo-EEG spectral maps: Difficulties and perspectives. Neuropsychobiology 1984; 11:264–272.

31. Lehmann, D. Human scalp EEG fields: Evoked, alpha, sleep and spike-wave patterns. In H.H. Petsche and M.A.B. Brazier, eds., Synchronization of EEG Activity in Epilepsies, Berlin: Springer, 1972; 301–325.

32. Lehmann, D. EEG phase differences and their physiological significance in scalp field studies. In E. Dolce and H. Kuenkel, eds., Computerized EEG Analysis, Stuttgart: Fischer, 1975; 102–110.

33. Lehmann, D. The EEG as scalp field distribution. In A. Rémond, ed., EEG Informatics, Amsterdam: Elsevier/North Holland, 1977; 365–384.

34. Lehmann, D., Meles, H.P., and Mir, Z. Scalp field maps of averaged EEG potentials evoked by checkerboard inversion. Biomed. Technik 1976; 21 (suppl.): 117–118.

35. Lehmann, D., and Skrandies, W. Multichannel mapping of spatial distributions of scalp potential fields evoked by checker-board stimuli to different retinal areas. In D. Lehmann and E. Callaway, eds., Human Evoked Potentials: Applications and Problems, London: Plenum, 1979; 201–214.

36. Koukkou, M., Lehmann, D., and Angst, J., eds. Functional States of the Brain: Their Determinants. Amsterdam: Elsevier, 1980.

37. Inouye, T., Shinosaki, K., and Yagasaki, A. The direction of spread of alpha activity over the scalp. Electroenceph. Clin. Neurophysiol. 1983; 55:290–300.

38. Petsche, H. EEG topography. In A. Rémond, ed. Handbook of Electroencephalography and Clinical Neurophysiology. Amsterdam: Elsevier, 1972; 58.

39. Childers, D. Evoked responses: Electrogenesis, models, methodology, and wavefront reconstruction and tracking analysis. Proc. IEEE, 1977; 65:611–626.

40. Pinson, L.J., and Childers, D.G. Frequency-wavenumber spectrum analysis of EEG multielectrode array data. IEEE Trans. Biomed. Eng. 1974; 21:192–206.

41. Duffy, F.H., Bartels, P.H., and Burchfiel, J.L. Significance probability mapping: An aid in the topographic analysis of brain electrical activity. Electroenceph. Clin. Neurophysiol. 1981; 51:455–462.

42. Duffy, F.H. Topographic display of evoked potentials: Clinical applications of brain electrical activity mapping. Ann. N.Y. Acad. Sci. 1983; 388:183–196.

43. Lehmann, D., and Skrandies, W. Visually evoked scalp potential fields in hemiretinal stimulation. Doc. Ophthalmol. Proc. Series, 1980; 23:237–243.

44. Brown, W.S., and Lehmann, D. Verb and noun meaning of homophone words activate different cortical generators: A topographical study of evoked potential fields. Exp. Brain Res. 1979; suppl. 2:159–168.

45. Lehmann, D., Meles, H.P., and Mir, Z. Average multichannel EEG potential fields evoked from upper and lower hemi-retina: latency differences. Electroenceph. Clin. Neurophysiol. 1977; 43:725–731.

46. Lehmann, D., and Skrandies, W. Multichannel evoked potential fields show different properties of human upper and lower hemiretinal systems. Exp. Brain Res. 1979; 35:151–159.

47. Adachi-Usami, E., and Lehmann, D. Monocular and binocular evoked average potential field topography: Upper and lower hemiretinal stimuli. Exp. Brain Res. 1983; 50:341–346.

48. Skrandies, W., Richter, M., and Lehmann, D. Checkerboard-evoked potentials:

Topography and latency for onset, offset and reversal. Prog. Brain Res. 1980; 54:291–295.

49. Skrandies, W., and Lehmann, D. Spatial principal components of multichannel maps evoked by lateral visual half-field stimuli. Electroenceph. Clin. Neurophysiol. 1982; 54:297–305.

4
EEG Topography and Mental Performance

Hellmuth Petsche, Helmut Pockberger, and
Peter Rappelsberger

The conjecture that types of mental performance are reflected in electrical brain activity is even older than the discovery of the electroencephalogram (EEG). In fact, this surmise was Berger's driving force in concentrating his efforts on the detection of traces of electrical brain activity on the human scalp, the existence of which had been known for almost half a century [1]. Berger's ultimate success in making such traces visible, nevertheless, as well as his lifelong exploration of the EEG in neurological diseases did not allow him proof of his conjecture; in those days, the technical equipment was far from sufficient to disclose specific traces of mental performance in the EEG. Only in the last decade has computerized EEG analysis enabled confirmation of Berger's initial ideas.

However, the number of papers dealing with EEG-related aspects of mental performance has considerably increased, mainly in research concerning hemispheric dominance, a phenomena only recently elucidated by cognitive studies on split-brain patients. Hitherto, however, the results of such studies have been far from consistent. A major source of these divergent results seems to be the different psychological paradigms and methods of EEG recording and processing. In many studies recording sites were restricted to temporal and parietal regions and seldom more than four electrodes were used for each hemisphere. Moreover, in many studies only hemispheric differences of alpha power or amplitude were heeded, the rest of the frequencies being neglected. In many studies, the power ranging between 0.5 and 30 Hz was considered as a composite to serve as the basis for comparison between hemispheres.

In order to increase the likelihood of finding evidence of mental processes, this study makes use of 19 electrodes placed according to the 10–20 system. Another reason for using this system as a standard montage is that it is used in current EEG practice and its electrodes are uniformly distributed over the whole scalp, thus enabling a complete topographic representation of the results.

Another issue involves the choice of the EEG parameters and their manner of presentation. Spectral analytical methods are applied to the EEG data to estimate power, frequency, and coherence parameters. By EEG segmentation and averaging of the spectra of the short epochs we are more or less independent of the duration of the mental tasks to be studied. Primary emphasis is placed on significant changes in the EEG at rest compared with the EEG during a mental task. Secondarily, interindividually common features are analyzed by plotting the results as probability maps.

METHODS

Experiments were performed on 32 healthy adults (27 male and 5 female) between the ages of 15 and 32 years. Nineteen electrodes were glued according to the 10–20 system to the scalp; the EEG was recorded on a 32-channel machine against connected earlobes as reference (cutoff frequency 30 Hz). All records were stored on analog tape and computed offline.

The subjects were comfortably seated in an armchair. The test situation was as follows: each mental task was performed for 1 minute; the tasks were separated one from another by a period of rest while the subject was allowed to move head and limbs with eyes open. During this rest interval, subjects were interrogated about their impression of the just-performed task. This not only yielded additional personal data on performance strategies for each task but also helped to maintain subjects in a state of alertness. Before and after each task 1-minute control records were made with eyes open or closed, during which the subjects were asked to relax.

Each experiment started with two control records, one with eyes open and one with eyes closed, to allow subjects to acquaint themselves with the situation. In the eyes open, relaxed condition, subjects were asked to fixate a black disk on a white wall 2 meters ahead. Then, the following mental tasks were examined, each for 1 minute: silently reading a newspaper text thought to be of interest to the subject, memorizing the content of this text with eyes open, viewing a highly detailed colored postcard, memorizing the content of the picture on the postcard (the subject had previously been asked to try to keep as many details of the postcard as possible in his memory). The following tasks were then performed with eyes closed: performance of mental arithmetic (continuously subtracting a two-digit number from a four-digit one), and listening to music (Mozart, KV 458 quartet,[1] first movement).

---

[1] KV means Köchel-Verzeichnis: This is the worldwide-used catalog of Mozarts works, edited by Mr. Köchel in the past century.

Each session took approximately a half hour. The sequence of tasks was changed at random among subjects. The 19 EEG traces were digitized at 256 Hz. Conspicuous artifacts were eliminated from computation by visual inspection. Fifteen sections of 2 seconds duration were selected from each trial for spectral analysis. Averaged power spectra and averaged coherence spectra between transversally adjacent electrodes and between electrodes on homologous regions of both hemispheres were calculated. From the spectra, broad-band parameters were selected for 5 frequency bands (theta; 4–7.5 Hz; alpha; 8–12.5 Hz; beta-1; 13–18 Hz; beta-2; 18.5–24 Hz; beta-3; 24.5–31.5 Hz). The broad-band parameters used were: natural logarithm of absolute power [2], median frequency and z-transformed mean coherence [3]. Together with these parameters, personal data for each subject were entered into a data bank.

In order to establish task-dependent changes in EEGs, confidence limits (95%) were estimated for the power and coherence parameters of the five selected frequency bands. Differences of median frequency of more than 0.5 Hz between control and task situation were arbitrarily taken as significant.

Subjects grouped by task and discrimination criteria (sex, handedness, etc.) were tested by means of paired *t*-tests, taking into consideration control before and after tasks.

For individuals, changes of power, frequency, and mean coherence parameters due to each task were presented for the five frequency bands schematically at the corresponding electrode positions as bars. Significant differences between control and task were marked by asterisks; reversible significant (s.r.) changes (control-task-control) were indicated by encircled asterisks.

The difference of the mean coherence spectra were entered between the two electrodes where they had been computed. The interhemispheric coherences were entered into a diagram of the brain as seen from the left side.

RESULTS

Since opening the eyes has long been known as the most effective means for eliciting a reorganization of the EEG pattern by sensory stimulation, the changes of power, median frequency, and coherence in EEG were studied using 1 minute of eyes closed readings as compared with 1 minute of eyes open readings in a group of healthy subjects [4]. Power decreases in all bands, particularly in the alpha band, a result known for a long time. Concomitant to these power changes when the eyes are opened, the EEG shows changes in median frequency. It particularly increases in the alpha and beta-3 bands. Beta-2 frequency decreases at most locations. Moreover, both transverse and interhemispheric coherence is reduced by opening the eyes, particularly in the lower frequency bands and on the anterior half of the skull, thus indicating a diminution of the degree of coupling between different cortical regions when the level of alertness is raised. Only in the posterior scalp did a few coherence values increase as a consequence of opening the eyes.

Intraindividual Changes in EEG during Mental Performance

We selected a 23-year-old healthy right-handed male student for analysis of intraindividual changes during mental activity. To better distinguish the five frequency bands in the following diagrams of EEG activity, the bars were marked with different symbols. Artifacts due to muscular activity may heavily influence the beta bands. To avoid this problem, we scrutinized every EEG trace and marked the corresponding electrode position in the diagrams with a capital "M" or a lower-case "m" according to content of muscle artifact. ("M" means heavy, "m" means slight muscle artifacts.)

Figure 4.1 presents the data obtained when the subject was asked to read a newspaper text to himself for 1 minute. The figure represents the differences in power, median frequency, transversal, and interhemispheric coherence (TRCOH and IHCOH) between the eye open and reading conditions. When reading, substantial muscle artifact was present in F7, and minor muscle artifact in T5, F8, and F1. These local results should therefore be neglected.

Alpha power shows considerable increase,particularly in regions around the vertex and at O2. In the beta band, a decrease occurs primarily in the beta-3 spectra during reading, most distinctly in both occipital, mid-temporal, parietal, and precentral regions, but also at Cz and Fz.

There are only minor frequency changes during reading, namely, an increase of median theta frequency at C3 and an increase of beta-3 frequency at T3 and O1. This frequency decreases at Fz and F2.

Among the TRCOH changes there is a considerable decrease registered at the frontal leads. Although muscle artifacts may contribute to these results, the decrease of beta-3 coherence between C3 and Cz and between Cz and C4 (s.r.) was found between electrodes free from muscle artifact. A decrease of beta-3 IHCOH was also found at all electrode sites. Only alpha coherence increased between F3 and F4 and C3 and C4.

When memorizing the same text while looking at a target (a black disk on a white wall in front of the subject) is compared with the condition eyes open before reading, alpha power increases even more than during mere reading in the parietal, posterior temporal, and frontal leads (Figure 4.2).

This alpha power increase is accompanied by a theta and beta-1 power increase. Beta-3 power, on the other hand, decreases in a manner similar to that during reading, but over a more extended area, most pronounced at the right temporal leads.

The difference in frequency shift are more conspicuous over the right hemisphere: the alpha frequency increases at T4 (s.r.) and a distinct beta-3 decrease in frequency is seen over the right hemisphere, particularly at Cz, C4 and P4.

The most distinct changes in TRCOH with respect to reading are an increase in alpha at the right anterior quadrant (s.r.) when memorizing.

IHCOH decreases while reading and memorizing the text between the frontopolar leads; the only noticable difference between these two tasks was found between F7 and F8: during reading, alpha coherence decreased (s.r.); during memorizing theta coherence increased (s.r.).

The changes are different when the same person is asked to look at a colored postcard with many details and to memorize as many of these details as possible (Figure 4.3). During this task the higher frequency bands of the electrodes F2, F7, and T5 should be ignored because of muscle artifact.

During viewing a remarkable asymmetry appears in the theta power: it decreases considerably at the right posterior quadrant of the skull, particularly at T6. Conversely, an s.r. alpha power decrease is found only on the left, at O1, T3, and probably also at T5, whereas, on the frontal half of the skull, alpha power increases (except at F1 and F2), particularly in the vertex region. In the beta bands, an s.r. reduction of power is found in the occipital and parietal regions and particularly at T3. As during reading, a decrease of beta-3 power was found during viewing, with almost the same spatial distribution. For median frequency, theta decreases across the whole scalp; s.r., in the parietal regions, at the vertex, and at O1; beta-1 frequency increases (s.r.) in the left frontal region. Beta-3 increases most noticably on the right temporo-occipital region while the picture is being contemplated. The coherence changes during viewing are similar to those observed during reading, that is, there is a marked change in the left temporal regions and a lesser change in the right temporal regions.

During 1 minute of memorizing the content of the picture with eyes open, a comparison with the resting condition with opened eyes just before viewing the picture yields the results shown in Figure 4.4. Alpha power increases over the whole skull; beta-1 increases in the frontal regions, beta-2 power decreases at the left and at both occipital leads (s.r.), but increases at both frontopolar leads (s.r.). The most distinct change involves beta-3 power, which decreases considerably at occipital leads (s.r.), at the right parietal lead (s.r.), and in the right temporal regions far more than in the left ones, whereas it increases at the right frontopolar lead (s.r.).

There is also an increase in alpha frequency (s.r. in P3, Pz and P4). Beta-2 frequency increases in the left (s.r. in T5) and decreases in the right hemisphere (s.r. in T4). As observed with power data, frequency changes are most pronounced in the beta-3 range, particularly in the frontal regions (s.r. in F1, Fz, and F4).

Listening to music for 1 minute concentrates the power changes in the theta- and beta-1 bands, whereas alpha power only decreases in mid-temporal

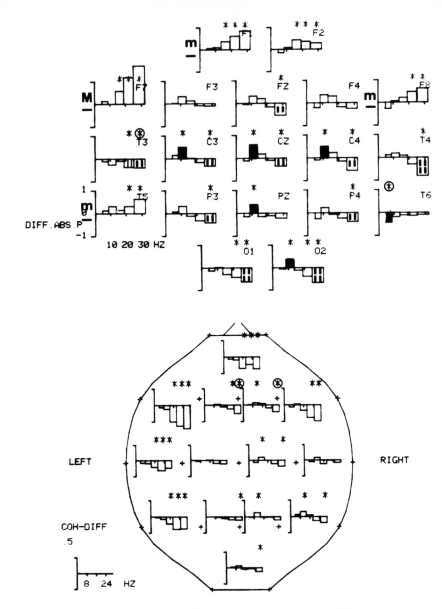

Figure 4.1. Changes of power (*top left*), median frequency (*top right*), transversal coherence (TRCOH), and interhemispheric coherence (IHCOH, *bottom*) during reading as compared with the previous control state (eyes open, relaxed) in one subject. In the upper diagrams, the five bars at the positions of the electrodes represent the five frequency

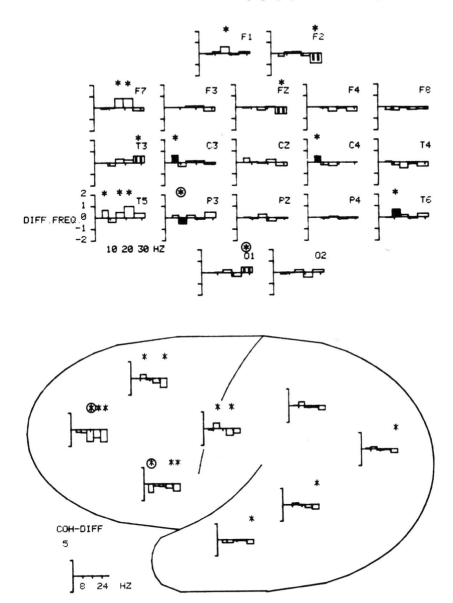

bands studied and indicate an increase or decrease of power and median frequency. Significant changes determined by 0.5% confidence intervals are marked by asterisks; for a better distinction, these bars are also marked by different symbols; encircled asterisks indicate significant reversible changes (control-task-control).

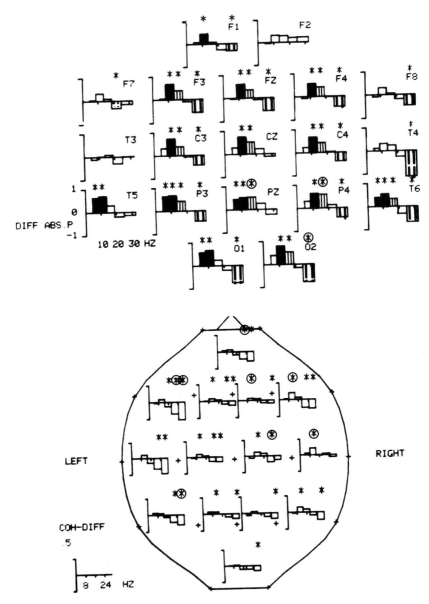

Figure 4.2. Changes caused by memorizing text. Same subject and representation as in Figure 4.1.

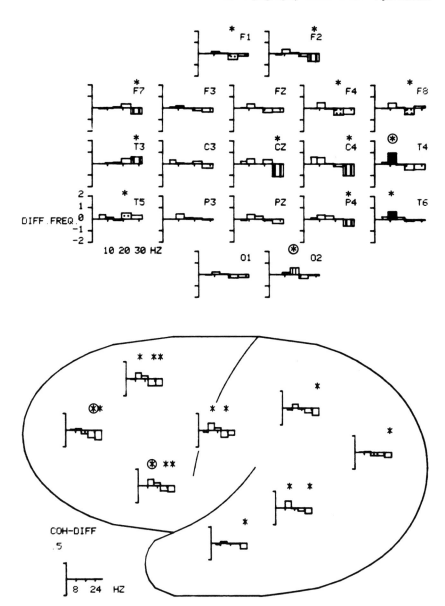

Figure 4.2 cont.

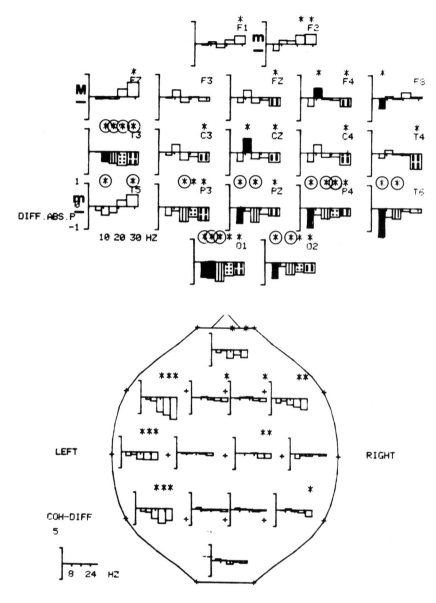

Figure 4.3. Changes caused by contemplating a picture. Same subject and representation as in Figure 4.1.

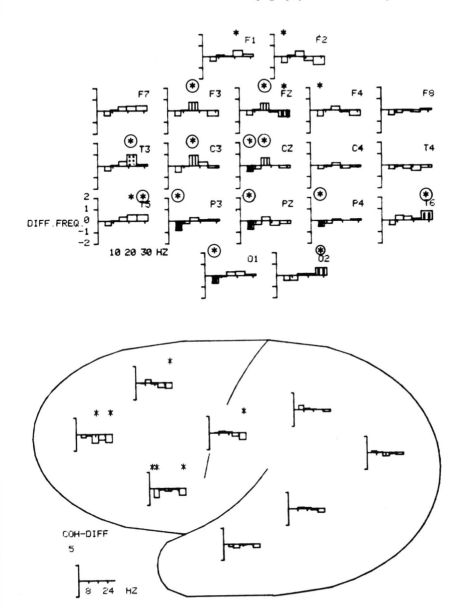

Figure 4.3 cont.

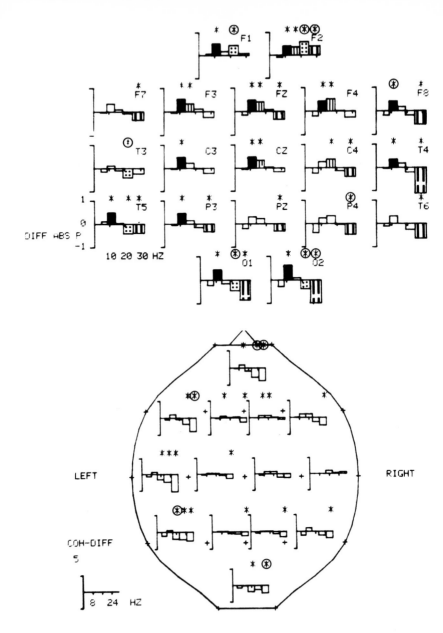

Figure 4.4. Changes caused by memorizing the content of a picture. Same subject and representation as in Figure 4.1.

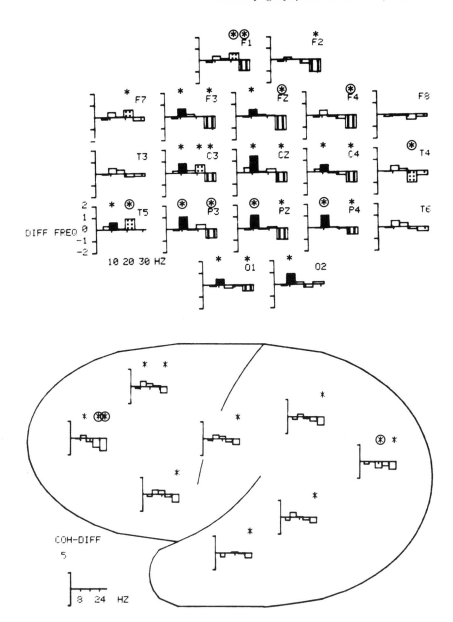

Figure 4.4 cont.

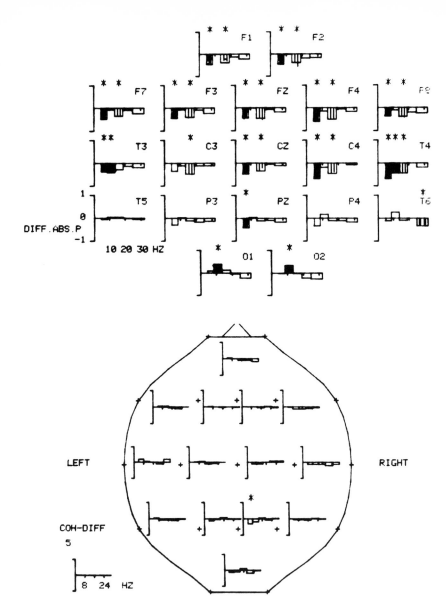

Figure 4.5. Changes caused by listening to music. Same subject and representation as in Figure 4.1.

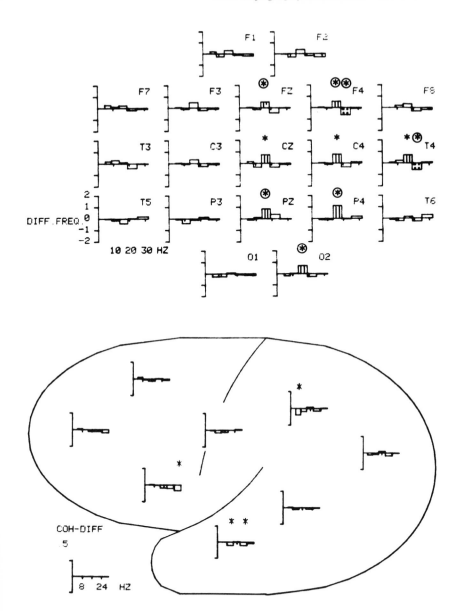

Figure 4.5 cont.

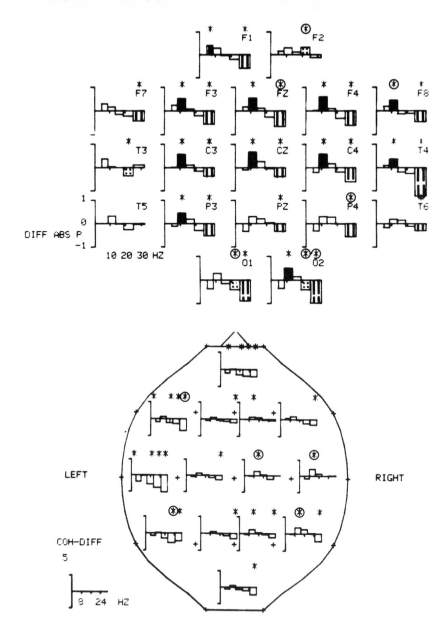

Figure 4.6. Changes caused by doing mental arithmetic. Same subject and representation as in Figure 4.1.

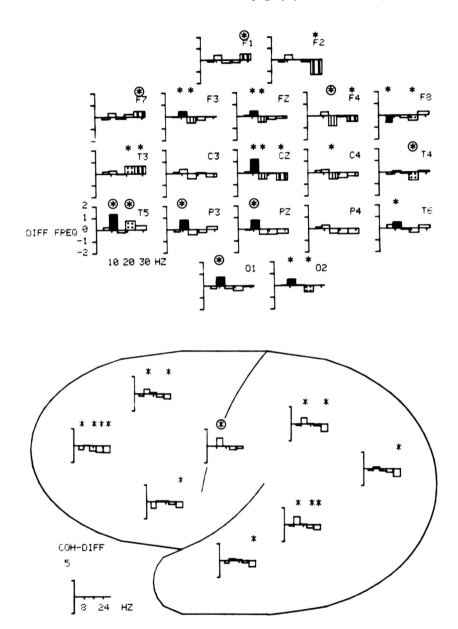

Figure 4.6 cont.

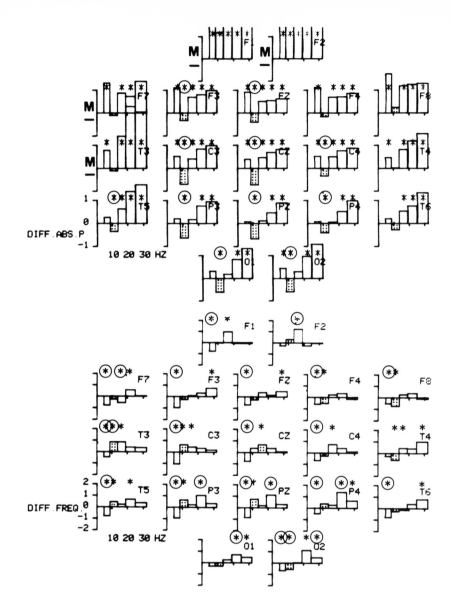

Figure 4.7. Changes of power and median frequency observed with a 32-year-old bilingual Japanese scientist when reading a Japanese (p. 80) and a German (p. 81) scientific text.

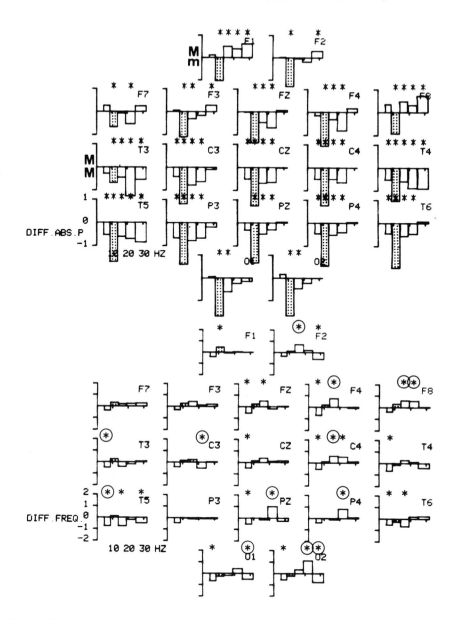

Figure 4.7 cont.

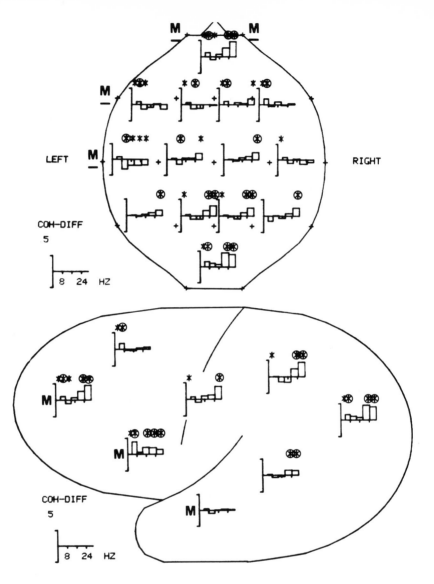

Figure 4.8. Transversal and interhemispheric coherence. Same subject as in Figure 4.7. Reading Japanese, p. 82; reading German, p. 83.

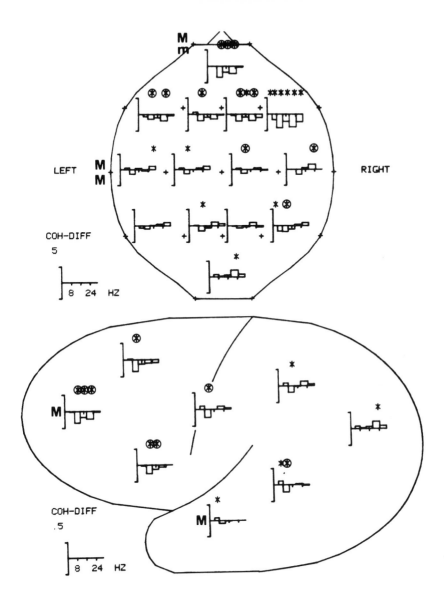

Figure 4.8 cont.

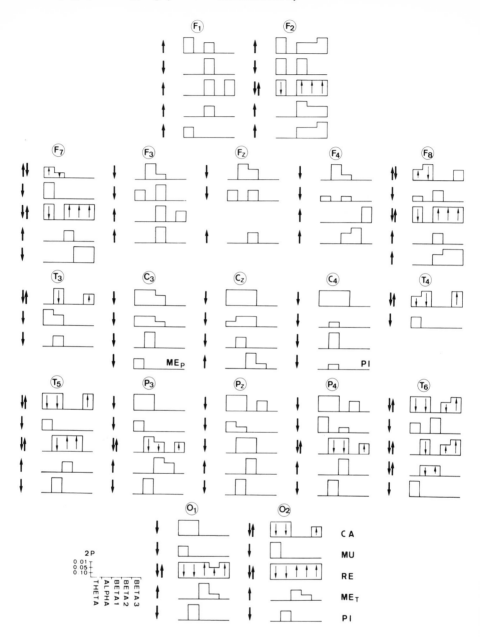

Figure 4.9. Topographic representation of the results of probability mappings of power changes for the following mental tasks: calculating (CA), listening to music (MU), reading (RE), memorizing text (ME$_T$), contemplating a picture (PI), and memorizing the content of a picture (ME$_P$) for the five frequency bands studied. Ordinate: changes according to the probabilities of error of $2P = 0.01$, 0.05, and 0.1. Abscissa: frequency bands. The arrows indicate increase or decrease of power.

areas (Figure 4.5). Conversely, an increase of alpha power is found at the occipital leads in both hemispheres. Theta power decreases considerably in the anterior skull and is more pronounced on the right side than on the left. Frequency changes while listening to music are only seen in the beta band and are almost entirely restricted to the right hemisphere, the beta-1 frequency augmenting and beta-2 abating at F4 and T4. Coherence changes are almost negligible in this task; they involve the temporal and parietal regions.

Brain electrical activity when doing mental arithmetic, as compared to eyes open shows an alpha increase over the whole skull (Figure 4.6). This task predominantly effects changes in beta-3 power, which decreases, together with beta-2, most distinctly at the two occipital leads (s.r.) and over large parts of the skull, with the exception of the left temporal leads T3 and T5.

The frequency changes while doing mental arithmetic as compared with the eyes open condition show dramatic asymmetric differences: alpha frequency increases predominantly at the left posterior quadrant of the skull (s.r.), beta-2 increases at T3 and T5 (s.r.), but decreases at T4 (s.r.), F8, and O2. Beta-3 increases at F1 (s.r.), F7 (s.r.), and T3, but decreases at F2, F4, and Oz.

Doing mental arithmetic, moreover, tends to decrease TRCOH on the left hemisphere, whereas alpha coherence is increased in the right hemisphere, the increase being most pronounced over the right posterior quadrant. Alpha coherence also increases between the hemispheres, particularly at C3-C4 (s.r.), but also at F3-F4, P3-P4, and T5-T6.

These findings for a single subject demonstrate that even a fairly uniform task such as reading involves large portions of the brain. Moreover, it turns out that the topography of the changes of the three parameters of power, median frequency, and coherence do not always coincide. This holds true for the five frequency bands.

That this method also turned out to be sensitive to differential mental processing in bilingual subjects is demonstrated by a 32-year-old Japanese colleague, who speaks fluent German. He was requested to read a German and a Japanese scientific text, written in Kanji (Figures 4.7 and 4.8). The differences were considerable: when reading Japanese, the power increased in all frequency bands except the alpha band, yet when reading German, there was, in almost all frequency bands, a decrease in power, most pronounced in the alpha band. Changes of median frequencies were also totally different and more conspicuous when reading Japanese than when reading German. There was some lateralization of the frequency changes; they concentrated more on the left hemisphere when reading Japanese, and more on the right when reading German. There were even more significant changes in coherence (Figure 4.9). Reading Japanese seemed to have slightly more influence on the left hemisphere, and reading German induced more changes on the right. Furthermore, reading Japanese generally increased the IHCOH, whereas, it decreased when reading German, most distinctly in the frontal and posterior temporal regions.

Common Group Properties during Mental Performance

The second part of our study dealt with the search for common features among groups of subjects performing the same mental tasks. For this purpose, the probabilities for changes were calculated for power and coherence (2 P = 0.01, 0.05, and 0.1). Only significantly reversible changes were taken into account. The following tasks were performed: mental arithmetic (CA), listening to music (MU), reading (RE), memorizing the text (ME$_T$), contemplating a picture (PI), and memorizing the content of the picture (ME$_P$). Only male right-handers were considered. The number of subjects performing each task was as follows: CA, 13; MU, 13; RE, 19; ME$_T$, 19; PI, 7; ME$_P$, 7.

Changes in Power

Figure 4.9 is a condensed representation of the power changes in electrical activity found during performance of these six mental tasks in our study group with respect to frequency bands, direction, and degree of significance. Generally, each task caused widespead power changes in one or several frequency bands. As a measure of the area of the skull experiencing change in electrical activity, calculating and listening to music caused power changes in all 19 leads, reading in 17, memorizing the text in 16, looking at a picture in 12, and memorizing the content of the picture in only 1 lead (Table 4.1). As Table 4.1 also demonstrates, the direction of changes differs according to the demand of each task.

The directions of task-dependent power changes are summarized in Table 4.2. During mental arithmetic both an increase and decrease of power was found in all frequency bands. Listening to music led to only a power decrease restricted within the theta to beta-1 range. Memorizing the content of the picture caused a power decrease limited to one lead (C3). All other tasks reduced power in the lower frequency bands and enhanced it in the higher frequency bands. The only exception to this finding was a theta increase at F1 during picture contemplation (see Figure 4.9), as well as at F7 and F8 during calculation (possibly due to eye artifact).

When looking for a possible anterior-posterior distribution of the directions of power changes, the following results are worth mentioning (see Figure 4.9):

- Mental arithmetic increased power at F1 and F2, but decreased it in other frontal, central, and parietal regions; in the lateral leads over both hemispheres, as well as at O2, both an increase and a decrease of power was observed, depending on frequency.
- Reading increased power at the frontal leads (F1, F2, F3, and F4) and decreased it at the central, parietal, and occipital leads. At F2, F8, and F7 as

well as at the posterior temporal, the parietal, and the occipital sites, alpha and theta power decreased, whereas beta power increased.

- Contemplating a picture increased power frontally and decreased it over the posterior portions of the skull.
- Listening to music did not show any topographic preference in the direction of power changes, nor did memorizing the text.

These findings supply only modest conclusions about lateralization of function (Figure 4.9):

- Mental arithmetic increased beta-2 and -3 power in the right anterior quadrant and beta-2 at Pz, P4, and T6, but not at P3 and T5.
- Reading decreased theta power at F2 yet not at F1, and increased beta-1 power at F3 yet not at F4. Alpha power decreased at T3, but not contralaterally.
- Memorizing the text increased beta-2 power at F2 and F4 but not contralaterally to these positions. Conversely, beta-2 power increased at P3 but not at P4.
- Contemplating a picture increased beta-1 and -3 power at F2 and theta power at F1 and decreased alpha power at C4.
- Memorizing the content of the picture only decreased theta power at C3.
- Listening to music decreased power in the beta-1 band at F8 and T6, but not at the corresponding contralateral leads.

On the basis of these findings and the relatively small subject sample, no definitive conclusions can be drawn about cerebral lateralization by means of the power spectrum of the EEG.

Changes in Transversal Coherence (TRCOH)

Among the mental tasks studied, TRCOH underwent several significant task-, area-, and frequency-dependent changes in both directions. These are summarized in Figure 4.10. Changes of TRCOH were most widespread during reading (in 8 out of 12 possible electrode pairs), followed by listening to music, memo-

Table 4.1 Number of Leads (*n*) in which Significant Power Changes were Found (Regardless of Frequency Bands)

		Direction of Power Change		
Task	*n*	↑	↓	↓ ↑
CA	19	2	10	7
MU	19	—	19	—
RE	17	3	5	9
ME$_T$	16	14	1	1
PI	12	4	8	—
ME$_P$	1	—	1	—

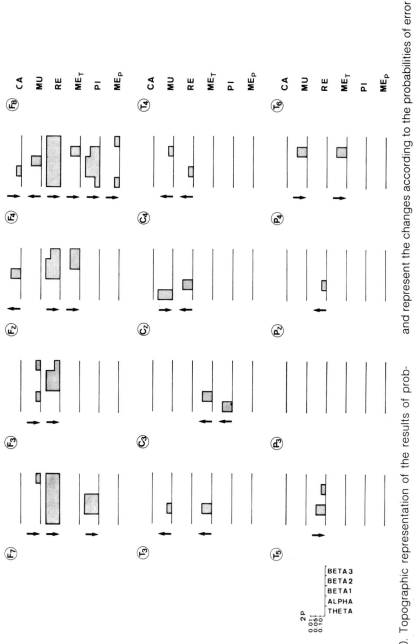

Figure 4.10. Topographic representation of the results of probablity mappings of transversal coherence (TRCOH) changes. The diagrams are arranged between the respective electrodes and represent the changes according to the probabilities of error of 2P (ordinate) and the frequency bands (abscissa) as in Figure 4.9.

Table 4.2   Direction of Power Change by Frequency Band and Task, Group Data

Task	Frequency Range				
	Theta	*Alpha*	*Beta-1*	*Beta-2*	*Beta-3*
CA	+	+	+	+	+
	−	−	−	−	−
MU					
	−	−	−		
RE			+	+	+
	−	−	−		
ME$_T$			+	+	+
	−	−			
PI	+		+	+	+
		−			
ME$_P$					
	−				

Table 4.3   Number of Electrode Pairs (*n*) in which Significant Changes in Transversal Coherence (TRCOH) Were Observed (maximum possible *n* = 12)

Task	*n*	*Left* ↑	↓	*Right* ↑	↓	*Total* ↑	↓
RE	8	—	3	3	2	3	5
MU	7	1	2	2	2	3	4
ME$_T$	5	2	—	—	3	2	3
PI	3	1	1	—	1	1	2
CA	1	—	—	—	1	—	1
ME$_P$	1	—	—	—	1	—	1
		4	6	5	10	9	16

rizing the text, and looking at a picture. The direction of change in TRCOH varied, with a distinctly more frequent occurrence of decrease in the right hemisphere (see Table 4.3).

Table 4.4 gives a survey of the frequency bands involved in changes of TRCOH during these six tasks. Reading caused decreases in all five bands and an increase only in the alpha band. The changes were quite similar when contemplating a picture. With subjects listening to music, in addition to a decrease in four frequency bands, TRCOH increased from theta to beta-2. The other tasks only caused changes in single bands.

Table 4.4 Frequency Bands Involved and Direction of Changes in Transverse Coherence (TRCOH), and Interhemispheric Coherence (IHCOH)

Task	(TRCOH) Frequency Band					(IHCOH) Frequency Band				
	Theta	Alpha	Beta-1	Beta-2	Beta-3	Theta	Alpha	Beta-1	Beta-2	Beta-3
CA			+			+	+	+	+	+
		−					−			
MU		+	+	+		+	+			
	−	−		−	−					
RE		+					+	+		
	−	−	−	−	−	−	−	−	−	−
ME$_T$		+					+			
		−		−						−
PI	+					+				
	−	−	−	−		−	−	−		
ME$_P$										
	−			−						

Table 4.5 Direction of Change in TRCOH in Transverse Electrode Rows

TRCOH	Increase		Decrease	
	Left	Right	Left	Right
F7-F3-Fz-F4-F8	0	2	5	7
T3-C3-Cz-C4-T4	4	3	0	1
T5-P5-Pz-P6-T6	0	1	1	2

As for a possible lateralization of functions, only mental arithmetic and memorization of the content of a picture demonstrated a tendency to right-sidedness. The other tasks proved to influence both hemispheres in different ways.

The direction of changes in TRCOH was not found to discriminate between the hemispheres, with the sole exception of memorizing the text, which turned out to enhance TRCOH on the left (T3-C3 and C3-Cz) and to cause a decrease on the right hemisphere (Fz-F4 and F4-F8). There was also no clearcut behavior of TRCOH with respect to the motor and sensory regions of the cortex. In both areas, the TRCOH was found to both increase and decrease. If, however, the three transverse electrode rows from which TRCOH was estimated are considered separately, differences become evident, an observation which may shed some light on the possible functions of the underlying cortical areas (Table 4.5).

As Figure 4.10 demonstrates, the area that seems most directly involved with all mental tasks under investigation is the right anterior quadrant of the skull. It is also the only area where changes of TRCOH in both directions were observed at the same recording site. Whether the preponderance of TRCOH changes over the right hemisphere is connected to the exclusive use of right-handers in this study is unclear.

Changes in Interhemispheric Coherence (IHCOH)

Mean group changes in interhemispheric coherence are summarized in Figure 4.11. In assessing the incidence of change across frequencies, reading, as with TRCOH, caused changes of IHCOH in all bands (see Table 4.4).

The greatest differences in effects on the defined frequencies measured as TRCOH, in contrast to IHCOH changes, was found during the calculating task, for which changes of IHCOH were evidenced in all frequency bands. Only the beta-1 band responded with a notable change in TRCOH. Another meaningful difference between TRCOH and IHCOH was observed in listening to music, a task that caused decreases only in TRCOH.

As for the direction of changes in IHCOH, the greatest difference was found between reading and calculating: during reading, IHCOH preponderantly decreased in contrast to mental arithmetic.

Table 4.6 gives a survey of the direction of changes in IHCOH with respect to brain regions: there was a general tendency of IHCOH to increase in the centro-parieto-temporo-occipital regions for calculating, reading, memorizing the text, and contemplating the picture. Exceptions were the decrease at T5-T6 during reading and at O1-O2 during memorizing text. In the frontal regions, IHCOH generally decreased during these tasks, the exception being mental arithmetic during which coherence decrease was only found in the beta-1 band and at F3-F4 and F7-F8. Otherwise coherence increased. Memorization of text followed this general trend of reading with the exception of O1-O2, but significant changes were found in fewer regions than when reading. Memorizing the content of the picture did not change IHCOH significantly. The changes during listening to music, on the other hand, turned out to fit to none of these patterns.

DISCUSSION

This study attempted to answer three questions. (1) Can evidence of mental processes be found in the EEG and be substantiated by statistical methods? To answer this a method was developed which, based on Fourier analysis, puts equal weights on an analysis of the ongoing EEG in time and space. (2) Can correlations be made between EEG findings and task- and personality-dependent brain conditions in an individual as a possible means of objectifying the ambiguous term "intelligence"? (3) What is the average brain electrical behavior of groups of subjects performing the same mental tasks?

The answer to the first question is yes. It turned out that several parameters chosen for this study exhibit significant changes during mental tasks that are significantly reversible if the task period is compared with the preceding and following control period.

A definite answer to the second question cannot yet be given, since too few subjects have so far been studied, not enough repetitions of the same task have been performed on single subjects, and no detailed psychological tests have been made to obtain closer insight into the subject's momentary psychological state. Therefore, we cannot yet be sure to what extent the changes of EEG parameters are due to the task alone or to additional emotional or other influences known to act upon the EEG [5–7]. However, the present findings encourage us to continue this study.

And finally, the answer to the third question is yes. As the above results demonstrate, both significant task- and brain-dependent changes in several parameters of electrical brain activity could be secured by statistical means.

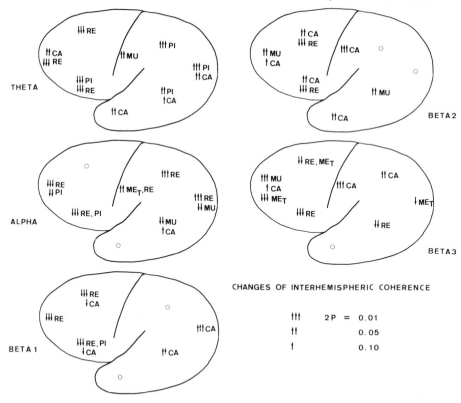

Figure 4.11. Topographic representation of the results of probability mapping of interhemispheric coherence (IHCOH) changes, indicated at the respective electrode positions. The number of arrows indicates the probability of error (three arrows, $2P = 0.01$; two arrows; $2P = 0.05$; one arrow; $2P = 0.1$).

Table 4.6 Direction of Regional IHCOH Changes

Task			Electrode Locations					
	F1-F2	F7-F8	F3-F4	C3-C4	T3-T4	P3-P4	T5-T6	O1-O2
CA	↑	beta-1 ↓ beta-2 ↑	beta-1 ↓ beta-2 ↑	↑	↑	↑	↑	↑
MU	↑	—	—	↑	—	—	alpha ↓ beta-2 ↑	↓
RE	↓	↓	↓	↑	—	↑	↓	↑
ME$_T$	↓	—	↓	↑	—	—	—	↓
PI	↓	↓	—	—	—	↑	↑	↑
ME$_P$	—	—	—	—	—	—	—	—

Before entering into a discussion of our data with regard to the literature, attention should be directed to the possible meaning of the parameters chosen and of their changes. With regard to power, one may be inclined to conclude from the power decrease observed when the eyes are opened that this is only due to an increase of the level of alertness, which initiates a larger number of cognitive processes and leads to a desynchronization of the EEG. This study, however, supplies sufficient data to abandon the simple conjecture that a decrease of alpha power is a general concomitant of increased mental efforts. Alpha power may increase or decrease conjointly with different mental performances, these changes occurring differentially over space as Figure 4.9 demonstrates. Neither does this study support the hypothesis that alpha is suppressed by that hemisphere which may be primarily responsible for information processing at any given time, as proposed by Robbins and McAdam [8]. A closer examination of the literature on hemisphere-specific changes of alpha resulted in the realization that our data cannot easily be compared with most of the data at hand for simple methodological reasons. Most authors prefer to talk about alpha percentage time, or use a right-left alpha index, or integrators, or record from only a few electrodes and neglect topographic aspects, or even record bipolarly. Many authors put more weight on sophisticated psychological paradigms than on meticulous EEG methodology.

Among the authors using Fourier analysis, the work by Stigsby et al. [9] is exemplary. They also provide a survey of the literature about alpha power changes in conjunction with mental tasks. Among the tests these authors use, the "visual reasoning test" is most like our visual task. They found a theta increase in the frontal area (in our data theta power increased only in F1, when contemplating a picture). Their increase in alpha in the temporal regions during the visual test could not be confirmed by our data, where the region of alpha decrease during picture contemplation was much larger. (Stigsby found a decrease in alpha only at the two occipital regions.)

Dolce and Waldeier [10] were not able to differentiate between mental arithmetic and reading, but reported a decrease in alpha intensity during both

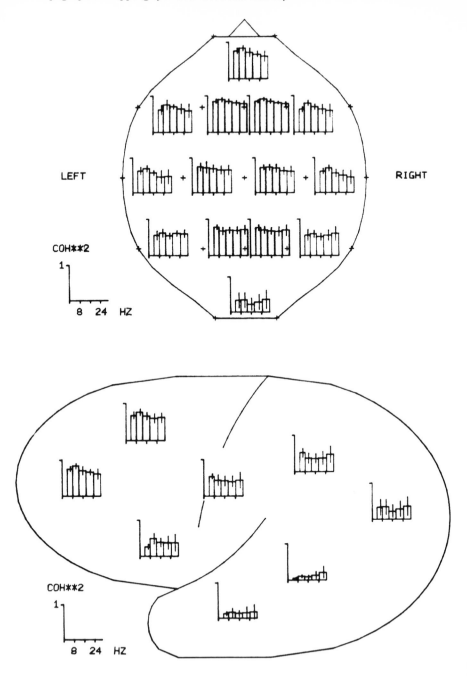

Figure 4.12. Average values of transversal and interhemispheric coherence of eight male right-handers under resting condition. Note the high values in the frontal and the low values in the temporal regions.

tasks as compared with the eyes open condition. However, they found an increased beta intensity during reading but not during mental arithmetic; these findings can be only partially confirmed by us since the beta increase depends on the site of the recording. We failed to confirm McLeod et al.'s [11] finding that frequency bands other than the alpha band did not supply significant results during verbal, arithmetic, visual, and musical tasks. These findings show that no general conclusions about power changes during these mental tasks can yet be made. Also, no interpretation of power changes in physiological terms can be supplied at the present time. The same holds true for the changes of median frequencies, changes which may be considerable and amount to more than 1 Hz, even in the low frequency bands. Very little correlation between the spatial distribution of power changes and the changes of median frequency was observed.

A few remarks concerning coherence are necessary, since this parameter has not yet found wide use in the EEG analysis. Shaw and Ongley [12] first emphasized the importance of coherence estimates for studying the functional organization of the cortex. In this connection also Livanov's [13] work has to be mentioned. He considered the topographic aspect to be of great import and recorded from as many as 50 electrodes. Unfortunately he did not give a clear enough description of his method of calculating correlations between areas, as such, a verification of his findings is hardly feasible.

Basically, coherence is a measure of the correlation of two signals as a function of frequency. Coherence thus indicates in which frequency ranges two brain regions become functionally more or less coupled during a certain mental task. The increased alpha coherence found by Shaw and Ongley during mental arithmetic in a right-handed group was confirmed in this study. Sklar et al. [14] found IHCOH in dyslexic children to be lower than in healthy children. Differences in IHCOH between right- and left-preference groups were also observed by Giannitrapani [15]. Beaumont et al. [16] found greater coherence changes over the right than over the left hemisphere in spatial tasks. Busk and Galbraith [17] concluded from their results with visuomotor tasks that task difficulty and practice influence the coherence level, which was found to decrease with increasing practice and to increase with increasing difficulty of the task. These authors also think that the number of fiber connections between two brain regions determines the basic level of coherence to a certain degree. This conjecture has been confirmed by our research [4]: lowest IHCOH levels are found in the mid-temporal region, which is known for its scanty fiber connections with contralateral structures.

For a reasonable evaluation of coherence changes under resting condition at all recording sites, it is desirable to measure the average values of coherence. These values show a fairly consistent topographic distribution. As already mentioned, IHCOH is smallest between T3 and T4 and between T5 and T6 and largest between F1 and F2. TRCOH is largest in the frontal, central, and parietal regions but considerably lower when estimated between the temporal and the paramedian electrodes (Figure 4.12). Because of the low level of temporal IHCOH under the resting condition, changes of these values should be evaluated with caution.

In contrast to opening the eyes, whereupon the changes of coherence are fairly equally distributed over both sides, considerable hemispheric differences were found during mental tasks. Most changes were observed over the frontal parts of the skull, and one may argue whether these changes are due to processes involving the frontal association areas of the cortex. Shaw and Ongley [12] suggested that a decrease in coherence could indicate that the area in question is involved in processing information. As plausible as this conjecture may appear, it is not sufficient to explain these findings since coherence is also occasionally increased in areas that are likely to be involved in the task.

Without a better neurophysiological explanation, coherence can be taken as an indicator of how strongly two brain areas are functionally connected over a frequency range during the performance of a task, be it by commissural fibers or subcortical structures. For the moment, the term "coherence" adequately describes some properties of ongoing brain activity, comparable to the two other parameters "power" and "frequency" whose true physiological significance are also still far from clear, although these two terms have long been used. The usefulness of these three parameters is enhanced by the finding that their changes during mental tasks show quite different topographic distributions.

Finally, attention should be directed toward consideration of the underlying brain regions that are involved in these changes. This issue is particularly difficult since no true 1:1 topographic correspondence exists between the electrical registrations at the scalp and the cortical regions producing these signals.

There are several reasons for this discrepancy, among them the differential thickness and composition of the tissues under the electrodes, differences which cause local differences in impedance. Another reason is the gyration of the generator layer for the EEG which may lead to heavy distortions not only of the shape of potentials but also of their local distribution. These require extreme caution in neuroanatomical interpretations of topographic findings. For this reason, we also preferred, for our diagrams, a representation of the calculated values at distinct electrode sites instead of contour maps. However, these data prove that mental tasks do not exclusively activate one distinct region but rather involve large regions of the cortex in a complex manner.

The aims of this study were as follows:

1. To develop a method to trace power, frequency, and coherence changes due to different types of mental performance by the 10–20 electrode montage and by calculation of broad-band parameters.
2. To test the changes of these parameters in individuals, and
3. To find group properties by means of probability mapping.

The results obtained show significantly reversible changes for any of these tested mental tasks, the spatial configuration of these changes being different for any task. These results indicate that any of the tasks tested involves large areas of both hemispheres in a complex way.

ACKNOWLEDGMENTS

This research was supported by the Fonds zur Förderung der Wissenschaftlichen Forschung in Österreich, Project Nr. S 25/01, and by the Herbert von Karajan Stiftung der Gesellschaft der Musikfreunde in Vienna. The authors wish to thank Mrs. E. Genner for her valuable assistance in recording the EEGs, in computation, and in production of figures. Moreover, we are grateful to Mrs. S. Etlinger, B.A., for her helpful linguistic comments and discussions.

REFERENCES

1. Caton, R. The electric currents of the brain. Br. Med. J. 1875; 2:278.
2. Gasser, Th., Bächer, P., and Möcks, J. Transformations toward the normal distribution of broad band spectral parameters of the EEG. Electroenceph. Clin. Neurophysiol. 1982; 53:119–124.
3. Jenkins, G.M., and Watts, D.G. Spectral Analysis and Its Applications. San Francisco: Holden-Day, 1969.
4. Petsche, H., Pockberger, H., and Rappelsberger, P. Vigilanz und kognitive Vorgänge. In J. Kugler and V. Leutner, eds. Vigilanz: Ihre Bestimmung und Beeinflussung. Basel: Editiones Roche, 1984; 127–142.
5. Wiet, S.G. Some quantitative hemispheric EEG measures reflecting the affective profile of students differing in university academic success. Biol. Psychol. 1981; 12:25–42.
6. Oltman, P.K., Semple, C., and Goldstein, L. Cognitive style and interhemispheric differentiation in the EEG. Neuropsychologia 1979; 17:699–702.
7. Schwartz, G.E., Davidson, R.J., and Maer, F. Right hemisphere lateralization for emotion in the human brain: Interactions with cognition. Science 1975; 190:286–288.
8. Robbins, K.I., and McAdam, D.W. Interhemispheric alpha asymmetry and imagery mode. Brain and Language 1974; 1:189–193.
9. Stigsby, B., Risberg, J., and Ingvar, D.H. Electroencephalographic changes in the dominant hemisphere during memorizing and reasoning. Electroenceph. Clin. Neurophysiol. 1977; 42:665–675.
10. Dolce, G., and Waldeier, H. Spectral and multivariate analysis of EEG changes during mental activity in man. Electroenceph. Clin. Neurophysiol. 1974; 36:577–584.
11. McLeod, S.S., and Peacock, L.J. Task-related EEG asymmetry: Effects of age and ability. Psychophysiology 1977; 14:308–311.

12. Shaw, J.C., and Ongley, C. The measurement of synchronization. In H. Petsche and M.A.B. Brazier, eds., Synchronization of EEG Activities in Epilepsies. New York: Springer, 1972; 204–214.

13. Livanov, M.N. Spatial Organization of Cerebral Processes. New York: John Wiley, 1977.

14. Sklar, B., Hanley, J., and Simmons, W.W. An EEG experiment aimed toward identifying dyslexic children. Nature 1972; 240:414–416.

15. Giannitrapani, D. Spectral analysis of the EEG. In G. Dolce and H. Künkel, eds., CEAN: Computerized EEG Analysis. Stuttgart: Gustav Fischer, 1975; 384–402.

16. Beaumont, J.G., Mayes, A.R., and Rugg, M.D. Asymmetry in EEG alpha coherence and power: Effects of task and sex. Electroenceph. Clin. Neurophysiol. 1978; 45:393–401.

17. Busk, J., and Galbraith, G.C. EEG correlates of visual-motor practice in man. Electroenceph. Clin. Neurophysiol. 1975; 38:415–422.

5

Event-Related Desynchronization Mapping: Visualization of Cortical Activation Patterns

Gert Pfurtscheller

One goal of the electroencephalographic (EEG) mapping technique should be the use of multiple scalp EEG recordings to obtain information about the function of underlying brain structures. Severe impairment of cortical tissue results in changes of EEG pattern. Such changes could include the disappearance of alpha activity and the appearance of slow wave activity. Mild impairment, however, can result in no detectible changes in the EEG. EEG mapping can be used not only to quantify severe brain damage, but also to help detect mild forms of cerebral dysfunction, even when the clinical EEG is visually scored as normal. Furthermore, EEG mapping should help to investigate cortical structures and interactions among them during conscious perceptions, motor behavior, spontaneous speech, and other forms of mental activity.

An important feature of EEG mapping is its reproducibility and reliability. Important considerations in ensuring reliability of results include the choice of electrode position, analysis time, number of recordings and analyzed parameters, and the control of the state of the brain during EEG recordings. In this last respect three different experimental situations have to be differentiated:

EEG processing during rest
EEG processing during continuous mental, sensory, or motor behavior
EEG processing during short-lasting event-related situations

EEG recording during rest, with eyes either closed or open, is the most common condition for EEG mapping [1–3]. This is a completely uncontrolled state of the brain and can never be reproduced. However, it is still the only way to generate EEG maps in patients with severe neurological impairment.

A typical example of continuous motor behavior is repetitive fist clenching over a period of minutes. In this situation the sensorimotor cortex is periodically activated at intervals of about 1 second. This EEG recording condition has been recommended by Harner (Chapter 18). Etevenon (Chapter 6) used continuous visual focusing or mental calculation over a period of 2 minutes. Ten different testing conditions such as speech, reading, and music were used in a dyslexia study by Duffy et al. [4]; approximately 3 minutes' EEG were recorded under each condition.

EEG recording during short-lasting single events requires sampling of EEG data restricted to the periods shortly before, during, and after the event. An example of such an event is a voluntary movement, a spoken word, or an exogenous stimulus. Voluntary, self-paced movement is, however, completely different from continuous, repetitive fist clenching or thumb movement. Intention, preparation for movement or "readiness to move," precedes each initiation of movement; the time period between the intentional process and the time when the movement actually begins covers an interval of 1-2 seconds [5]. A similar situation holds for voluntary, self-paced speech [6]. Repetitive fist clenching is an automatic process that requires no intention and planning for each individual movement and a minimum of conscious mental effort. Repetitive movement can be done in parallel to another mental task, unlike self-paced voluntary movement, which needs full mental concentration when performed carefully. Self-paced motor behavior such as finger movement or spontaneous speech is therefore an excellent possibility for reproducing the state of the brain within a period of about 1-2 seconds. Another, more complex way to do this is the use of the contingent negative variation (CNV) paradigm as introduced by Walter [7].

Short-lasting EEG processing during a well-defined event, i.e., during a reproducible mental state, is the only way to generate EEG maps characteristic of specific cortical activation patterns. To obtain statistically reliable maps, the event must be repeated 40–60 times and the averaging technique used. The aim of this chapter is to introduce a technique for computing maps during short-term, well-defined, and reproducible mental states, thus permitting visualization of the cortical activation pattern. This technique is called event-related desynchronization (ERD) mapping.

PHYSIOLOGICAL BASE FOR ERD MAPPING

Jasper and Penfield [8] reported that special cortical areas generate their own rhythmic activity (intrinsic rhythm) which appears as a short amplitude attenuation (blocking, desynchronization) when the underlying cortical generator structure is activated. Activation by voluntary movement seems to block the central beta rhythm in a manner similar to the blocking of occipital alpha rhythm in response to visual stimuli. The latter is known as alpha blocking after eyes opening [9] or light stimulation [10]; the former as blocking of the central mu rhythm [11,12] or central beta rhythm [13,14]. We can assume that the speech centers (Broca's area, Wernicke's area) and the auditory cortex also generate their own intrinsic rhythms that are desynchronized during speech and hearing, respectively. Frontal intrinsic activity is desynchronized during expectancy, decision making, and similar processes occurring during a CNV paradigm [15].

QUANTIFICATION OF ERD IN THE TIME DOMAIN

The desynchronization or blocking of the occipital alpha rhythm after short light stimulation can easily be seen in raw EEG data from the occipital and parietal areas, regardless of the type of recording used. The magnitude and exact time course of the desynchronization (blocking) of the alpha rhythm can be measured with different methods in the time domain [16–18]. These techniques demonstrate that the blocking phenomenon is phasic (1–2 seconds) and maximal over the occipital pole. In comparison to alpha blocking after light stimulation, blocking of central mu and beta rhythm during sensorimotor activation is rarely seen in the raw EEG. Studies on large groups reported a blocking in only 0–30% of subjects (see review in [19]). Using quantitative EEG this percentage is increased; Storm van Leeuwen et al. [20] found a blocking of central mu rhythm in 60% of their subjects and Schoppenhorst et al. [21] in 57% during repetitive opening and closing of the hand. Pfurtscheller and Aranibar [22] found in 90% of volunteers a blocking of mu rhythm with voluntary, self-paced movements. This demonstrates that the reactivity of central intrinsic rhythms to sensorimotor activation is a physiological phenomenon found in nearly every subject, when an appropriate experimental setup and a special recording and analyzing technique are used.

EXPERIMENTAL SETUP FOR ERD MAPPING

An example of an appropriate experimental setup is the recording during an event (finger movement, fist clenching, etc.) that is voluntary, self-paced, and repeated with intervals longer than 8 seconds. In our study we used 40–60 EEG epochs of 6 seconds each with 4 seconds preceding the movement or speech onset. In the case of externally paced events (stimulation), the sampled prestimulus interval was 3 seconds. This technique is so sensitive that voluntary, self-paced thumb movements resulted in a measurable EEG desynchronization starting 1–2 seconds prior to movement onset in all 10 subjects investigated [22]. After quantification of the ERD by calculating the curve of average alpha power against time, the exact time course of the phasic blocking response became visible (Figure 5.1).

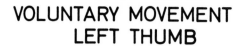

VOLUNTARY MOVEMENT
LEFT THUMB

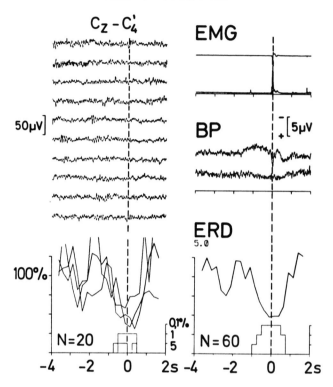

Figure 5.1. ERD and slow potentials in right central-vertex area, contralateral to voluntary, self-paced left thumb movement. EMG from left thenar eminence. BP; *Bereit-schaftspotential* (readiness potential). In the abscissa, $t = 0$ second and indicates triggering by button pressing. Left ordinates of the ERD curve; percentage of alpha power; right ordinates; statistical significance level (nonparametric Wilcoxon test). From Pfurtscheller and Aranibar [22], reprinted with permission.

ELECTRODE MONTAGE AND ERD

In addition to the experimental design, the type of EEG recording is another important consideration. To demonstrate this problem, EEG recordings were made from Cz with different electrode distances; the smallest distance was 18 mm and the greatest 180 mm (Cz-A2). The results of the measurements during voluntary self-paced thumb movements are displayed in Figure 5.2 and can be summarized as follows: Bipolar derivations with closely spaced electrodes (channels 1 and 2 in Figure 5.2) are more appropriate to measure ERD than widespread montages (e.g., Cz-A2). With increasing interelectrode distance, the power (amplitude) increases but ERD decreases. As early as 1938, Jasper and Andrews [13] recommended such bipolar derivations with closely spaced electrodes for studying localized blocking phenomena.

The ear or the mastoid is not always an advantageous position for reference electrodes, because these can experience large-amplitude alpha rhythm. For example, one can readily measure the potential on the mastoid with an averaged intracerebral reference in the frontal brain [23]. Therefore, referential recordings to the ear (mastoid) are unsuitable for ERD studies over the sensorimotor cortex.

Examples of different intrinsic rhythms within the alpha band in central and temporal areas can be seen in Figure 5.3. Some rhythms (8.6 and 10.2 Hz) are reactive to eyes opening (spectra during eyes opened are not displayed in Figure 5.3), some (9.2 Hz) to voluntary finger movement. This demonstrates that there is not only one alpha rhythm but a variety of alpha band rhythms. The existence of more than one alpha band rhythm makes it, however, problematical to study topographic scalp distributions of amplitude or phases of alpha waves in single trials.

ERD MEASUREMENT IN THE FREQUENCY DOMAIN

The use of digital filtering and averaging techniques allows calculation of the exact time course of the phasic blocking reaction (ERD in Figures 5.1 and 5.4). This procedure allows an ERD measurement in time intervals at least equal to the sample interval (e.g., 12 msec sample frequency with 64 Hz); ERD maps can then be computed in intervals of milliseconds. A disadvantage of this tech-

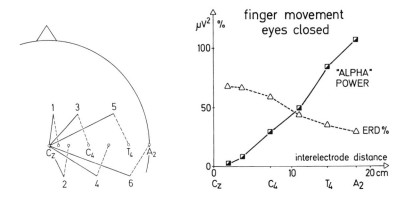

Figure 5.2. Alpha power (uv²) and ERD (%) during voluntary, self-paced movement in different bipolar recordings. Recording scheme upper panel, eyes closed.

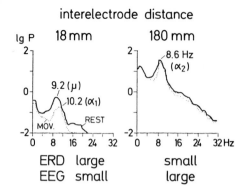

interelectrode distance

Figure 5.3. Two-second logarithmic spectra measured with closely spaced (*left-side*, derivation 1 in Figure 5.2, *upper panel*) and widely spaced (*right-side*, derivation 6 in Figure 5.2) electrode positions. Full-line spectra calculated before (and stippled-line spectra during) voluntary, self-paced thumb movements. The "alpha" peak frequencies are marked. Note the different peak frequencies.

nique is the large amount of computation time. For on-line computation a faster method that can be used is ERD measurement in the frequency domain. This method is based on two short-time spectra (1 or 2 seconds), one calculated in the activity period (close to the event) and the other in the reference period before the event. The exact choice of the activity period depends on whether there are self-paced (movement) or externally paced (exogenous stimulation) events. The logarithmic spectra calculated in both periods can differ significantly in the alpha and beta bands. These differences are measurements for ERD and are equivalent to ERD values obtained in the time domain (Figure 5.4). The short-time spectra can also be used to calculate EEG maps for different frequency bands or to calculate frequency maps.

ERD is a normalized measurement in percentage, where the power in the reference period is assumed to be 100%; +100% ERD means complete blocking, 0% ERD means no change, and negative ERD means an event-related alpha (beta) provocation (e.g., alpha spindles). The ERD scale can thus contain both positive and negative values.

MAP COMPUTATION AND DISPLAY

We used two methods for depicting the two-dimensional distribution of the EEG parameters over the head surface: First, the solution of the potential equation (partial differential equation of the second order) with 16 (32) parameters as supporting values, located between the electrode position for bipolar derivations. The potential equation is solved for a 48-x-80 matrix by an iterative algorithm, requiring approximately 5 seconds computation time on a PDP 11/23 computer. Second, the approximation of a three-dimensional head surface by triangles, linear interpolation within the triangles, and projection in two lateral views and one top view. For gray-scale presentation we use a matrix printer; for color output, a high-resolution graphics terminal. Examples of colored maps are shown in Plate 3; black white maps are displayed in Figures 5.5 and 5.6.

Besides the ERD and band power, the alpha peak frequency and the alpha mean frequency (center of gravity of the alpha power), respectively, can also be displayed in the form of maps. Frequency maps are especially suitable in studying patients with unilateral cerebral ischemia; the alpha frequency is very often slowed over the affected region [24].

RESULTS

Plate 3 demonstrates representative examples of ERD maps. The maps display the transient percentage decrease of alpha band (7–12 Hz) power during different experimental conditions. In the lower left panel the effect of visual stimulations on the occipital alpha rhythm is seen; it is noteworthy that blocking of the alpha rhythm only occurs over the occipital cortex. The region with the largest activation is marked in red.

In Plate 3 (upper left panel), the extent of the ERD during self-paced movement of the left hand is shown. It is obvious that the ERD pattern is almost symmetrical over both hemispheres with a maximum over the sensorimotor areas. This pattern is, however, different from the activation pattern obtained during speech performance (Plate 3, upper right panel). Evidently the local blocking phenomenon covers an area much wider than that of hand movement and also involves the left first frontal gyrus, an area known as Broca's area that is important for the pure motor performance of speech. The ERD map is slightly different when the subject is asked to count voluntarily from 1 to 10 (Plate 3, lower right panel). Local blocking covers the central region symmetrically with an extension, however, over the supplementary speech area of the upper third of the first frontal gyrus of the left hemisphere.

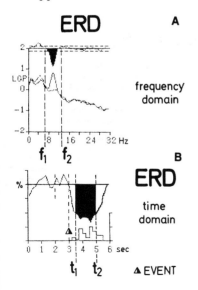

Figure 5.4. *A*: Power spectra calculated in the reference (full-line) and the activity (stippled-line) period. The black area indicates the integral over the difference of the two spectra in the frequency band limited by f_1 and f_2, used as ERD parameter for topographic presentation. *B*: Power versus time curve calculated for the frequency band f_1-f_2. The black area within the time window t_1 and t_2 can be used as measurement for ERD. Statistical significance of the power decrease (*black area*) is indicated by the step function to be read on the right vertical scale ($p < 10^{-2}$, 10^{-6}, and 10^{-10}). From Pfurtscheller et al. [24], reprinted with permission from Elsevier Biomedical Press, Amsterdam).

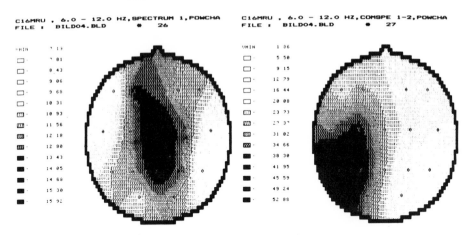

ALPHA

C16MRU , 6.0 - 12.0 HZ,SPECTRUM 1,POWCHA
FILE : BILDO4.BLD   #   26

'MIN   7 13
□ ·   7 81
□ ·   8 43
□ ·   9 06
□ ·   9 68
□ ·   10 31
▦ ·   10 93
▩ ·   11 56
▩ ·   12 18
▨ ·   12 80
■ ·   13 43
■ ·   14 05
■ ·   14 68
■ ·   15 30
■ ·   15 92

MOVEMENT

C16MRU , 6.0 - 12.0 HZ,COMSPE 1-2,POWCHA
FILE : BILDO4.BLD   #   27

'MIN   1 86
□ ·   5 50
□ ·   9 15
□ ·   12 79
□ ·   16 44
▣ ·   20 08
▣ ·   23 73
▦ ·   27 37
▩ ·   31 02
▨ ·   34 66
■ ·   38 30
■ ·   41 95
■ ·   45 59
■ ·   49 24
■ ·   52 88

R. M. 59a
ICA subtotal stenosis right
CS

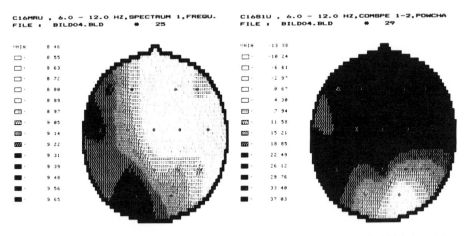

FREQUENCY

C16MRU , 6.0 - 12.0 HZ,SPECTRUM 1,FREQU.
FILE : BILDO4.BLD   #   25

'MIN   8 46
□ ·   8 55
□ ·   8 63
□ ·   8 72
□ ·   8 80
□ ·   8 89
▣ ·   8 97
▦ ·   9 05
▩ ·   9 14
▨ ·   9 22
■ ·   9 31
■ ·   9 39
■ ·   9 48
■ ·   9 56
■ ·   9 65

SPEECH

C16S1U , 6.0 - 12.0 HZ,COMSPE 1-2,POWCHA
FILE : BILDO4.BLD   #   29

'MIN   -13 38
□ ·   -10 24
□ ·   -6 61
□ ·   -2 97
□ ·   0 67
▣ ·   4 30
▣ ·   7 94
▦ ·   11 58
▩ ·   15 21
▨ ·   18 85
■ ·   22 49
■ ·   26 12
■ ·   29 76
■ ·   33 40
■ ·   37 03

Figure 5.5. Alpha map displaying the square root of power within the 6–12-Hz band (*upper left*), frequency map (*lower left*), and ERD maps calculated during voluntary fist clenching right (*upper right*) and during the voluntary speech (*lower right*). ERD map scale in percentage, frequency map scale from 8.5 to 9.7 Hz, and alpha map scale in μV. Sixteen-channel monopolar recording according to the international 10-20 system with linked earlobe reference. Patient with completed stroke (CS) and subtotal stenosis of the right internal carotid artery (ICA).

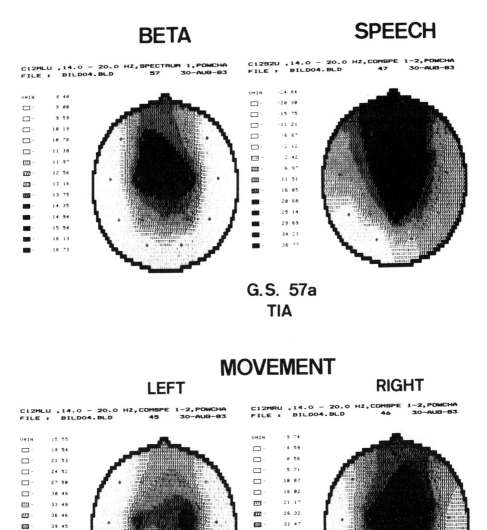

Figure 5.6. Beta map displaying the square root of power within the 14–20-Hz band (*upper left*) and ERD maps calculated during voluntary speech (*upper right*) and movement (*lower panel*) in a patient with transitory ischemic attack (TIA). For further explanation see Figure 5.5. Note the different localization and spread of the ERD during hand movement and speech.

EEG, ERD, and frequency maps from a 59-year-old patient (R.M.) with a left hemiparesis after a stroke are displayed in Figure 5.5. The EEG map demonstrates a bilaterally symmetrical alpha distribution; the ERD map, however, shows normal reactivity only over the left centroparietal region and a lack of reactivity over the right hemisphere. The frequency map demonstrates a reduced frequency of 8.5 Hz over the right central area in comparison to 9.5 Hz over the left hemisphere, and the ERD map shows widespread reactivity over the frontal and central areas during spontaneous speech. Although the alpha map is symmetrical and therefore normal, the frequency and ERD maps indicate cerebral dysfunction in the right hemisphere. From the alpha frequency we know that interhemispheric frequency differences of more than 0.4 Hz are abnormal [25].

A 57-year-old patient (G.S.) had a transitory ischemic attack (TIA) with left-sided sensory deficit. The beta map was symmetrical and the ERD maps (reactivity in the beta band) showed bilaterally symmetrical blocking response to movement and to spontaneous speech four weeks after the TIA (Figure 5.5). The alpha map was also symmetrical, but the corresponding ERD map displayed reduced reactivity over the right hemisphere [26]. This example shows that beta activity can also be used to study cortical activation patterns.

DISCUSSION

ERD mapping is a promising new technique in applied brain research and clinical electroencephalography. There are, however, problems to be solved. One problem concerns the question of monopolar versus bipolar derivations. Since the aim of ERD mapping is the investigation of localized phenomena, the monopolar derivation can be a disadvantage, because the reference point has an unknown potential. Nevertheless the use of monopolar derivations is of great interest since all possible bipolar derivations can easily be calculated. In our opinion, closely spaced electrodes, as recommended by Jasper and Andrews [13], give satisfying results in ERD mapping. However, the use of the source derivation technique remains an alternative possibility [27].

Another problem is establishing the number of channels that can be used for the calculation of ERD maps. To coordinate regions with localized ERD to the right anatomical structure more than 16 channels (e.g., 32) have to be used (beginning in 1985 we will have available a 32-channel system).

Finally, it should be emphasized that the question of intersubject reproducibility and validity remains a problem, especially when individual finger movements or spontaneous speech are performed. Nevertheless ERD mapping is a new, inexpensive technique that does not use radioactive isotopes and thus, can be repeated many times on one subject and used in every modern EEG laboratory. Taken together, ERD mapping is a further development of

EEG mapping offering interesting new potential for the psychological and neurophysiological investigation of the human brain.

In summary, ERD is the name given to the phasic blocking reaction of physiological EEG rhythms in association with an event. Such an event may be an external stimulation, but can also be an internally paced voluntary movement or spontaneous speech. The ERD map consists of the topographic scalp distribution of this localized blocking phenomenon. ERD mapping can therefore be used to visualize cortical activation patterns during various types of sensory, motor, or mental activity and is a further development of EEG mapping during short-lasting, controlled, and reproducible states of the brain. The application of ERD mapping offers interesting prospects for the psychological and neurophysiological investigation of the human brain and also can be used in clinical electroencephalography.

ACKNOWLEDGMENT

Supported by the Fonds zur Förderung der Wissenschaftlichen Forschung, project number 5240. I thank Dr. Maresch and Dr. Köpruner for writing the computer programs, Dr. Vollmer for suggestions for the experimental setup, and Dr. Ladurner for the clinical data.

REFERENCES

1. Lehmann, D. Multichannel topography of human alpha EEG fields. Electroenceph. Clin. Neurophysiol. 1971; 31:439–449.
2. Nagata, K., Mizukami, M., Araki, G., Kawase, T., and Hirano, M. Topographic electroencephalograhic study of cerebral infarction using computed mapping of the EEG. J. Cereb. Blood Flow Metab. 1982; 2:79–88.
3. Buchsbaum, M.S., Rigal, F., Coppola, R., Cappelletti, J., King, C., and Johnson, J. A new system for gray-level surface distribution maps of electrical activity. Electroenceph. Clin. Neurohysiol. 1982; 53:237–242.
4. Duffy, F.H., Denckla, M.B., Bartels, P.H., and Sandini, G. Dyslexia: Regional differences in brain electrical activity by topographic mapping. Ann. Neurol. 1980; 7:412–420.
5. Kornhuber, H.H., and Deecke, L. Hirnpotentialänderungen beim Menschen vor und nach Willkürbewegungen, dargestellt mit Magnetbandspeicherung und Rückwärtsanalyse. Pflügers Arch. Ges. Physiol. 1964; 281:52.
6. Grözinger, B., Kornhuber, H., and Kriebel, J. EEG investigation of hemispheric asymmetries preceding speech: The R-wave. In C. McCallum and J. Knott, eds., The Responsive Brain, Bristol: J. Wright, 1976; 103–107.
7. Walter, W.G. Electrical signs of association, expectancy and decision in the human brain. Electroenceph. Clin. Neurophysiol. 1967; 25:309–322.
8. Jasper, H.H., and Penfield, W. Electrocorticograms in man: Effect of voluntary movement upon the electrical activity of the precentral gyrus. Arch. Psychiat. Z. Neurol. 1949; 183:163–174.

9.   Berger, H. Über das Elektroenkephalogramm des Menschen. Arch. Psychiat. Nerven Kr. 1933; 100:301–320.

10. Morrell, L.K. Some characteristics of stimulus-provoked alpha activity. Electroenceph. Clin. Neurophysiol. 1966; 21:552–561.

11. Gastaut, H. Etude électrocorticographique de la réactivité des rhythmes rolandiques. Res. Neurol. 1952; 87:176–182.

12. Chatrian, G.E., Petersen, M.C., and Lazarte, J.A. The blocking of the rolandic wicket rhythm and some central changes related to movement. Electroenceph. Clin. Neurophysiol. 1959; 11:497–510.

13. Jasper, H.H., and Andrews,H.L. Electro-encephalography. III. Normal differentiations of occipital and precentral regions in man. Arch. Neurol. Psychiat. 1938; 39:96–115.

14. Pfurtscheller, G. Central beta rhythm during sensorimotor activities in man. Electroenceph. Clin. Neurophysiol. 1981; 51:253–264.

15. Pfurtscheller, G., and Aranibar, A. Occipital rhythmic activity within the alpha band during conditioned externally paced movement. Electroenceph. Clin. Neurophysiol. 1978; 45:226–235.

16. Grünewald, G., Grünewald-Zuberbier, E., and Netz, J. Event-related changes of EEG alpha activity in relation to slow potential shifts. In G.Pfurtscheller, P. Buser, F. H. Lopes da Silva,and H. Petsche, eds., Rhythmic EEG Activities and Cortical Functioning: Developments in Neuroscience. Amsterdam: Elsevier, 1980; 10:235–248.

17. Pfurtscheller, G., and Aranibar, A. Event-related cortical desynchronization detected by power measurements of scalp EEG. Electroenceph. Clin. Neurophysiol. 1977; 42:817–826.

18. Aranibar, A., and Pfurtscheller, G. On and off effects in the background EEG activity during one-second photic stimulation. Electroenceph. Clin. Neurophysiol. 1978; 44:307–316.

19. Chatrian, G.E. The mu rhythm. In G.E. Chatrian and G.C. Lairy, eds., The EEG of the Waking Adult: Handbook of EEG and Neurophysiology. Amsterdam: Elsevier, 1976; 6A:46–69.

20. Storm van Leeuwen, W., Wieneke, G.,Spoelstra, P., and Versteeg, H. Lack of bilateral coherence of mu rhythm. Electroenceph. Clin. Neurophysiol. 1978; 44:140–146.

21. Schoppenhorst, M., Brauer, F., Freund, G., and Kubicki, S. The significance of coherence estimates in determining central alpha and mu activities. Electroenceph. Clin. Neurophysiol. 1980; 48:25–33.

22. Pfurtscheller, G.,and Aranibar, A. Evaluation of event-related desynchronization (ERD) preceding and following voluntary self-paced movement. Electroenceph. Clin. Neurophysiol. 1979; 46:138–146.

23. Pfurtscheller, G., and Cooper, R. Frequency dependence of the transmission of the EEG from cortex to scalp. Electroenceph. Clin. Neurophysiol. 1975; 38:93–96.

24. Pfurtscheller, G., Ladurner, G., Maresch, H., and Vollmer, R. Brain electrical activity mapping in normal and ischemic brain. In G. Pfurtscheller, J. Jonkman, and F. Lopes da Silva, eds., Brain Ischemia: Quantitative EEG and Imaging Techniques. Amsterdam: Elsevier, 1984; 287–302.

25. Van Huffelen, A.C., Poortveiet, D.C.J., and Van der Wuep, C.J.M. Quantitative electroencephalography in cerebral ischemia: Detection of abnormalities in "nor-

mal" EEGs. In G. Pfurtscheller, J.Jonkman, and F. Lopes da Silva, eds., Brain Ischemia: Quantitative EEG and Imaging Techniques. Amsterdam: Elsevier, 1984; 3–28.

26. Pfurtscheller, G., and Ladurner, G. ERD mapping in cerebral ischemia. Proc. Int. Joint Alpine Symp. Silver Spring: IEEE Comp. Soc. Press, 1984; 89–93.

27. Hjorth, B. An online transformation of EEG scalp potentials into orthogonal source derivations. Electroenceph. Clin. Neurophysiol. 1975; 39:526–530.

6
Applications and Perspectives of EEG Cartography

Pierre Etevenon

Electroencephalograph (EEG) cartography can be traced retrospectively through the entire history of EEG research and development. Three years after Berger's discovery of the human EEG [1], Dietsch [2] applied Fourier analysis to the EEG. Chweitzer et al. [3,4], together with Liberson [5] studied mescalinic intoxication by computing instantaneous amplitude histograms. In 1937 and 1938 Drohocki [6,7] introduced new quantitative EEG analyses: integrated and rectified amplitude analysis and also a first-frequency analysis named electrospectrography. Gibbs [8] and Grass and Gibbs [9] applied the Fourier transform to the analysis of EEG. Bertrand and Lacape [10] published a book on EEG modeling, considering ranks of harmonics in the EEG and addition of sinusoidal waves.

Grey Walter built a low-frequency analyzer in 1943 [11] and in 1951, with Shipton [12], a new toposcopic display system. In 1952 Zee Zang Zao et al. [13] described the electrical field of the eye. The same year Rémond and Offner [14] presented the first topographic studies of occipital EEG, and Petsche [15] proposed the vector EEG method. In 1954, Petsche and Marko [16] built the photocell toposcope, and Lilly [17] proposed electrical figures during responses of spontaneous activity. Since 1955 Rémond and his associates [18–25] developed topographic studies. In 1956 Ananiev [26] introduced the electroencephaloscope. Cooper et al. [27] presented "spatial and temporal identification of alpha activities in relation to individual mental states, by means of the 22-channel helical scan toposcope." Saltzberg and Burch [28] introduced the period analysis of EEG. Rémond and Delarue [22] proposed the unchallenged EEG montage using 58 recording electrodes.

Adey, D.O. Walter, and their associates [29–35] applied Fourier analysis based on fast Fourier transform (FFT) and phase analysis to EEG signals. This was the starting point of computerized spectral analysis. Petsche and Stumpf [36] published on "topographic and toposcopic study of origin and spread of the regular synchronized arousal pattern in the rabbit." Petsche in 1962 [37] presented the spike and wave propagation studied by toposcopic methods. Goff et al. [38–40] presented scalp topographic studies of evoked responses. Bechtereva et al. [41] localized focal brain lesions by EEG studies, anticipating EEG cartography. This pioneering research was followed by a growing number of findings and new analyses [42–67].

Models of EEG electrogenesis provided the theoretical framework for the chronotopographic and toposcopic findings. The first important contribution was made by Bertrand and Lacape [10] in 1943 in Paris who proposed an EEG classification of spindles, delta, alpha, and beta activities and spike and waves, based upon graphically computed Fourier analyses. Grey Walter [68] in 1959 was already proposing models in EEG. Lesèvre et al. [69] presented in 1967 the alpha average rhythm, followed by Rémond [20,23,70] with an "alpha average" theoretical model, Joseph et al. [71] with models of alpha rhythm and Ragot et al. [72]. Elul [73,74] also presented an EEG model based on amplitude histograms of EEG. Vaughn and Ritter [75] determined the sources of evoked responses. Cracco in 1972 [76] considered the human scalp-recorded evoked responses as traveling waves. Creutzfeldt in 1974 [58] published a review on the neuronal generation of the EEG. Further contributions in EEG modeling were made by Zetterberg [77,78], Lopes da Silva et al. [79], and Childers [80]. In 1977 we proposed a radio electrical model of EEG based on Hilbert transform of EEG [81,82]. In 1981, Saïto and Harashima [83] considered the causal analysis of EEG, following Gersch [56], Gersch and Tharp [57], and our own findings [81]. Watanabe and Shikata [84] studied by contour maps the stability of alpha rhythm, and Suzuki [85] published on temporospatial changes of alpha rhythm and coherence changes. Naitoh and Lewis [86] studied the statistics of extracted EEG features. Petsche et al. [87,88] proposed a model of current-source-density method for the analysis of field potentials: the micro-EEG method. Tucker [89] presented new findings on asymmetries of coherence topography. We proposed [90] a model of intra- and inter-hemispheric relationships based on four quadrants dividing the scalp where stimulation and inhibition processes are applied. This model has been clinically validated. Thus EEG mapping is well grounded, both theoretically [67,91–93] and experimentally.

EEG cartography started with Lehmann's article [51] on multichannel topography of human alpha EEG fields (followed by Lehmann [94–96] and Skrandies and Lehmann [97]). Ueno et al. [98] published on topographic computed display of abnormal EEG activities in patients with CNS diseases. Ragot and Rémond [99] published in 1978 on EEG field mapping, a year before the first publication of Duffy et al. [100]. Since that time, Duffy and his associates have published a growing number of articles [101–113]. They were followed by Duff [114], Coppola et al. [115–117], Buchsbaum et al. [118–122], Terao et al. [123], Nagata et al. [124], Etevenon et al. [125–130], Pidoux et al. [131], Persson and Hjorth [132], Maresh et al. [133], Gaches [134], Gaches and Etevenon

[135], Sebban and Debouzy [136], Debouzy et al. [137], Pfurtscheller and Lad-urner [138], and Itil et al. [139].

The utilization of microprocessors specialized in EEG analysis [140] and presently in EEG cartography is also very well documented [126, 127,129,132,134–137,141–144]. The domain of EEG cartography appears like a diaspora and there is growing usage of EEG cartography among classical elec-troencephalographists. Moreover, EEG mapping has been correlated by Duffy, Buchsbaum, Etevenon, Gaches, and others, with other imaging techniques such as computed tomography (CT) scans, emission tomography, and local ce-rebral circulation [145].

ISSUES IN EEG CARTOGRAPHY

Six issues currently confronting EEG researchers are given in Table 6.1. The first issue, the choice of number of electrodes, is a difficult one. Too many elec-trodes are better than too few, but what is the minimum number? It seems that this question has no absolute answer but it is more a question of protocol and of definition of the purpose of the study. In their early research Rémond and Delarue [22] used 58 electrodes; later Ragot and Rémond [99] and Lehmann [51] used 48 electrodes. Duffy and his school are using 20 EEG electrodes. Du-binsky and Barlow [146], Coppola et al. [115,116], Buchsbaum et al. [120–122], Etevenon et al. [125], and Pidoux et al. [131] are using 16 electrodes over each hemisphere. Persson and Hjorth [132] are using a 21-channel polygraph and applying the source derivation technique, but only 8 of the 21 EEG channels are shown on an EEG topogram. More recently, Sebban et al. [136], Debouzy et al. [137], Etevenon et al. [126,127], Gaches [134], and Gaches and Etevenon [135] have recorded 16 electrodes over the entire scalp for microcomputer real-time EEG cartography of neurological patients. At the Collegium Internation-ale Neuropsychopharmacologicum (CINP) meeting in Florence, Itil et al. [139] argued for the use of 8 EEG leads for representing hemispheric dynamic EEG brain maps. Furthermore, in the grid sector analysis developed by Duffy [102],

---

Table 6.1 Issues in EEG Cartography

1. Choice of number of electrodes [4,8,12,16,20,32,48,58]
2. Position of electrodes
3. Choice of reference: common average reference, monopolar, bipolar
4. Choice of interpolation algorithm: weighting function ($1/d$, , $1/d^2$, $1/d^3$); interpolation: triangular, quadrilateral, extended to all the electrodes; spatial filtering, splines, etc.
5. Choice of spectral parameters
6. Choice of statistics: statistical strategy of Duffy et al., nonparametric Fisher permutation tests prior to EEG maps?

---

diffuse abnormalities were shown to be differentiated from focal lesions using statistics (Z-value histograms) on the finest grid based on brain electrical activity mapping from 20 EEG channels, on a medium grid (64 sectors instead of the original 4096 pixels, or picture elements, or 8-x-8 sectors), and on the coarse grid (16 sectors or 4-x-4 areas over the scalp). The coarse grid, in terms of EEG mapping, is very similar to a recording with 16 electrodes over the scalp, or 8 over each hemisphere. Samson-Dollfus (personal communication, 1984) is using 12 electrodes over the scalp for mapping purposes. We published [90] a model of inter- and intrahemispheric relationships, applying two dynamic processes of excitation and inhibition into quadrants, dividing the scalp (and the cortex underneath) into four areas separated by the sensory motor rolandic area and the midline (right and left hemispheres). This minimal model provides 16 possible states which have been correlated with psychopathology and already applied on a group of depressed schizophrenic patients [147] before and after treatment with clomipramine. This can be considered as the lower limit of the grid sector analysis of Duffy. Finally, Tucker [89] has published on asymmetries of coherence topography, recording only 8 EEG channels referenced to linked ears. However, 28 unique coherences were computed between these channels and intra- and interhemispheric coherence images were computed and nicely displayed using spatial smoothing based on splines function (from Hermite orthogonal functions). This last article illustrates the fact that the number of electrodes chosen depends on research goals.

The second issue is linked to the first one. The position of electrodes over the scalp is crucial for meaningful topography of computed EEG maps. This positioning depends on the choice of the number of electrodes. Generally, the 10–20 system is chosen as a basic grid for EEG electrode locations [120,148]. When using 16 electrodes over one hemisphere this is not as significant a problem because there are more electrodes than the 10–20 grid system. However, it becomes increasingly difficult as the number of electrodes is decreased. Again, this is a question of protocol and of experimental situation grounded to research goals. For instance, Duff [114] has been able to describe the topography of scalp-recorded potentials evoked by stimulations of the digits placing the EEG electrodes in an optimal setting according to his purpose. With few electrodes, "holes" can be present on the montage and the EEG mapping will present distortions in comparison to the greater density packing of other EEG electrodes. Ueno et al. [98] attempted to solve this problem of gaps between electrodes by interpolating experimental adjacent values and then replacing the "hole" by the averaged interpolated value prior to applying the grid and contouring algorithm used to create the EEG map.

The third issue is also important and very often neglected. It concerns the choice of electrode reference. This question is extensively treated in D.O. Walter et al. [144]. Following Lehmann [51,94–96,149], the best known choice is the common average reference (instead of the monopolar technique). We have computed EEG maps with different computerized references, and we have also

Table 6.2 10 EEG Spectral Parameters Used in Generating Topographic Maps

3 means: f_{Hz}, $a_{\mu V}$, a%
3 dispersions: CV (f), CV (a), s (a%)
1 form coefficient: k% (resonance)
2 asymmetry coefficients: L/R, (L − R)/(L + R)
1 ratio: theta/alpha

L/R, left/right.

recorded the same subjects, under the same conditions, eyes closed, with different reference electrodes (ear contralateral to the recorded hemisphere, linked ears, vertex, common average reference). We observed that with the use of monopolar reference, the spontaneous EEGs presented lower amplitudes near the monopolar positioning of the reference. However, in practice, the dominant rhythm is usually well represented topographically, despite the choice of electrode reference. This is, however, not the case with the less important activities (in terms of magnitudes or amplitude modulus) such as theta or beta rhythms.

We have also been dealing with the fourth issue [144], the choice of interpolation algorithm. Buchsbaum and Coppola, as well as Duffy and co-workers, are applying a weighting function inverse to the distance of the proximal experimental measured EEG values (triangular interpolation for Duffy and quadrilateral for Buchsbaum and Coppola). We showed with D.O. Walter [144] that for such an interpolation algorithm, the computed EEG map seems unlikely to represent the true scalp field. According to the practice of geophysicists and also the laws of electromagnetic wave propagation, we chose to use a nonlinear interpolation algorithm, that is, the inverse cubic distance of the interpolated point from the four experimental nearest electrodes inside a quadrilateral polygon. This subtle computational difficulty may be important when we consider that computed EEG maps may be used as aids to diagnoses in neurosurgery, neurology, and even in emergency rooms using brain EEG monitoring. Other authors have chosen other ways of interpolating between points such as spatial filtering [98] and splines functions for spatial smoothing [89]. Debouzy et al. [137] and Sebban et al. [136] applied an inverse quadratic distance to the 16 electrode values recorded over the scalp. We compared this interpolation algorithm with our own (quadrilateral inverse cubic distance) and found quite similar EEG maps starting from the same 16 EEG spectral values. Another difference between maps is the definition of the EEG map in terms of elementary areas or pixels, as well as the number of levels of gray scales, or of pseudocolors, or hues of colors, and also the dimensions of the computed and printed or photographed EEG mappings.

Table 6.2 presents 10 spectral parameters that we compute to describe in quantitative terms an EEG recording giving birth to 90 different maps. Usually, EEG cartographers use few spectral parameters, the most commonly computed being absolute power values or relative percentage power values for the raw EEG and different spectral frequency bands. Ueno et al. [98] computed square roots of average power values over desirable spectral frequency bands in power spectra of 40-second EEG data. These RMS (root-mean-square) absolute amplitude values, expressed in microvolts, are our second spectral parameter: a μV. This parameter [81] is similar to the "activity" used by Persson and Hjorth [132] in their EEG topograms. This mean amplitude value is better than its squared power value because D.O. Walter demonstrated that the power value is similar to a chi-square variable with two degrees of freedom. Therefore the RMS mean amplitude value is like a gaussian variable normally distributed. Our first parameter is the mean frequency (f: according to the centroid computation of Lehmann, [94–96,149]) a variable that is similar to the "mobility" of Hjorth [81]. Our third parameter is the relative percentage amplitude: a% [81,150]. These three spectral parameters are completed by what we have named (with de Barbeyrac in 1969) the "resonance coefficient," k% [81]. This coefficient of resonance is a form coefficient, independent of frequency, phase, or amplitude, equal to unity for a pure sinusoidal wave and to 0.1 for a pure white noise [81]. This spectral coefficient is, in terms of signal analysis, an inverse rectangular spectral window, easy to compute (the square of k is the integral of the square absolute power spectrum divided by the squared integral of the absolute power spectrum). Practically speaking, this coefficient of resonance is an index of monomorphism/polymorphism of a tracing, like the "complexity" coefficient of Hjorth but with fewer biases.

We also compute the dispersions around the first three coefficients using the coefficient of variation (CV) of the mean centroid frequency, and of the mean absolute amplitude, the standard-deviation of the relative amplitude %.

We also compute the ratio theta/alpha. With the exception of this last coefficient, all the other coefficients are computed for the five frequency bands: delta (1.56 to 4.52 Hz), theta (3.91 to 7.42 Hz), alpha (7.81 to 14.06 Hz), beta-1 (14.45 to 28.13 Hz), beta-2 (28.52 to 49.61 Hz), and certain coefficients (f, a μV, k%, asymmetries) are computed for the raw EEG. All these parameters are computed over the 32 EEG channels (right and then left hemisphere) with the exception of the two asymmetries represented over one hemisphere. This provides 90 EEG maps for one EEG topographic recording.

The last issue is the choice of pertinent statistics. Duffy et al. [104,105] have presented their statistical strategy in four steps: (1) topographic mapping, (2) cartooning, (3) significance probability mapping (SPM): Z-transform SPM, t-statistic SPM, cartooning of t and Z images, other statistical tests, serial applications of statistical transforms, and (4) grid sector analysis (GSA). A confusion may occur between the theoretical validity of Z or t SPM images and spectral parameter images, in such a way that if power or RMS amplitude EEG maps [144] are related to basic electromagnetic wave propagation there are no t or Z statistical propagating waves. Therefore, these statistical images should be compared and validated with more basic statistics defined from the set of experimentally computed spectral values extracted from the recorded EEG channels.

For this purpose, we use the nonparametric permutation test of Fisher, using the algorithm of extreme configurations on the set of experimental EEG spectral parameters. This test, created by Fisher in 1935, has been well documented by Lebart et al. [151] and programmed in FORTRAN. We have implemented this test on our Hewlett-Packard minicomputer, microprogrammed in FORTRAN. Its statistical efficiency is 100%. We have applied it to compare two recorded situations (eyes closed versus mental arithmetic eyes closed, eyes closed versus eyes open, mental arithmetic versus eyes open), the two hemispheres recorded successively (right before left), and the two subgroups of men and women within the same recorded situation.

Against this background of the historic development of EEG cartography, I would like to present some of my own findings and address some of the critical issues which continue to require further study. I will begin with a detailed discussion of my research methodology in a recently completed study.

METHODS

Protocol

Table 6.3 describes the group of 20 volunteers recorded for the present study. The subjects were matched in terms of age (28.1 mean age), gender (10 men, 10 women), handedness (right-handers, according to the Annett questionnaire (Annett, M. A clarification of hand preference by association analysis. Brit. J. Psychol. 1970; 61: 303–321.)), sociocultural status (students) and ethnic origin (Caucasian). Moreover, the subjects were matched so that the total group was composed of 10 subjects defined as "low alpha" averaged amplitude and 10 subjects defined as "high alpha" averaged amplitude for the right occipital O2 EEG channel. The threshold of 40 μV was chosen from previous studies of normal subjects for discriminating between low and high alpha amplitudes [81,126,127].

We have presented the protocol of recordings elsewhere. For this study [129,130,131,150] we present results based on three recorded situations: eyes

Table 6.3   Group Studied

Gender	Mean Age ± SD	High Alpha	Low Alpha
Masculine	27.6 ± 6.4	4	6
Feminine	28.6 ± 7.2	6	4
Total	28.1	10	10

closed and relaxed, eyes open with visual fixation of a cartoon, and mental arithmetic, eyes closed. We were aware of four problems of protocol: (1) no rejection of artifacts; (2) right hemisphere recording prior to left hemisphere recording, and median line recorded twice; (3) gender differences; (4) small sample size.

Equipment

EEG signals were recorded by a 16-channel polygraph (REEGA 16, Alvar) linked simultaneously to both mini and microcomputer systems. Table 6.4 presents the compared specifications of both systems. The minicomputer system (Hewlett-Packard) was composed of a fast Fourier analyzer (HP 5451 C, microprogrammed FFT, 64 K words of 16 bits memory), triggered by a 16-channel multiplexer (SOPEMEA), coupled with a fast FORTRAN programming minicomputer (HP 1000, 21 MX F, 192 K words of 16 bits memory). This first system used two digital magnetic tapes (800 bpi) and two hard-disc peripheral memories (5M and 20M words of 16 bits), six different consoles (two graphic units), one alphanumeric and graphic printer, and a modem line.

Table 6.4   Comparative Specifications of Computer Systems

Minicomputer	Microcomputer
HP 5451C	REEGA 2000
+ HP 1000 21 MXF	Alvar Electronic
ADC 10 bits	ADC 8 bits
anti-aliasing 48 db/octave	48 db/octave
Sample and hold multiplexer (SOPEMEA); 16 channels	16-channel multiplexer
Epoch: 60 × 2.56s	epoch: variable 3-sec units
Sampling 200 Hz	Sampling 128 Hz
Spectral resolution 0.38 Hz	Resolution 1 Hz
Spectral analysis: 10 parameters × 5 frequency bands + raw EEG	3 spectral parameters, variable frequency and intensity scales
90 maps per EEG record for each hemisphere	manually defined maps
Common average reference	common average reference
16 electrodes/hemiscalp	16 electrodes/hemiscalp
	16 electrodes over the scalp
Contour maps: hemispheric	hemispheric
	bihemispheric
Maps: 10 gray levels; 4260 pixels of 5×6 points	9 gray levels
	700 pixels of 8×8 points
Interpolation: $1/d^3$ inside quadrilateral	$1/d^2$ extended to the contour

The second microcomputer system (REEGA 2000, Alvar Electronic) was controlled for the EEG sampling by a microprocessor (Intel 8085), coupled to the polygraph by a 16-channel multiplexer and an FFT microprogrammed board triggered by a microcomputer system (based on a Commodore 8000, 32 K RAM, 16 K ROM bytes of memory), equipped with a semigraphic console, two floppy discs (1M bytes each), and a graphic thermal printer.

EEG Recordings and EEG Mapping

EEG recordings were obtained from both control subjects and patients. A number of situations were recorded under the same conditions: eyes closed, eyes open looking at a cartoon, mental arithmetic task (14 successive multiplications of three digit numbers by 1 digit, recorded on audiotape and transmitted through an amplifier), different motor tasks, etc. Twenty-seven silver electrodes were glued with collodion according to the 10–20 system as suggested by Coppola [116], Coppola et al. [115], and Buchsbaum et al. [122]: Oz, Pz, Cz, Fpz, Fcz for the mid-line (recorded twice during the first sequence for the right hemisphere and during the second sequence for the left hemisphere), and O1, O2, P3, P4, C3, C4, F3, F4, Fpl, Fp2, F7, F8, Ftc L and R, Tcp L and R, T5, T6, T3, T4, Cbl, Cb2 on both right and left hemiscalps. All EEG channels were recorded with a common average reference, according to Lehmann [95,96] and D.O. Walter et al. [144]. Detailed protocols can be found elsewhere [125–127,150]. In each situation, the right hemiscalp was recorded first for 153.6 seconds (60 x 2.56 seconds). This first sequence was followed by a second sequence similarly recorded over the left hemiscalp.

On the minicomputer system, 323 sequences recorded over both hemispheres have been stored into a cartography data base (IMAGE 1000, Hewlett Packard). More than 100 sequences have been recorded from the microcomputer system and stored. Ten Topo-EEGs have been recorded simultaneously on both systems, using control subjects and patients. We also recorded well-defined white noises and fed the output signals into both EEG mapping systems. Each recorded sequence provided 90 maps of right and left hemispheres.

RESULTS: STUDY OF A CONTROL GROUP

Table 6.5 indicates the trends in brain electrical activity as measured by four spectral EEG parameters for our group of 20 subjects during visual fixation on a cartoon, eyes opened, as compared to the previously relaxed situation, eyes closed. The arrows indicate that during the opening of the eyes, the activation of the EEG tracings is statistically validated by the Fisher tests, especially by the following results [152]:

Table 6.5   Eyes Closed versus Eyes Open

Parameters	f Hz	a μV	a%	k%
Raw EEG	↓(↑)	↓	—	↓(↑)
Delta	↓	↑	↑	↑
Theta	↓	↓(↑)	↑	↑(↓)
Alpha	↑	↓	↓	↓
Beta-1	↑(↓)	↓(↑)	↑	↓
Beta-2	↑	↑	↑	↑

Significant Fisher permutation tests; $n = 20$, 32 EEG channels, $p \leq 0.05$ and 0.01.

Table 6.6   Mental Arithmetic Eyes Closed versus Eyes Open

Parameters	f Hz	a μV	a%	k%
Raw EEG	↓(↑)	↓	—	↓(↑)
Delta	↑	↑	↑	↑
Theta	↓	↓(↑)	↑	↑
Alpha	(↓)	↓	↓	↓
Beta-1	↑	↓(↑)	↑	↓
Beta-2	↑	↑↓	↑	↓

Significant Fisher permutation tests; $n = 20$, 32 EEG channels, $p \leq 0.05$ and 0.01.

Table 6.7   Eyes Closed versus Mental Arithmetic with Eyes Closed

Parameters	f Hz	a μV	a%	k%
Raw EEG	↓(↑)	↓(↑)	—	↓
Delta	↓	↑	↑	↑(↓)
Theta	↓	↓	↓	↓
Alpha	↑	↓	↓	↓
Beta-1	↑	↑(↓)	↑(↓)	↓
Beta-2	↑	↑	↑	↑

Significant Fisher permutation tests; $n = 20$, 32 EEG channels, $p \leq 0.05$ and 0.01.

- The mean frequency (f) decreases for the raw EEG, the delta and theta frequency bands and increases for the alpha, beta-1, and beta-2 fast activities.
- The mean absolute amplitude in microvolts (a μV) decreases for the raw EEG and the theta, alpha, and beta-1 spectral frequency bands.
- The mean relative amplitude (a%) decreases for the alpha rhythm.
- The resonance coefficient (k%) decreases for the raw EEG, the alpha and beta-1 fast activity.

Table 6.6 presents the results of the comparison between brain activation during performance of a mental arithmetic task, eyes closed, and the opening of the eyes with visual fixation of a cartoon for the group of 20 subjects. Table 6.6 is very similar to Table 6.5 because the activation by the visual arousal reaction is much greater than the mental arithmetic task, which is undertaken with eyes closed.

The most interesting findings are presented in Tables 6.7 and 6.8, which compare the eyes closed situation with the mental arithmetic task under eyes closed condition. When Table 6.7 is compared with Tables 6.5 and 6.6, it appears that the mental arithmetic task induces an EEG activation which is similar to that resulting from the opening of the eyes after an eyes closed situation.

Table 6.8 presents the secondary spectral parameters of the topographic EEG: the dispersions of the averaged values of mean frequency, absolute and relative amplitude, and coefficient of resonance. Table 6.8 is complementary to Table 6.7. In general, the dispersions around mean frequencies and absolute and relative amplitudes present the same trends, statistically validated by the Fisher tests, when mental arithmetic activation is compared to basic EEG recording with eyes closed, the subjects being relaxed with uncontrolled attention and in a state of diffuse vigilance. The left versus right amplitude ratios present a decrease for the raw EEG and the alpha, beta-1, and beta-2 spectral frequency bands, indicating a greater activation for the left hemisphere during mental arithmetic. Since the coefficients of asymmetries present the same trends as the

Table 6.8 Eyes Closed versus Mental Arithmetic, Eyes Closed

Parameters	CV (f)	CV (a μV)	s (a%)	L/R	Theta/Alpha
Raw EEG	—	—	—	↓	↑ (L)
Delta	↓ ↑	↑	↑	↓	—
Theta	NS	↓ ↓	↓	↑	—
Alpha	↑	↑ ↓	(↑)	↓	—
Beta-1	↓	↑	↑	↓	—
Beta-2	(↑)	↑	↑	↓	—

Significant Fisher permutaton tests; $n = 20$, 32 EEG channels, $p \leqslant 0.05$ and 0.01; L/R, left/right.

Table 6.9 Comparisons between Sequences: Right Hemisphere (First Sequence) versus Left Hemisphere (Second Sequence)

Alpha	f Hz	a μV	a%	k%
Eyes open	(NS)	7 ↑	3 ↑	7 ↑
Eyes closed	8 ↑	3 ↓	2(↓)	6 ↓
Calculation: eyes closed	11 ↑	3 ↓	1(↑)	6 ↓

Numbers significant or not (NS); Fisher permutation tests: $p \leqslant 0.05$, 0.01; 32 EEG channels statistically tested.

left to right ratios, this is not represented in Table 6.8. The theta/alpha ratios increase over the left hemisphere because of the activation over the left hemisphere during mental arithmetic. This effect is even more obvious in the results presented in Table 6.11.

Table 6.9 presents the results of comparisons between sequences (that is, between hemispheres). We have restricted these results to the main four spectral parameters and to the major frequency band of alpha. It appears that during visual fixation, eyes opened, the left hemisphere presents a "habituation," probably because of the monotony of looking for a long time at the same cartoon. However, a pattern of activation for the left hemisphere is observed under the eyes closed condition and during the mental arithmetic task, despite the fact that the left hemisphere (second sequence) was recorded after the right hemisphere (first sequence). This activation of the left hemisphere is statistically validated by an increase of mean frequency, a decrease of mean amplitude and, a decrease of the resonance coefficient for the alpha rhythm.

Table 6.10 presents a comparison between men and women when splitting the group of 20 subjects according to gender. There is no difference between subgroups for the eyes open situation. Under the eyes closed condition, the amplitude in microvolts is increased for the women's subgroup; this may be a result of the small number of subjects. As indicated in Table 6.3, the women's subgroup had six high alpha subjects as compared to four high alpha subjects in the men's subgroup. This small difference may be enough to explain the fact that six Fisher tests (over 32 tested for the 32 EEG channels) were statisti-

Table 6.10   Comparisons between Subgroups: Men versus Women ($n = 10$)

Alpha	f Hz	a μV	a%	k%
Eyes open	(NS)	(NS)	(NS)	(NS)
Eyes closed	(NS)	6 ↑	(NS)	(NS)
Calculation: eyes closed	(NS)	21 ↑	6 ↑	1(↑)

Numbers significant or not (NS); Fisher permutation tests: $p \leqslant 0.05, 0.01$; 32 EEG channels statistically tested.

Table 6.11   Comparisons between Situations for the Alpha Rhythm: Eyes Closed (EC), Eyes Open (EO), Mental Arithmetic, Eyes Closed (MA) ($n = 20$)

Alpha	f Hz	a μV	a%	k%
EC versus EO	8 ↑	32 ↓	32 ↓	32 ↓
MA versus EO	2(↓)	32 ↓	32 ↓	31 ↓
EC versus MA	4 ↑	23 ↓	32 ↓	2(↓)

Numbers significant or not (NS); Fisher permutation tests: $p \leqslant 0.05, 0.01$; 32 EEG channels statistically tested.

cally significant for the absolute amplitude spectral parameter. However, during mental arithmetic, the women's subgroup appears less activated than the men's subgroup, based on the amplitude parameters and the coefficient of resonance.

Table 6.11 presents a summary, for the three situations, compared two by two with statistical Fisher tests of the main parameters considered for the alpha rhythm. In the three comparisons, the pattern of activation is almost the same, especially for the absolute and relative amplitudes which are decreased in the eyes open situation or following mental arithmetic. The coefficient of resonance is also decreased, indicating EEG signals which present more harmonics and are closer to desynchronized background noise. The mean frequency also increased for the alpha rhythm over the left hemisphere, despite the fact that it was recorded in the second sequence following the first sequence recording over the right hemisphere.

RESULTS OF EEG MAPS OF THE CONTROL GROUP STATISTICALLY VALIDATED

Figure 6.1 represents EEG mean frequency maps for the control group ($n = 20$). In this figure the two upper images present the frequency maps averaged between subjects for the eyes closed situation (EC); the lower part presents the same averaged maps for the mental arithmetic (MA) task with eyes closed. The two maps on the right side represent the right hemisphere; the two maps on the left side represent the left hemisphere. The small black dots over two EEG channels on each frequency map concerning the mental arithmetic task indicate that these channels are statistically significant when compared to the eyes closed situation (Fisher tests significant at $p = 0.01$). Note that during mental arithmetic the mean frequencies of P3 and T5 are statistically increased compared to the eyes closed situation.

Figure 6.2 gives the mean absolute amplitude EEG maps in microvolts for the entire group. Observe that the occipital alpha rhythm presents a larger intense area around O2 than O1 in the eyes closed situation as well as during mental arithmetic. However, the black dots indicate that the mean amplitude is decreased significantly (significant Fisher tests; small black dots, $p = 0.05$; large black dots, $p = 0.01$) during the mental arithmetic task performed with eyes closed compared to the eyes closed situation.

Figure 6.3 represents the mean alpha relative amplitude % EEG maps for the group, for the same comparison as that in Figure 6.1 and 6.2. The activation of tracings after mental arithmetic is obvious, with a general decrease of relative amplitudes over all EEG channels.

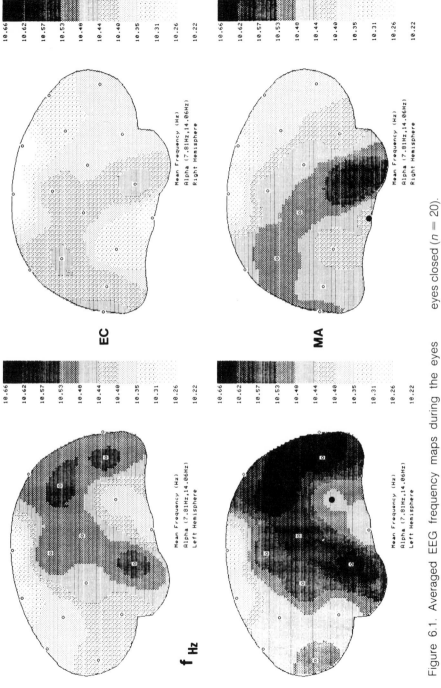

Figure 6.1. Averaged EEG frequency maps during the eyes closed situation (EC) and the mental arithmetic task (MA) with eyes closed (*n* = 20).

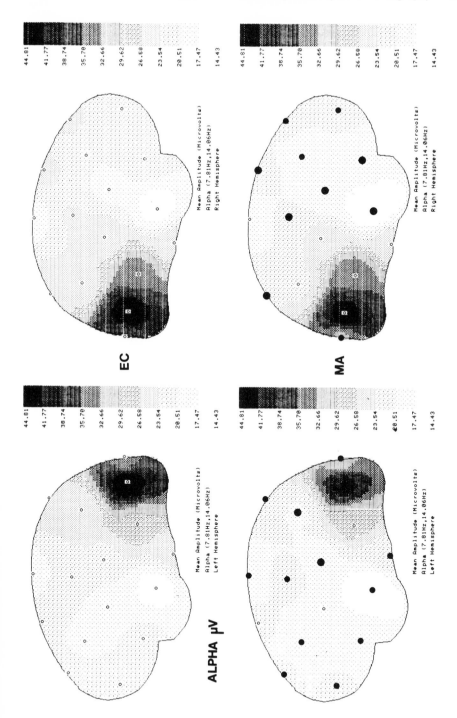

Figure 6.2. Mean absolute amplitude EEG maps in microvolts. Same group and activity comparison as in Figure 6.1.

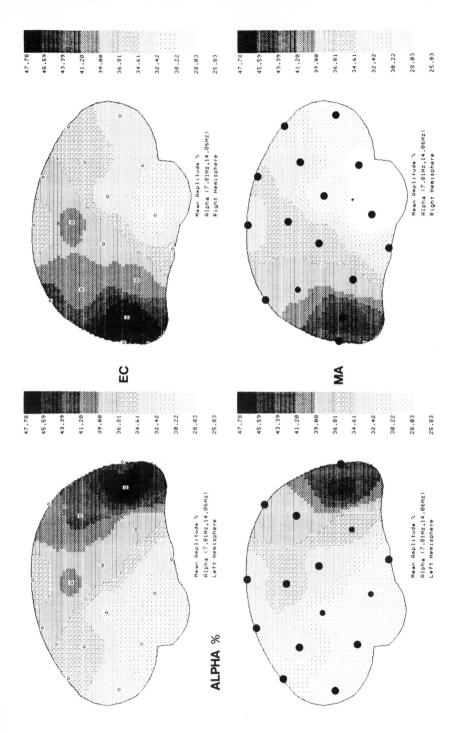

Figure 6.3. Mean relative amplitude EEG maps (%). Same group and activity comparison as in Figure 6.1.

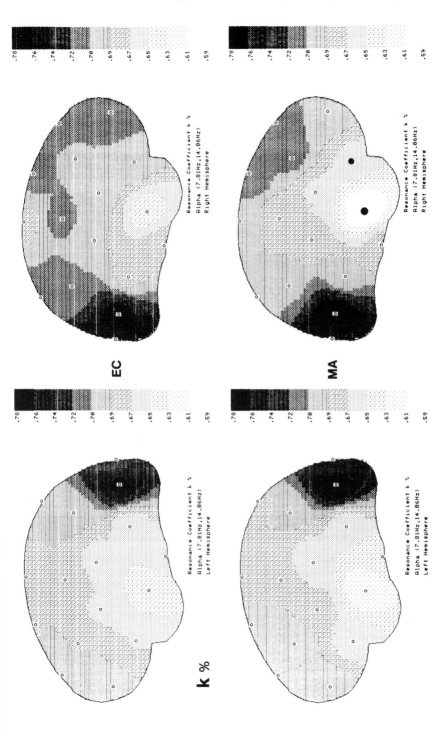

Figure 6.4. Mean coefficient of resonance k% EEG maps. Same group and activity comparison as in Figures 6.1–6.3.

Figure 6.4 represents the coefficient of resonance (k%) EEG maps for the group, for the same comparison as that in Figures 6.1, 6.2, and 6.3. Contrary to the two preceding figures dealing with mean amplitudes, Figure 6.4 does not show significant statistical changes except on T4 and F8 on the right hemisphere where an activation can be discerned because the coefficients of resonance are statistically significantly lower during mental arithmetic than during the resting eyes closed situation.

DISCUSSION

It is better to apply nonparametric statistical tests, like the Fisher permutation tests, on the sets of experimental EEG values which are used for computing EEG maps. The naked eye observes more differences when comparing EEG maps for different situations, even when the maps are drawn with the same gray shade scales. Do these maps distinguish between them or not? When we have computed nonparametric tests between the experimental sets of EEG values, we can respond rather soundly to this basic question. Indeed, what we have found in this example is that Fisher permutation tests provide much less significant changes between sets of EEG channels than we may hypothesize by looking at only the averaged EEG maps.

Nevertheless, even the use of such powerful Fisher tests has some limitations. For instance, Table 6.5 of our results implies that the computation of 736 Fisher tests (four parameters x five spectral frequency bands plus raw EEG x 32 EEG channels) and the set of tables of our results (Tables 6.5–6.11) represents a computation of more than 10,000 Fisher tests. We know that our data bank of experimental values is based on 20 subjects recorded twice (right and then left hemisphere) under three successive situations. The experimental variables are not independent. If statistical changes are due to sampling error, general conclusions cannot be drawn from this pilot study. However, we may consider that testing men against women's subgroups is not substantially different from duplicating the study with subgroups of 10 individuals. We should never say that our results are statistically true with a probability of falsehood defined in advance. Therefore, the best way to deal with such a general statistical problem of validating results would be to compare, variable by variable and test by test, results obtained from different topographic mapping laboratories under the same conditions and to compare the results. Thus, I would argue in favor of a reliability study with the object of developing an international atlas of brain electrical activity mapping.

For improvement of EEG cartography, we have investigated in 1982 with D.O. Walter, issues of the griding and contouring processes as well as the interpolation algorithm and the choice of reference electrode. Presently we record 16 EEG channels over each hemisphere in two successive sequences of 153.6 seconds (60 x 2.56 seconds). We use the average common electrode instead of linked ears or other monopolar reference electrodes. We have adopted Buchsbaum and Coppola EEG electrode placement montage. We use a nonlinear interpolation between the four EEG channels which are the nearest electrodes to the interpolated point. After studying the effects of weighting the inverse distance on the spatial resolution and aspects of EEG mappings, we have applied an inverse cubic distance algorithm instead of quadratic or linear inverse distance algorithms which produce more irregularities in gray scale boundaries.

We have also, with J. Gaches, been able to compare EEG cartography from our minicomputer system (HP Fourier Analyzer 5451C and HP 1000 21MX F) to topography from a microcomputer system (REEGA 2000, Alvar Electronic). We recorded well-defined white noises (into the junction box of the polygraph REEGA 16, Alvar) and fed the output signals into both EEG mapping systems to record 10 normal subjects and 10 patients. We were able to conclude from this reliability study that the microcomputer system, working on real time, with 16 FFT circuits following the multiplexer, is a very efficient EEG mapping system. We recorded more than 220 EEG sequences on the minicomputer and 50 on the microcomputer system. Clinical applications have been made and cases have already been published of neurological patients (brain strokes, brain tumors, epilepsy, etc.). We are presently obtaining homogeneous groups of EEG quantified records for cartography of patients and of matched controls from human volunteers. Each sequence on the minicomputer provides ninety maps of right and left hemisphere, from 10 spectral parameters applied to raw EEG or five frequency bands: mean frequency, RMS amplitude and amplitude %, coefficients of variation or standard deviation, left/right ratios and asymmetries, coefficient of resonance which is an index of monomorphism/polymorphism, and theta/alpha ratio.

Along these lines, we compared groups of men and women, recorded under different situations including eyes closed and relaxed, eyes open looking at a cartoon, mental arithmetic task, and different motor tasks. We presented results where we have studied statistically the first three situations by using the nonparametric permutation Fisher test. It already appears that the mental arithmetic task undertaken with eyes closed activates the EEG even more for P3, T5, than the visual fixation of a cartoon.

Finally, we would like to propose a multicentric study based on similar EEG tests, such as the ones already used by Duffy, in order to realize an international standardization of EEG mapping protocols. This may lead to the publication of an international atlas of EEG mapping.

ACKNOWLEDGMENTS

This review of research and development in EEG cartography resulted from teamwork. Therefore, we would like to thank the following co-workers who have published with us since 1972: C. Benkelfat, D. Campistron, C. Debouzy,

P. Deniker, J. Gaches, B. Gueguen, S. Guillou, J.C. Jouffre, P. Peron-Magnan, B. Pidoux, D. Tortrat, G. Verdeaux, B. Wendling. This chapter presents results of research undertaken at the Laboratoire d'EEG quantitative, Centre Hospitalier Sainte-Anne, by the Equipe de Recherche Recommandée, Université René Descartes, Paris V. We are grateful to the French I.N.S.E.R.M. (contrats de recherche externe n°490 and 848010), to the D.R.E.T., to the French Mission des Universités and to the Faculté de Médecine Cochin Port-Royal, Paris V, for research grants which have supported this research since 1972.

REFERENCES

1. Berger, H. Uber das Elektrenkephalogramm des Menschen. Arch. Psychiat. Nervenkr. 1929; 87:527–570.
2. Dietsch, G. Fourier-Analyse von Elektrenkephalogramment des Menschen. Arch. Ges. Physiol. 1932; 230:106–112.
3. Chweitzer, A., Geblewicz, E., and Liberson, W. Etude de l'électroencéphalogramme humain dans un cas d'intoxication mescalinique. Ann. Psychol. (Paris), 1936; 37:94–119.
4. Chweitzer, A., Geblewicz, E., and Liberson, W. Action de la mescaline sur les ondes alpha (rhythme de Berger) chez l'homme. C.R. Soc. Biol. 1937; 124:1296–1299.
5. Liberson, W. Les recherches sur les EEG transcraniens de l'homme. Travail humain. 1937; 5:431–463.
6. Drohocki, Z. Die spontane elekstrische Spannungsproduktion der Grosshirnrinde im Wach- und Ruhezustand. Pfluegers. Arch. Ges. Physiol. 1937; 239:658–679.
7. Drohocki, Z. L'électrospectrographie du cerveau. C.R. Soc. Biol. 1938; 129:889–893.
8. Gibbs, F.A. Regulation of frequency in cerebral cortex. Am. J. Physiol. 1937; 119:317–318.
9. Grass, A.M., and Gibbs, F.A. A Fourier transform of the electroencephalogram. J. Neurophysiol. 1938; 1:521–526.
10. Bertrand, I., and Lacape, R.S. Théorie de l'électroencéphalogramme: Etats élémentaires. Paris: Doin, 1943.
11. Walter, W.G. An automatic low frequency analyser. Electronic Eng. 1943; 11:237.
12. Walter, W.G., and Shipton, H.W. A new toposcopic display system. Electroenceph. Clin. Neurophysiol. 1951; 3:281–292.
13. Zee Zang Zao, Gelbin, and Rémond, A. Le champ électrique de l'oeil. Sem. Hop. Paris 1952; 28, 36:1–8.
14. Rémond, A., and Offner, F. A new method for EEG display. Electroenceph. Clin. Neurophysiol. 1952; 7:453.
15. Petsche, H. Das Vektor-EEG, line neuerweg zur Zlärung hirnelektrisher Vorgänge. Wien. Z. Nervenheilkd. 1952; 5:304–320.
16. Petsche, H., and Marko, A. Das Photozellentoposkop, eine einfache Methode zur

Bestimmung der Feldverteilung und Ausbreitung hirn elektrischer Vorgänge. Arch. Psychiatr. Zschr. Neurol. (D) 1954; 192:447–462.

17. Lilly, J.C. Instantaneous relations between activities of closely spaced zones on cerebral cortex: Electrical figures during responses of spontaneous activity. Ann. J. Physiol. 1954; 176:493–504.

18. Rémond, A. Orientations et tendances des méthodes topographiques dans l'étude de l'activité électrique du cerveau. Rev. Neurol. 1955; 93(2):399–432.

19. Rémond, A. Intégration temporelle et intégration spatiale à l'aide d'un même appareil. Rev. Neurol. 1956; 95(6):585–586.

20. Rémond, A. The importance of topographic data in EEG phenomena and an electrical model to reproduce them. Electroenceph. Clin. Neurophysiol. 1968; suppl. 27:29–49.

21. Rémond, A. Automatique et informatique en électroencéphalographie. Rev. EEG Neurophysiol. 1976; 2:145–154.

22. Rémond, A., and Delarue, R. Le système EHP 58: Électrodes, harnais, placement a 58 électrodes d'enregistrement électroencéphalographique. Rev. Neurol. 1959; 101(3):261–262.

23. Rémond, A., Lesèvre, N., Joseph, J.P., Rieger, H., and Lairy, G.L. The alpha average, I: Methodology and description, II: Quantitative study and the proposition of a theoretical model. Electroenceph. Clin. Neurophysiol. 1969; 26(1):245–265, (II):350–360.

24. Rémond, A., Lesèvre, N., and Torres, F. Etude Chrono-topographique de l'-activité occipitale moyenne recueillie sur le scalp chez l'homme en relation avec les déplacements du regard. Rev. Neurol. 1965; 113(3):193–226.

25. Rémond, A., and Torres, F. A method of electrode placement with a view to topographical research. I Basic concepts. Electroenceph. Clin. Neurophysiol. 1964; 17:577–578.

26. Ananiev, V.M. The electroencephaloscope. Fiziol. Zh. 1956; 42:981–988.

27. Cooper, R., Shipton, H.W., Shipton, J., Walter, V.J., and Walter, W.G. Spatial and temporal identification of alpha activities in relation to individual mental states, by means of the 22-channel helical scan toposcope. Electroenceph. Clin. Neurophysiol. 1957; 9:375.

28. Saltzberg, B., and Burch, N.R. A new approach to signal analysis in electroencephalography. I.R.E. Trans. Biomed. Eng. 1957; 8:24–30.

29. Adey, W.R., Dunlop, C.W., and Hendrix, C.E. Hippocampal slow waves: Distribution and phase relations in the course of approach learning. A.M.A. Arch. Neurol. 1960; 3:74–90.

30. Adey, W.R., Walter, D.O., and Hendrix, C.E. Computer techniques in correlation and spectral analyses of cerebral slow waves during discriminative behavior. Exp. Neurol. 1961; 3:501–524.

31. Adey, W.R., and Walter, D.O. Application of phase detection and averaging techniques in computer analysis of EEG records in the cat. Exp. Neurol. 1963; 7:186–209.

32. Walter, D.O. Analysis of cerebral neuroelectric waves, and their possible relation to memory processes. Ph.D. dissertation, U.C.L.A., 1962.

33. Walter, D.O. Spectral analysis for electroencephalograms: Mathematical determination of neurophysiological relationships from records of limited duration. Exp. Neurol. 1963; 8(2):155–181.

34. Walter, D.O., and Adey, W.R. Spectral analysis of EEGs recorded during learning in the cat, before and after subthalamic lesions. Exp. Neurol. 1963; 7:481–501.

35. Walter, D.O., Berkhout, J.I., Bushness, R., Kram, E., Rovner, L., and Adey, W.R. Digital computer analysis of neurophysiological data from biosatellite III, Biosatellite III results. Aerospace Med. 1971; 42(3):314–321.

36. Petsche, H., and Stumpf, S.L. Topographic and toposcopic study of origin and spread of the regular synchronized arousal pattern in the rabbit. Electroenceph. Clin. Neurophysiol. 1960; 12:589–600.

37. Petsche, H. Pathophysiologie und Klinik des Petit Mal. Toposkopische Untersuchungen zur Phänomenologie des Spike-Wave Musters. Wien. Z. Nervenheilkd. 1962; 19(4):345–442.

38. Goff, W.R., Rosner, B.S., and Allison, T. Distribution of cerebral somatosensory evoked responses in normal man. Electroenceph. Clin. Neurophysiol. 1962; 14:697–713.

39. Goff, G.D., Matsumiya, Y., Allison, T., and Goff, W.R. The scalp topography of human somatosensory and auditory evoked potentials. Electroenceph. Clin. Neurophysiol. 1977; 42:57–76.

40. Goff, W., Allison, T., Willamson, P., and Van Gilder, J. Scalp topography in the localization of intracranial evoked potential sources. Proc. 4th Intl. Cong. Event-Related Slow Potentials of the Brain. EPA-600/9-77-042, 1978; 526–532.

41. Bechtereva, N.P., Vvedenskaia, I.V., Dubikaitis, Y.V., Stepanova, T.S., Ovnatov, B.S., and Usov, V.V. Localization of focal brain lesions by electroencephalography. Electroenceph. Clin. Neurophysiol. 1963; 15:177–196.

42. Gotman, J., and Gloor, P. Automatic recognition and quantification of interictal epileptic activity in the human scalp EEG. Electroenceph. Clin. Neurophysiol. 1966; 41:513–529.

43. De Mott, D.W. Cortical micro-toposcopy. Med. Res. Eng. 1966; 5:23–29.

44. Pozo-Olano, J.D., Mezan, I., and Rémond, A. Les relations de phases orthogonales en EEG. Montage en croix. Rev. Neurol. 1967; 117(1):136–141.

45. Gavrilova, N.A., and Aslanov, A.S. Application of electronic computing techniques to the analysis of clinical electroencephaloscopic data. In M.N. Livanov and V.S. Rusinov, eds., trans. J.S. Barlow: Mathematical Analysis of the Electrical Activity of the Brain, Cambridge: Harvard Univ. Press, 1968; 53–64.

46. Mezan, I., Lesèvre, N., and Rémond, A. Etude chrono-topographique de la réponse somesthésique évoquée moyenne recueillie sur le scalp par stimulation électrique du nerf médian. Rev. Neurol. 1968; 119(3):288–295.

47. Harris, J.A., and Bickford, R.G. Spatial display and parameter computation of the human epileptic spike focus by computer. Electroenceph. Clin. Neurophysiol. 1968; 24:281.

48. Gaches, J., and Supino, V. Variations fonctionnelles de l'EEG. Codification quantitative de l'analyse des tracés. Fol. Neuropsychiat. 1969; 12:463–476.

49. Bourne, J.R., Childers, D.G., and Perry, N.W. A spatio-temporal representation of the visual evoked response, Proc. 8th Int. Cong. Biomed. Eng. Chicago, 1969; 149.

50. Bourne, J.R., Childers, D.G., and Perry, N.W. Topological characteristics of the visual evoked response in man. Electroenceph. Clin. Neurophysiol. 1971; 30:423–436.

51. Lehmann, D. Multichannel topography of human alpha EEG fields. Electroenceph. Clin. Neurophysiol. 1971; 31:439–449.
52. Bickford, R.G., Billinger, T.W., Fleming, N.I., and Stewart, F. The compressed spectral array (CSA). A pictorial EEG. Proc. San Diego Biomed. Symp. 1972; 11:365–370.
53. Bickford, R.G. New trends in clinical electroencephalography. Practitioner. 1976; 217:100–107.
54. Bickford, R.G. A combined EEG and evoked potential procedure in clinical EEG (automated cerebral electrogram—ace test). In N. Yamaguchi and K. Fujisawa, eds., Recent Advances in EEG and EMG Data Processing. Amsterdam: Elsevier, 1981; 217–235.
55. Petsche, H., and Shaw, J.C. EEG topography. In A. Rémond, ed., Handbook of Electroencephalography and Clinical Neurophysiology, Vol. 5B, Amsterdam: Elsevier, 1972.
56. Gersch, W. Causality or driving in electrophysiological signal and analysis. Math. Biosci. 1972; 14:177–196.
57. Gersch, W., and Tharp, B.R. Spectral regression/amount of information analysis of seizures in humans. In P. Kellaway, ed., Quantitative Analytic Studies in Epilepsy. New York: Raven Press, 1976; 509–532.
58. Creutzfeldt, O. Electrical activity from the neuron to the EEG and EMG, Vol. 5, Parte: The neuronal generation of the EEG. In A. Rémond, ed., Handbook of EEG and Clinical Neurophysiology, Amsterdam: Elsevier, 1974.
59. Gotman, J., Gloor, P., and Ray, W.F. A quantitative comparison of traditional reading of the EEG and interpretation of computer extracted features in patients with supratentorial brain lesions. Electroenceph. Clin. Neurophysiol. 1975; 38:623–639.
60. Bostem, F. A system of acquiring and treating neurophysiological information for synoptic representation. In G. Dolce and H. Künkel, eds., CEAN, Computerized EEG Analysis. Stuttgart: Gustav Fischer, 1975; 403–420.
61. Bostem, F. Postprocessing techniques. On-line vs. Off-line processing. Presentation and evaluation of the results. Display methods and techniques. Simple statistical treatment. In A. Rémond, ed., EEG Informatics: A Didactic Review of Methods and Applications of EEG Data Processing. Amsterdam: Elsevier, 1977; 171–192.
62. Bostem, F., and Degossely, M. Spectral Analysis of Alpha Rhythm during Schultz's Autogenic Training. In W.A. Cobb and H. van Duijn, eds., Contemporary Clinical Neurophysiology (EEG suppl. 34), Amsterdam: Elsevier, 1978; 182–190.
63. Kunkel, H., Luba, A., and Niethardt, P. Topographic and psychosomatic aspects of spectral EEG analysis of drug effect. In P. Kellaway and I. Petersen, eds., Quantitative Analytic Studies in Epilepsy. New York: Raven Press, 1976; 207–223.
64. Harner, R.N., and Ostergren, K.A. Progress in computerized EEG topography, Electroenceph. Clin. Neurophysiol. 1976; 41:541.
65. Harner, R.N., and Ostergren, K.A. Computed EEG topography. Electroenceph. Clin. Neurophysiol. 1978; suppl. 34:151–161.
66. Harner, R.N. EEG Analysis in the time domain. In A. Rémond, ed., EEG Infor-

matics: A Didactic Review of Methods and Applications of EEG Data Processing. Amsterdam: Elsevier, 1977; 57–82.

67. Livanov, M.N. Spatial Organization of Cerebral Processes. New York: Wiley and Sons, 1977.

68. Walter, W.G. Intrinsic rhythms of the brain. In J. Field, ed., Handbook of Physiology, Sect. I, Washington, D.C.: American Physiological Society, 1959; 279–298.

69. Lesèvre, N., Rieger, H., and Rémond, A. Le rythme alpha moyen et son aspect topographique, définition et intérêt. Rev. Neurol. 1967; 117(1):130–136.

70. Rieger, J. H., Rémond, A. Essai de modèle théorique du rythme alpha moyen. Rev. Neurol. 1967; 117 (1):208–211.

71. Joseph, J.P., Rieger, H., Lesèvre, N., and Rémond, A. Mathematical simulations of alpha rhythms recorded on the scalp. In H. Petsche and M.A.B. Brazier, eds., Synchronization of EEG Activity in Epilepsies. Vienna: Springer Verlag, 1972; 327–346.

72. Ragot, R., Cecchini, A., and Rémond, A. Les possibilités de la saisie topographique et du traitement cartographique des signaux EEG. Rev. EEG Neurophysiol. 1976; 6(2):278–284.

73. Elul, R. Amplitude histograms of the EEG as an indicator of the cooperative behavior of neuron populations. Electroenceph. Clin. Neurophysiol. 1967; 23:87.

74. Elul, R. Gaussian behavior of the electroencephalogram: Changes during performance of mental task. Science, 1969; 164(3877):328–331.

75. Vaughn, H.G. Jr., and Ritter, W. The sources of auditory evoked responses recorded from the human scalp. Electroenceph. Clin. Neurophysiol. 1970; 28:360–378.

76. Craco, R.Q. Travelling waves of the human scalp recorded somatosensory evoked responses: Effects of differences in recording technique and sleep on somatosensory and somatomotor responses. Electroenceph. Clin. Neurophysiol. 1972; 33:557–566.

77. Zetterberg, L.H. Stochastic activity in a population of neurons: A systems analysis approach, Report 2.3.153/1, TNO. Utrecht: Medisch.-Fysisch Instituut, 1973.

78. Zetterberg, L.H. Experiments with a model for a neuron population. Electroenceph. Clin. Neurophysiol. 1977; 43(4):480.

79. Lopes Da Silva, F.H., Hoeks, A., Smits, H., and Zetterberg, L.H. Model of brain rhythmic activity, the alpha-rhythm of the thalamus. Kybernetik, 1974; 15: 27–37.

80. Childers, D.G. Evoked responses: Electrogenesis, Models, Methodology, and Wavefront Reconstruction and Tracking Analysis. Proc. IEEE, 1977; 65(5): 611–626.

81. Etevenon, P. Etude méthodologique de l'électroencéphalographie quantitative. Application à quelques exemples. Thèse doctorat ès-Sciences Paris: Copedith Pub., 1978.

82. Etevenon, P., Giannella, F., and Abarnou, F. Modèle d'EEG par modulation radioélectrique d'amplitude et de phase. Conséquences sur l'aspect morphologique du signal. Rev. EEG Neurophysiol. 1980; 10(1):69–80.

83. Saito, Y., and Harashima, H. Tracking of informations within multichannel EEG record: Causal analysis in EEG. In N. Yamaguchi, K. Fujisawa, eds., Recent Advances in EEG and EMG Data Processing. Amsterdam: Elsevier, 1981; 133–146.

84. Watanabe, S., and Shikata, Y. Stability of alpha rhythm. In N. Yamaguchi and K. Fujisawa, eds., Recent Advances in EEG and EMG Data Processing. Amsterdam: Elsevier, 1981; 87–94.

85. Suzuki, H. Variations of the regional relationships in waking EEG. In N. Yamaguchi and K. Fujisawa, eds., Recent Advances in EEG and EMG Data Processing. Amsterdam: Elsevier, 1981; 209–214.

86. Naitoh, P., and Lewis, G.W. Statistical analysis of extracted features. In N. Yamaguchi and K. Fujisawa, eds., Recent Advances in EEG and EMG Data Processing. Amsterdam: Elsevier, 1981; 179–194.

87. Petsche, H., Pockberger, H., and Rappelsberger, P. The assessment of dependence of electrical activities on cortical morphology by the micro-EEG. J. J. EEG-EMG 1981; suppl: 39–48.

88. Petsche, H., Pockberger, H., and Rappelsberger, P. The Micro-EEG: Methods and application to the analysis of the antiepileptic action of benzodiazepines. In W.M. Herrmann, ed., EEG in Drug Research. Stuttgart: Gustav Fischer, 1982; 159–182.

89. Tucker, D.M. Asymmetries of coherence topography: Structural and dynamic aspects of brain lateralization. In P. Flor-Henry and J. Gruzelier, eds., Laterality and Psychopathology. Amsterdam: Elsevier, 1983; 349–362.

90. Etevenon, P. A model of intra and inter-hemispheric relationships. In P. Flor-Henry, J. Gruzelier, eds., Laterality and Psychopathology, Amsterdam: Elsevier, 1983; 291–300.

91. Freeman, W.J. Mass Action in the Nervous System. New York: Academic Press, 1975.

92. Robinson, A.H., and Petchenik, B.B. The Nature of Maps. London: Chicago Press, 1976.

93. Nunez, P. Electrical Fields of the Brain. New York: Oxford Press, 1981.

94. Lehmann, D. The EEG as scalp field distribution. In A. Rémond, ed., EEG Informatics: A Didactic Review of Methods and Applications of EEG Data Processing. Amsterdam: Elsevier, 1977; 365–384.

95. Lehmann, D. Spatial analysis of evoked and spontaneous EEG potential field. In N. Yamaguchi, K. Fujisawa, eds., Recent Advances in EEG and EMG Data Processing. Amsterdam: Elsevier, 1981; 117–132.

96. Lehmann, D. EEG assessment of brain activity: spatial aspects, segmentation and imaging. Intl. J. Psychophysiol. 1984; 1:267–276.

97. Skrandies, W., and Lehmann, D. Occurrence time and scalp location of components of evoked EEG potential fields. In W.M. Herrmann, ed., EEG in Drug Research. Stuttgart: Gustav Fischer, 1982; 183–191.

98. Ueno, S., Matsuoka, S., Mizoguchi, T., Nagashima, M., and Cheng, C.L. Topographic computer display of abnormal EEG activities in patients with CNS diseases. Memoirs Fac. Eng., Kyushu Univ. 1975; 24(3):196–209.

99. Ragot, R.A., and Rémond, A. EEG field mapping. Electroenceph. Clin. Neurophysiol. 1978; 45:417–421.

100. Duffy, F.H., Burchfiel, J.L., and Lombroso, C.T. Brain Electrical Activity Mapping (BEAM): A method for extending the clinical utility of EEG and evoked potential data. Ann. Neurol. 1979; 5:309–321.

101. Duffy, F.H. Brain Electrical activity mapping (BEAM): Computerized access to complex brain function. Int. J. Neurosci. 1981; 13:55–65.

102. Duffy, F.H. Topographic display of evoked potentials: Clinical applications of brain electrical activity mapping (BEAM). Ann. N.Y. Acad. Sci. 1982; 388: 183–196.

103. Duffy, F.H., Denckla, M.B., Bartels, P.H., and Sandini, G. Dyslexia: Regional differences in brain electrical activity by topographic mapping. Ann. Neurol. 1980; 7:412–420.

104. Duffy, F.H., Denckla, M.B., Bartels, P.H., Sandini, G., and Kiessling, L.S. Dyslexia: Automated diagnosis by computerized classification of brain electrical activity. Ann. Neurol. 1980; 7:421–428.

105. Duffy, F.H., Bartels, P.H., and Burchfiel, J.L. Significance probability mapping: An aid in the topographic analysis of brain electrical activity. Electroenceph. Clin. Neurophysiol. 1981; 51:455–462.

106. Duffy, F.H., Jensen, F., Erba, G., Burchfiel, J.L., and Lombroso, C.T. Extraction of clinical information from electroencephalographic background activity: The combined use of brain electrical activity mapping and intravenous sodium thiopental. Ann. Neurol. 1984; 15:1.

107. Duffy, F.H., Albert, M.S., McAnulty, G., and Garvey, A.J. Age-related differences in brain electrical activity mapping of healthy subjects. Ann. Neurol. 1984; 16:430–438.

108. Duffy, F.H., Albert, M.S., and McAnulty, G. Brain electrical activity in patients with presenile and senile dementia of the Alzheimer's type. Ann. Neurol. 1984; 16:439–448.

109. Lombroso, C.T., and Duffy, F.H. Brain Electrical Activity mapping as an adjunct to CT Scanning. In R. Canger, F. Angeleri, and J.K. Penry, eds., Advances in Epileptology, XIth Epilepsy Intl. Symp. New York: Raven Press, 1980; 83–88.

110. Lombroso, C.T., and Duffy, F.H. Brain electrical activity mapping in the epilepsies. In H. Akimoto, H. Kazamatsuri, M. Seino, and A. Ward, eds., Advances in Epileptology: The XIIIth Epilepsy Intl. Symp. New York: Raven Press, 1982; 173–179.

111. Morihisa, J.M., Duffy, F.H., Mendelson, W.B., and Wyatt, R.J. The use of brain electrical activity mapping (BEAM) as an exploratory technique to delineate regional differences between schizophrenic patients and control subjects. In P. Flor-Henry and J. Gruzelier, eds., Laterality and Psychopathology. Amsterdam: Elsevier, 1983; 339–347.

112. Mortsyn, R., Duffy, F.H., and McCarley, R.W. Altered P 300 topography in schizophrenia. Arch. Gen. Psychiatry. 1983; 40:729–734.

113. Morstyn, R. Duffy, F., and McCarley, R. Altered topography of EEG spectral content in schizophrenia. Electroenceph. Clin. Neurophysiol. 1983; 56:263–271.

114. Duff, T.A. Topography of scalp recorded potentials evoked by stimulation of the digits, Electroenceph. Clin. Neurophysiol. 1980; 49:452–460.

115. Coppola, R., Buchsbaum, M.S., and Cappelletti, J. Presentation of Multilead EEG by Topographic Maps of Electrical Activity. Proc. 9th Ann. Bioenging. Conf., New York: Pergamon Press, 1981.

116. Coppola, R. Topographic methods of functional cerebral analysis. IEEE Frontiers of Engineering in Health Care, 1982; 71–78.

117. Coppola, R., Salb, J., and Chassy, J. Topographic analysis of epileptiform discharges. Abstract, 15th Epilepsy Int. Symp. Am. Epilepsy Soc. Meeting, 1983.

118. Buchsbaum, M.S., Coppola, R., Gershon, E.S., Van Kammen, D.P., and Nurnberger, J.I. Evoked potential measures of attention and psychopathology, Adv. Biol. Psychiat., 1981; 6:186–194.

119. Buchsbaum, M.S., Rigal, F., Coppola, R., Cappelletti, J., King, C., and Johnson, J. A new system for gray-level surface distribution maps of electrical activity. Electroenceph. Clin. Neurophysiol. 1982; 53:237–242.

120. Buchsbaum, M.S., King, A.C., Cappelletti, J., Coppola, R., and Van Kammen, D.P. Visual evoked potential topography in patients with schizophrenia and normal controls. Adv. Biol. Psychiat. 1982; 9:50–56.

121. Buchsbaum, M.S., Mendelson, W.B., Duncan, W.C., Coppola, R., Kelsoe, J., and Gillin, J.C. Topographic cortical mapping of EEG sleep stages during daytime naps in normal subjects. Sleep, 1982; 5(3):248–255.

122. Buchsbaum, M.S., Coppola, R., and Cappelletti, J. Positron emission tomography, EEG and evoked potential topography: New approaches to local function in pharmaco-electroencephalography. In W.M. Herrmann, ed., EEG in Drug Research. Stuttgart: Gustav Fischer, 1982; 192–207.

123. Terao, A., Nomura, N., Fukunaga, H., Moriyasu, M., and Shiota, J. The scalp topographic mapping of human somatosensory evoked potentials. Kawasaki Med. J., 1981; 7(1):37–45.

124. Nagata, K., Mizukami, M., Araki, G., Kawase, T., and Hirano, H. Topographic electroencephalograhic study of cerebral infarction using computed mapping of the EEG. J. Cereb. Blood Flow Metab. 1982; 2:79–88.

125. Etevenon, P., Peron-Magnan, P., Verdeaux, G., Gaches, J., and Deniker, P. Electroencéphalographie quantitative en neurologie et psychiatrie: Images topographiques d'EEG, effets d'agents psychotropes, typologie de la schizophrénie. Colloque Nat. Génie Biol. Méd. 1982; 43:422, 473A.

126. Etevenon, P., Gaches, J., Debouzy, C., Gueguen, B., and Peron-Magnan, P. EEG cartography. I. By means of mini or micro-computers. Reliability and interest of this electrical non-invasive brain imagery. Neuropsychobiology, 1985; 13: 141–146.

127. Etevenon, P., Tortrat, D., and Benkelfat, C. EEG cartography II. By means of statistical group studies. Activation by visual attention. Neuropsychobiology, 1985; 13:69–73.

128. Etevenon, P. Cartograhie EEG. Une nouvelle méthode d'imagerie médicale non-invasive. Exemple détaillé d'un cas d'accident vasculaire cérébral. In Pr. Cambier, ed., Nouvelles explorations atraumatiques en pathologie vasculaire cérébrale. Paris: Spécia, 1984; 103–109.

129. Etevenon, P., and Gaches, J. Electroencéphalographie quantitative et procédé de cartographie d'images d'EEG quantitative sur ordinateur dans l'étude de la sénescence et des accidents ischémiques cérébraux. In J. Cahn, A. Agnoli, F. Cohadon, S. Hoyer, and H. Lechner, eds., Drugs and Cerebrovascular Diseases, Médicaments et les Maladies Cérébrovasculaires. London: John Libbey, Eurotext, 1983.

130. Etevenon, P., and Gaches, J. Quantitative EEG maps in Neuro-Psychiatry. Problems and Perspectives. Proc. 14th C.I.N.P. Congress, Florence, June 19–23, 1984. In Clinical Neuropharmacology, 7, suppl. 1. New York: Raven Press, 1984; 122–123.

131. Pidoux, B., Etevenon, P., Campistron, D., Peron-Magnan, P., Bisserbe, J.C., Verdeaux, G., and Deniker, P. Topo-Electroencephalographie quantitative par ordinateur (T.E.Q.O.). Rev. EEG Neurophysiol. 1983; 13(1):27–34.

132. Persson, A., and Hjorth, B. EEG topogram: An aid in describing EEG to the clinician. Electroenceph. Clin. Neurophysiol. 1983; 56:399–405.

133. Maresh, H., Pfurtscheller, G., and Kopruner, V. Topographical presentation of EEG parameters by colour graphic. Part I. Third Europ. Cong. EEG Clin. Neurophysiol. Basel, Sept. 12–14, 1983, Poster 8.

134. Gaches, L. Representation cartografica del EEG quantificado aplication en clinica neurologica. Simp. Int. Adv. Neurofisiol. Clin. 1984; 111:39.

135. Gaches, J., and Etevenon, P. Topographie loco-régionale du spectre EEG chez l'homme: Cartographie de deux cas d'accident vasculaire cérébral (Dont l'un suivi sous sommeil). In N.A. Lassen, J. Cahn, eds., Maladies et Médicaments, Drugs and Diseases. Paris: John Libbey, 1984; 1:1.

136. Sebban, C.L., Debouzy, C.L., and Berthaux, P. EEG quantifié et cartographie numérisée. In N.A. Lassen, and J. Cahn, eds., Maladies et Médicaments, Drugs and Diseases, Paris: John Libbey, 1984; 1:1.

137. Debouzy, C., Etevenon, P., Sebban, C., Gueguen, B., and Gaches, J. Cartographie EEG. Exemples d'applications cliniques. Rev. EEG Clin. Neurophysiol. (submitted for publication).

138. Pfurtscheller, G., and Ladurner, G. ERD mapping in cerebral ischemia. Proc. IEEE. 1985; in press.

139. Itil, T.M., Shapiro, D., Itil, K.Z., Eralp, E., and Bergamo, M.L. Psychotropic drug evaluation using an integrated computer data bank and dynamic brain mapping, 14th CINP Congress, Florence, 1984.

140. Baillon, J.F., and Rémond, A. Analyse et description de l'EEG par décompositon en éléments simples à l'aide d'un micro-ordinateur. Rev. EEG Neurophysiol. 1976; 6(2):271–277.

141. Etevenon, P., Peron-Magnan, P., Benkelfat, C., and Deniker, P. Application of quantitative EEG and EEG cartography in neuropsychology, psychiatry and neuro-pharmacology. First maps of state I of sleep and paradoxical sleep. Cong. Int. Trait. Sig. EEG. 1985 (in press).

142. Etevenon, P., and Debouzy, C. Principes et difficultés de la cartographie EEG sur mini et micro-ordinateurs. Cong. Int. Trait. Sig. EEG, 1985 (in press).

143. Gaches, J., Etevenon, P., and Gueguen, B. Applications de la cartographie EEG à la pratique neurologique. Cong. Int. Trait. Sig. EEG, 1985 (in press).

144. Walter, D.O., Etevenon, P., Pidoux, B., and Tortrat, D., Guillou, S. Computerized topo-EEG spectral maps: Difficulties and perspectives. Neuropsychobiology, 1986;11:264–272.

145. Ingvar, D.H., Rosen, I., and Johannesson, G. EEG related to cerebral metabolism and blood flow. Pharmakopschiatrie, 1979, 12:200–209.

146. Dubinsky, J., and Barlow, J.S. A simple dot-density topogram for EEG. Electroenceph. Clin. Neurophysiol., 1980; 48:473–477.

147. Etevenon, P., and Tortrat, D. First application of a model of intra and inter-hemispheric changes in psychotic patients before and after treatment by clomipramine. Adv. Biol. Psychiatry 1983; 13:135–141.

148. Coppola, R., Buchsbaum, M.S., and Rigal, F. Computer generation of surface dis-

tribution maps of measures of brain activity. Comput. Biol. Med. 1982; 12(2): 191–199.

149. Lehmann, D. EEG phase differences and their physiological significance in scalp field studies. In G. Dolce and H. Künkel, eds., CEAN, Computerized EEG Analysis. Stuttgart: G. Fischer, 1975; 102–110.

150. Pidoux, B., Etevenon, P., Campistron, D., Peron-Magnan, P., Verdeaux, G., and Deniker, P. Aspects topographiques des rythmes rapides médicamenteux en électroencéphalographie quantitative. Rev. EEG Neurophysiol; 1983; 13(1):35–41.

151. Lebart, L., Morineau, A., and Fenelon, J.L. Traitement des données statistiques. Paris: Durod, 1982.

152. Etevenon, P., Tortrat, D., Guillou, S., and Wendling, B. Cartographie EEG au cours d'une tâche visuo-spatiale. Cartes moyennes et statistiques de groupes. Rev. EEG Neurophysiol. 1985 (in press).

7

Selected Applications of a Topographic Approach to Event-Related Potentials

Nicole Lesèvre and Antoine Rémond

The principal characteristic of all topographic analyses applied to scalp-recorded electroencephalograms (EEG) is that they all use interpolation methods in order to try to smooth out the spatial discontinuities of electrophysiological data; indeed, these discontinuities still remain, however numerous might be the electrodes placed on the scalp. The spatiotemporal mapping display conceived by one of us (Antoine Rémond) years ago, and utilized ever since in our laboratory for research purposes, is based upon a simple spatial interpolation method [1–5]. We attempt to illustrate its usefulness by giving a synthetic overview of some of the recent results this approach has enabled us to obtain in the field of evoked potential research, and discuss the possibilities as well as the limits of such an approach. The spatiotemporal mapping display has been extensively used in our research group in order to address two entirely different research objectives. The first concerns the localization of the underlying generators of the sensory components of evoked potentials; the second, in the domain of psychophysiology, is the identification of functional components, in other words, the identification of the event-related potential components reflecting information processing stages and task variables.

For the first objective, we have used spatiotemporal mapping to provide information (or at least clues) concerning the intracranial sources of the visual evoked potential obtained in response to stimulation of various parts of the visual field, be it to flash stimuli [6] or pattern [7–13]. Spatial distribution on the scalp is then considered as an independent variable in terms of anatomical structures [14]. Hypotheses concerning the most probable sites of origin of these various components have been proposed by our team on the basis of topography and polarity changes obtained from analysis of many normal subjects and patients experiencing changes in stimulus location in the visual field. These data have been interpreted, as has the research of other authors [15–20],

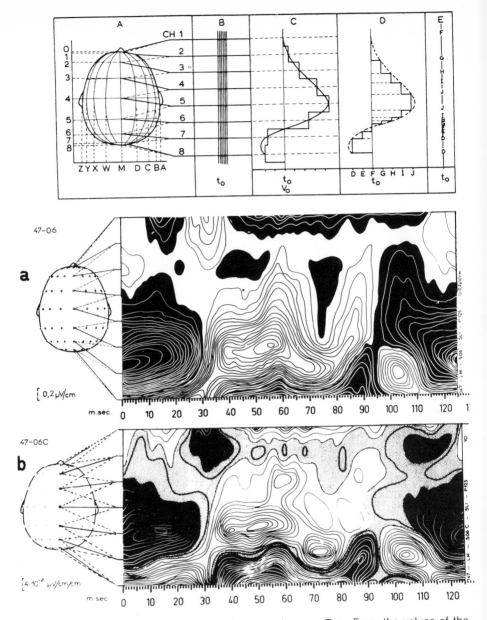

Figure 7.1. Method used to produce spatiotemporal maps. *Top*: From the values of the signals obtained from eight bipolar derivations (*A*), at one instant (*B*), a distribution histogram is constructed (*C*) and a smooth distribution curve is obtained by a second-order interpolation (*C*). The amplitude dimension is marked off in increments corresponding to a value in microvolts chosen by program for the spacing of the isopotential (or isogradient) lines (*D* and *E*). *Bottom*. Contour maps are constructed after the potential distribution obtained for a succession of time instants. *a*. Map of gradients corresponding to bipolar recordings (positive gradients appear in white, negative in black). *b*. Current density map, obtained by calculating the first derivative of gradients according to space, showing the distribution of sinks (*in black*) and sources (*in white*).

by referring to classical simplified dipole sheet models of the visual cortex [11–13].

More recently, spatiotemporal mapping has been used in our group as a method enhancing the identification of functional components and establishment of their relation to psychological variables, with the intent of elucidating the elements of human information processing. Spatial distributions are then considered as dependent variables, i.e., variables dependent upon sensory, motor, and cognitive processes, as has been emphasized by many psychophysiologists [14,21]. In such a view one is only interested in the functional significance of a component, whatever its generator, and topography is then only one of the dependent variables of a component. According to Donchin et al. [21] the very definition of a component is that "it varies systematically as a function of some independent experimental variable." We shall further insist upon this characterization of "scalp distribution" as a dependent variable, by illustrating some of the recent results we have obtained in the field of mental chronometry through the use of the missing stimulus paradigm and analysis of the single-trial spatiotemporal maps of each individual omission evoked response [22–27].

THE SPATIOTEMPORAL MAPPING DISPLAY

Contour mapping is one of the most efficient ways of overcoming the problem of discrete sampling in space and has been used for several years as an EEG analytic technique [1–3,5,28–36].

Rémond's spatiotemporal mapping procedure [2–5] is based upon contour plotting and linear amplitude distribution. This display (Figure 7.1) corresponds to a classical contour map in which the abscissa represents time and the ordinate a dimension in space along a linear array of electrodes. The amplitude variations are represented in the form of a series of isopotential lines (or isogradient lines in the case of bipolar recordings) as a function of time and of electrode location; amplitude values between two successive electrodes are obtained by a second-order interpolation using a sliding window over three neighboring and simultaneous recorded values. For the successive time instants, the amplitude dimension is given as increments of a given value chosen by program for the spacing of the equipotential lines that are drawn by a computer on a paper chart.

This display makes it possible to identify at a glance the location of peaks and dips of potential (or of potential gradients in the case of bipolar recordings as in the upper map of Figure 7.1 or of current density when calculating the second derivative of potential according to space, as shown in the lower map of Figure 7.1) along the spatial axis as well as their occurrence along the time axis. It may allow the pinpointing of subtle changes between two adjacent channels in different experimental conditions at the same instant or for the same experimental condition at different moments. Moreover, this mapping display makes it possible to visualize certain nonaveraged components of single-trial evoked potentials which would have been difficult to identify using a standard set of amplitude versus time traces.

It is true that such spatiotemporal maps do not permit as accurate a representation of potential distribution over the scalp as whole-brain maps that deal with two-dimensional spatial data [31,32,37–39]. But contrary to such whole-brain maps, which are plotted at discrete time intervals, such spatiotemporal displays have the advantage of directly representing time-space relationships.

LOCALIZATION OF THE UNDERLYING GENERATORS OF THE VARIOUS COMPONENTS OF THE PATTERN ONSET EVOKED RESPONSE

It is well known that theoretically a given potential distribution on a surface such as the scalp, enclosing a volume such as the brain, can be generated by an infinite variety of underlying source configurations. Therefore it is evident that however sophisticated a topographic analysis of scalp-recorded evoked potentials might be, this analysis cannot give precise information concerning the site and orientation of the multiple underlying generators. However, valuable clues regarding the most probable sites of some of these sources can be obtained whenever such topographic analyses are applied, provided that the researcher takes into account the complex geometry of the sensory cortex and isolates some of the different overlapping components of the response.

The whole-field pattern onset response (Figures 7.2–7.5) is a complex response made up of many components. Some components are easy to recognize since they peak at different times and on different regions of the scalp, but others, overlapping in space and time, can only be individualized by the manipulation of experimental variables such as those related to the part of the visual field being stimulated, or such as luminance and contrast variables. We give a few examples of such component identifications obtained using our spatiotemporal display. In particular we demonstrate the existence of laterally located components and their reactivity according to the part of the retina stimulated.

The type of pattern onset response under study was obtained from a large population of over 60 normal subjects and recorded under the same experimental conditions as the stimuli characteristics described by Lesèvre [13]. The montage used for our studies consisted of at least nine electrodes in two lines forming a "cross montage," the center of the cross being located on the midline, 4 cm above the inion. The interelectrode distance was usually either 4 cm (Figures 7.2–7.7) or 2 cm. The longitudinal part of the cross was on the midline, going from the inion to a point 16 cm above, i.e., near the vertex; the transverse branch crossed the midline 4 cm above the inion and extended 8 cm or 16 cm away from the midline, on both hemispheres, in the direction of the upper part of the ears. The reference electrode was usually placed on the linked earlobes, but in several cases a systematic study of the influence of the reference electrode on the spatiotemporal organization of the response was made by simultaneously using three different references: linked earlobes, Fz, and the sternovertebral, noncephalic reference.

The pattern full-field onset response is made up of not only four successive components peaking on the midline a little above the inion, namely, the four classical N60, P100, N140, and P200, but also two components peaking more laterally (at least 4 cm away from the midline on both hemispheres) and more anteriorly (approximately 8 to 10 cm above the inion, a little lower than the vertex). We have labeled these two positive and negative lateral-anterior components as LP120 and LN150, since they usually peak 10 to 20 msec later than the preceding midline peaks of like polarity (Figures 7.2, 7.4A, and 7.5).

When only the lower half-field was stimulated, this spatiotemporal image remained practically the same (despite amplitude changes), either on the longitudinal or on the transverse axis (Figure 7.3). However, it must be noted that on the lower field transverse maps for some individuals the lateral components were not as well differentiated from the midline components as in the full-field response, peaking a little earlier and closer to the midline (Figure 7.3).

In contrast, the space and time image of the upper field response (Figure 7.3) changes entirely on both axes, a classical finding about which all authors agree [9,11,16,40,41]. On the longitudinal part, one sees that P100 becomes much more posterior, often peaking lower than the inion; therefore, a large N100 replaces the midline P100 between the inion and the parietal region. This polarity change has been classically interpreted as a dipole sheet orientation effect. On the transverse montage, no such polarity change can be observed for the lateral components when changing from lower to upper field stimulation (Figure 7.3). This finding indicates that these lateral components take their origin in a cortical area different from the one where the midline positive component originates, which then reverses polarity when changing from lower to upper field stimulation.

The relative importance of these lateral components varies to a large extent from one normal subject to another (Figure 7.4A). In many cases, the midline and lateral components overlap and mingle together in such a way that for some subjects only the midline components manifest themselves, whereas for others only the lateral components are clearly seen [11]. But for over 50% of our population the posterior-midline components and the anterior-lateral components were clearly differentiated in both the full-field and the lower field response (Figures 7.2–7.5).

When the right or left hemifield of these subjects was stimulated, the response clearly showed that it was only the anterior-lateral components (LP120 and LN150) that became asymmetrical, peaking on the hemisphere contralateral to the stimulated field, whereas the midline posterior components P100

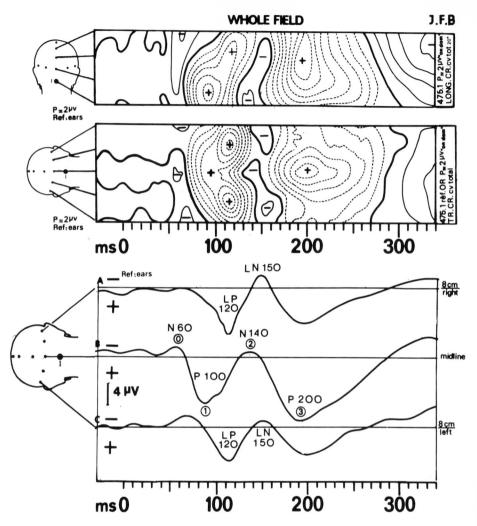

Figure 7.2. Typical average whole-field (20-degree checkerboard) pattern onset evoked response (central fixation), obtained from a normal subject, on the two branches of a cross-montage. Linked earlobes reference. On this map (and maps of following figures) the positive potentials are represented by broken lines, the negative ones by plain thin lines, zero potential being marked by a thick plain line. Each peak of potential is indicated at the exact place where it occurs by a plus or minus sign according to polarity. On this map, isopotential lines increase by steps of 2 µV. Derived from the above data, the amplitude versus time curves under the maps are obtained from three electrodes of the transverse branch placed 8 cm on the right, on the midline, 4 cm above the inion, and 8 cm on the left. Note the presence of symmetrical positive (LP120) and negative (LN150) waves peaking, 20 to 10 msec later than the midline-posterior components of same polarity, 4 cm away from the midline (transverse branch) and 8 cm above the inion (longitudinal branch). Reproduced by permission of the publisher from Lesèvre, Le Moyennage et son utilisation à l'étude des potentiels évoqués en clinique. Rev. EEG. Neurophysiol. 1976; 6 (2):155–167.

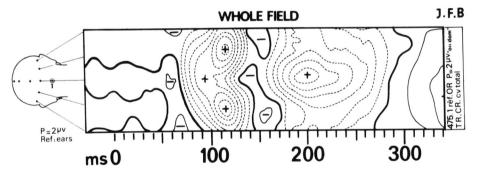

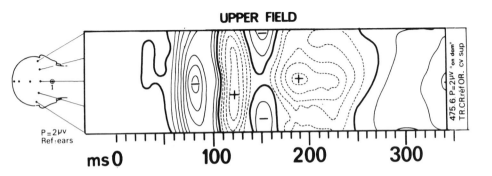

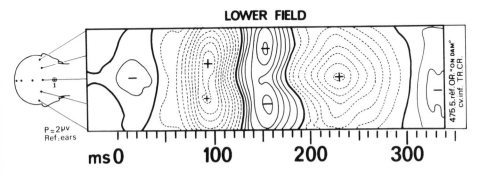

Figure 7.3. Average pattern onset evoked response obtained from whole-field (20-degree checkerboard), upper half-field, and lower half-field stimulation, on the transversal branch of a cross-montage (same subject as that of Figure 7.2). Linked earlobes reference. Isopotential lines increase in steps of 2 μV. Compared to the whole-field response, the upper field response shows a polarity reversal for the midline P100 but not for the lateral LP120. The lower field response is very similar to the whole-field response but its positive lateral waves are not as well differentiated.

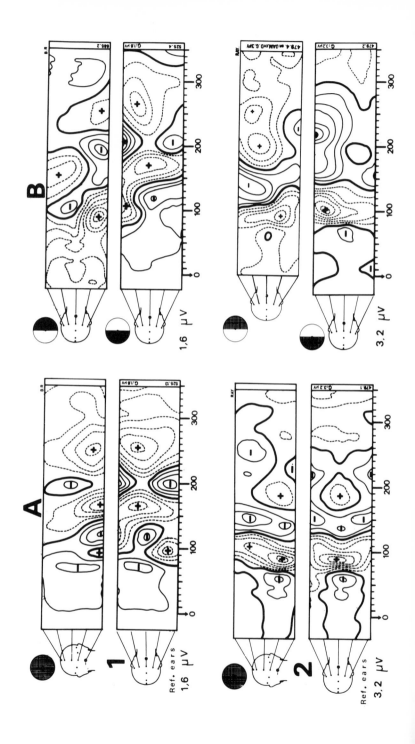

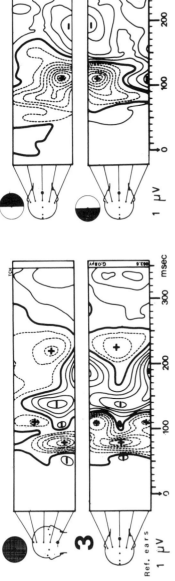

Figure 7.4. Whole-field (*A*) and right and left half-field (*B*) average pattern onset evoked responses obtained, on both branches of the cross-montage, from three normal subjects (different from those of Figures 7.2 and 7.3). Linked earlobe reference. Isopotential lines increase in steps of 1.6 μV for subject 1, 3.2 μV for subject 2, and 1 μV for subject 3. This figure illustrates: (1) The interindividual variability of the whole-field pattern onset response: the lateral positive components LP120 are more important (subject 1) or less important (subject 2) than the midline posterior P100. The lateral anterior components LP120 are as important as the midline posterior P100 (subject 3); (2) The controlateral topography of LP120 and LN150 when the right or left hemifield is stimulated. It must also be noted that when the controlateral LP120 is very important it pushes aside the midline N140 which appears as ipsilateral. Reproduced with the permission of the publisher from Lesèvre. Chronotopographical analysis of the human evoked potential in relation to the visual field. Ann. N.Y. Acad. Sc: 1982; 388:156–181.

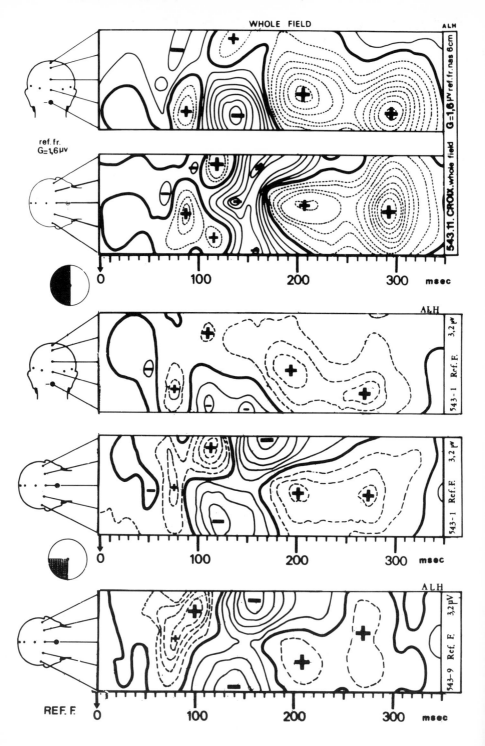

Figure 7.5. (*opposite page*) Average pattern onset evoked response obtained from a normal subject (different from those of other figures) to whole-field (*upper maps*), left half-field (*middle maps*), and left lower quadrant (*lower map*) stimulations. Frontal reference (Fz). Isopotential lines increase in steps of 1.6 µV on the two whole-field response maps and in steps of 3.2 µV on the three other maps. For this subject, it is clear that when the left half-field or left lower quadrant is stimulated, the posterior midline P100 remains on the midline whereas the anterior lateral LP120 becomes asymmetrical, peaking on the right hemisphere.

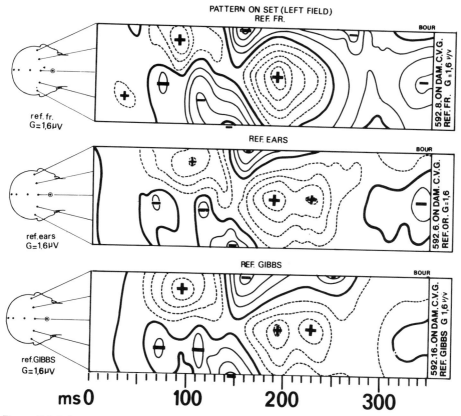

Figure 7.6. Influence of the reference electrode. Three maps of left half-field pattern onset average evoked response obtained, on the transversal branch of the cross-montage, from the same subject (different from those of other figures), with three different reference electrodes. *Upper map*: Frontal reference (Fz); *Middle map*: Linked earlobe reference; *Lower map*: Noncephalic sternovertebral reference. Isopotential lines increase in steps of 1.6 µV. On the three maps, whatever the reference electrode, the first positive component and LN150 peak on the controlateral (right) hemisphere whereas the late P200 wave remains on the midline. Similar ipsilateral negativities appear on the three maps. Reproduced by permission of the publisher from Lesèvre and Joseph, Modifications of the pattern-evoked potential in relation to the stimulated part of the visual field. Electroenceph. Clin. Neuropysiol. 1979; 47:183–203.

and N140 remained more or less on the midline (Figure 7.5). This result concerning the predominantly contralateral distribution of these positive and negative components of the pattern onset response is in agreement with the findings of several authors [20,42–44].

It must be emphasized that in contrast to its large intersubject variability the overall space and time organization of the pattern (evoked) response obtained in a given visual field condition is remarkably reproducible within one subject over months or even years, despite changes in amplitude, insofar as all experimental variables remain unchanged. Therefore, this space and time image constitutes an individual characteristic in much the same way as does a fingerprint [11,13].

Before considering the possible origin of the lateral components as compared to that of the midline components, we questioned the validity of such a description. In particular we systematically analyzed the influence of the reference electrode on such a spatiotemporal organization. In spite of changes in amplitude and latency, these lateral components were obtained with a similar topographic organization regardless of the reference electrode (ears, Fz, noncephalic sternovertebral; Figure 7.6). In particular, the same asymmetrical organization was found at approximately 120 msec, i.e., a positive peak on the hemisphere contralateral to the stimulated hemifield. This rules out for these peaks an artifactual origin caused by the choice of reference electrode. This contralateral predominance of both LP120 and LN150 was confirmed by maps of gradient corresponding to bipolar recordings, on which the phase reversal that indicates the maximum of potential was clearly situated on the hemisphere contralateral to the stimulated field [9,10,13], and also by maps of current density by calculating the second derivative of potential according to space.

Since it was noticed that for some subjects these lateral waves peaked in the lower field response a little earlier and closer to the midline than they did in the full-field response (Figure 7.3), it was suggested that the latency and topography characteristics of the full-field lateral components could be due to the presence of the negative upper field response N100. Whenever this upper field N100 was particularly important it would split the midline P100 of the lower field response into two and thus create artifactual peaks, 4 to 8 cm from the midline. But an artifactual origin in relation to the upper field component was ruled out after analyzing the maps obtained by systematic stimulation of the right or left lower quadrant. Indeed, for most subjects, these lateral-anterior-positive components, labeled LP120, still appeared as distinct components in these lower quadrant responses, still peaking on the contralateral hemisphere (Figure 7.5).

These various findings therefore support the existence of two positive components having different latencies, different reactivities according to half-field stimulations, and different scalp distributions, thus originating in different cortical areas and probably having different functional significance.

As to their functional significance, a comparison of the responses to pattern onset, to pattern reversal, and to blank-field onset for each subject (all other conditions remaining the same) demonstrated that, in contrast to the midline-posterior P100, these lateral positivities were mainly related to luminance changes and not to spatial contrast since they were not obtained in the pattern reversal response (Figure 7.7) and were increased in the pure luminance response [8,9,11]. This finding explains why we, in agreement with Shagass and co-workers [43], observed that the pattern reversal responses to right or left hemifield stimulation were much less lateralized than the pattern onset responses, suggesting that the underlying generators of pure spatial contrast responses are located nearer to the midline than those of luminance responses. However this does not explain why, in contradiction to the findings of Halliday and his group [45], we never observed, whatever the reference electrode, an ipsilateral predominance of the P100 pattern reversal component.

What do these findings suggest about the possible generators of these lateral-anterior components? In some of our previous work [11–13] and in agreement with Halliday and Michael [16,17], several arguments were given in favor of an area 18 origin for the midline-posterior P100, rather than the area 17 origin claimed by Jeffreys [46] and Jeffreys and Axford [19]. In contrast, the topography and latency characteristics of the lateral components labeled LP120 and LN150 (characterized by their peaking 10 msec later than the midline components of same polarity, in regions more laterally and more anteriorly situated) support a theory of their origin in area 19 rather than in area 18 as probably does midline P100. This theory is further supported by finding that, contrary to the midline posterior P100, they did not change polarity when changing from lower to upper field stimulation and became asymmetrical when the right or left half-field was selectively stimulated.

However, very little is known about retinotopic organization across the various regions of area 19 in humans; it is evident that such spatiotemporal mapping findings, obtained with a limited number of electrodes along two short spatial axes, do not permit much speculation about generator location.

IDENTIFICATION OF FUNCTIONAL LATE COMPONENTS RELATED TO INFORMATION PROCESSING

Since 1975, several experiments have been undertaken in our laboratory in order to study, through their electrophysiological correlates, the mechanisms underlying the various stages that take place between a relevant stimulus and a response, in situations implying choice or decision for the subject [22–27,47].

The brain response to a relevant stimulus which delivers information that the subject has to process in order to perform a task (in particular, a motor

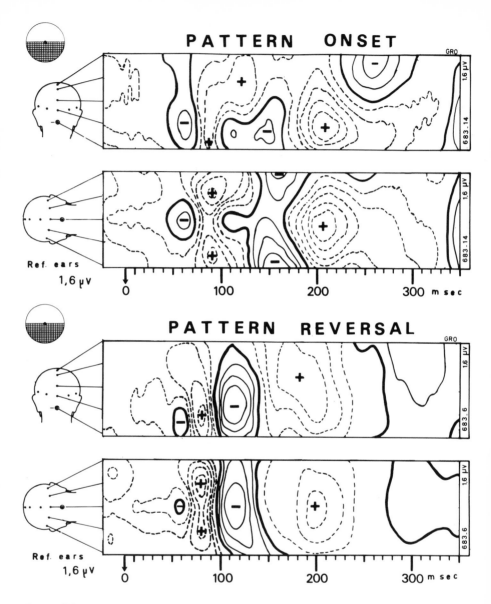

Figure 7.7. Average pattern onset (*upper maps*) and pattern reversal (*lower maps*) evoked responses to lower half-field stimulation, obtained on a cross-montage, from the same normal subject (different from those of other figures). Linked earlobe reference. Isopotential lines increase in steps of 1.6 μV. The anterior lateral LP120s seen on the pattern onset maps are not seen on the pattern reversal maps. For this subject, the P100 of both pattern onset and pattern reversal responses is made up of a posterior component on the longitudinal montage and of two symmetrical waves peaking away from the midline on the transversal montage.

task) is a complex response made up of a number of stimulus and motor-related components, followed or overlapped by slow components that are considered to be chiefly related to cognitive processes. These slow components include, in particular, the so-called P300 wave that is preceded by a negative component, N200. N200 is difficult to analyze since it occurs at the same time as the P200 stimulus-related component that usually has so large an amplitude and so wide a topographic distribution on the scalp that not only does it hide N200 but sometimes also mingles with P300.

For this reason, we have used the "missing stimulus" paradigm for such studies. This requires a motor (or a mental) response from the subject whenever the stimulus is omitted. This experimental situation is particularly suitable for studying the preparatory stage of perception and the role of memory templates; moreover, with such a paradigm the electrical correlates of the various task-related cognitive processes are not distorted by the stimulus-related potentials.

Several studies have established that the potentials associated with expected but missing stimuli are also made up of at least two components, a negative one followed by a positive one apparently assimilated to P300 since it has the same parietal topography and varies in amplitude according to the probability of the missing stimulus [22,48–53]. It has also been demonstrated that the topography of the negative component varies according to the sensory modality of the expected stimulus, whereas the topography of the positive component does not [22–25,50,52]. In fact, as has been demonstrated by spatiotemporal mapping displays, the actual process description is still more complex; in response to an unpredictable task-relevant omitted stimulus, two different types of positive and negative components have been distinguished according to topographic criteria and related to different psychophysiological processes [22,23,50].

To study this missing stimulus response we first utilized the following GO/NO-GO paradigm: during three runs of 450 visual stimuli on each subject (pattern onset of 20 msec duration delivered at fixed intervals), 10% of the stimuli were randomly omitted. Subjects were asked: (1) to respond as quickly as possible to the missing stimulus with a finger displacement, (2) to withhold their response to the missing stimulus and respond to pattern onset, and (3) to count mentally the missing stimuli [22].

The moment the stimulus should have occurred but did not served as the time trigger to obtain the average omission response (Figure 7.8). On the corresponding maps the first negative component peaked in the parietal region and was followed by two positive components, the first one peaking near the vertex, the second one, a little later, peaking on the parietal region. On these average maps no negative vertex component was clearly seen.

In order to overcome the latency variability in single trials that characterizes this sort of response (due to the absence of a precisely timed external stimulus), these omission responses were topographically analyzed trial by trial,

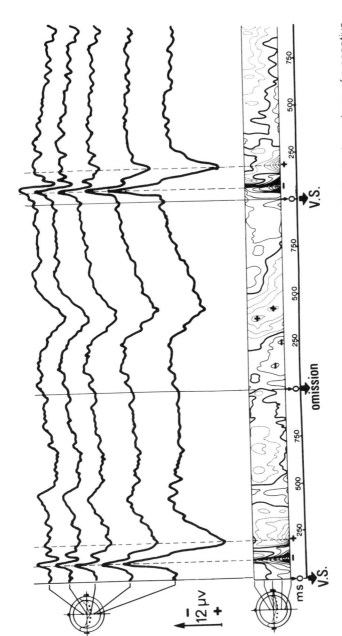

Figure 7.8. Average emitted response obtained from a normal subject, with five midline electrodes going from 4 cm above to 12 cm below the vertex, to 45 missing visual stimuli. The subject was asked to count mentally the missing stimuli. On the time scale, 0 indicates either the occurrence of the visual stimulus (*V.S.*) or its omission. Linked earlobe reference. From one isopotential line to the next, potentials increase in 2 μV steps. The re-sponse to the omitted stimulus is made up of a negative component peaking in the posterior region followed by a positive wave peaking first near the vertex, later in the preoccipital region (see text, experiment 1). Reproduced by permission of the publisher from Renault and Le-sèvre, in A. Otto, ed., Multidisciplinary Perspectives in Event-Related Brain Potential Research, Washington, D.C.: U.S. Government Printing Office, 1978.

using the spatiotemporal mapping method to help visualize components. It must be pointed out that this type of trial-by-trial study is particularly time-consuming. For this study, approximately 250 maps corresponding to 2.5 seconds of nonaveraged EEG preceding and following an omission were analyzed for each experimental condition. For each subject, the averaged responses time-locked to the omission were used as templates for visual identification of each component. This visual identification was performed independently by two scorers. Only those identifications for which both scorers agreed were accepted for further analysis. Approximately 190 single-trial maps were thus taken into account for this study, since approximately 25% of these maps were rejected because of a poor signal-to-noise ratio.

By this method we were able to differentiate three types of omission responses (Figure 7.9): (1) the "vertex type," composed of two successive waves of short duration, first negative, second positive, both peaking in the vertex region; (2) the "parietal type," made up of a long duration negative wave in the parietal region followed by a long duration positive wave in the same region; (3) a "mixed type," representing 65% of all trials, which consisted of one negative wave beginning in the parietooccipital region and a later, overlapping negative wave in the central region, followed by two positive components, the first one peaking at Cz, the second one at Pz (Figures 7.9 and 7.10).

Latencies, topographies, and amplitudes of these different types supported the hypothesis that the "mixed type" resulted from the addition of the vertex and parietal types of emitted responses. The vertex type appeared more frequently during the GO/NO-GO tasks than during the counting, whereas in the GO condition, both the number of parietal types and the ratio between the parietal and the vertex positive waves amplitude increased with the mean value of the reaction time. These results demonstrated the existence of different kinds of emitted potentials. Moreover, they suggested that a shift in brain activity from the central to the parietal region was linked to the motor (GO/NO-GO) or sensory (mental counting) task and, in a motor task, to the level of performance [24]. On the other hand, it appeared that the negative components always occurred before the motor response, whereas the positive components began either a little before or a little after the motor response was achieved, their latency showing a lower correlation with the reaction time than did the negative components.

A second experiment was then designed in order to better understand the time relationships between these various components of the missing stimulus response, the reaction time (RT), and the subject's time estimation of the moment that the omitted stimulus should have occurred [23,26]. Indeed, it was hypothesized that this "estimated time" could be the internal event upon which depended both the reaction time and the latency of the negative components. For this experiment subjects were asked to tap the rhythm at the same frequency as that of the visual stimuli, and whenever a stimulus did not occur, to give an additional motor response as quickly as possible. Each tap in the rhythm was considered an index of when the subject expected the stimulus to occur, with the additional motor response being a measure of reaction time [23,26].

The grand mean across subjects of the averaged omission-triggered response, either on the moment of the omission, or on the tap of the rhythm, which represented the subjects' estimated time of this moment, once again showed clearly two foci of activity, one parietal, the other toward the vertex, for both negative and positive components [23,27].

A trial-by-trial analysis was once more performed and confirmed that the response associated with missing visual stimuli is made up of four distinct components, two of long duration (negative-positive) peaking near the parietal region, and two of shorter duration (negative-positive) peaking near the vertex (Figure 7.10). Furthermore, these single-trial studies showed that this kind of "mixed response" is observed quite frequently, even for subjects who had an average response (triggered by the moment of the omission) with only one focus of negative-positive activity; indeed the trial-by-trial examination of the omission responses of these subjects showed that the two foci of same polarity seen on the averaged maps of the other subjects were, in their case, so closely located in space and time that they mingled in the averaged data and thus appeared as one focus.

The timing of these different components and their relationship with the estimated time of the stimulus and with the motor response provided some clues regarding their functional significance. Across subjects, all single-trial reaction times were divided into quartiles as a function of their duration, and the corresponding single-trial omission responses were then averaged together as a function of the RT quartiles (Figure 7.11). A significant relation was then found between the duration of RTs and the duration of the negative parietal component: the longer the RT, the longer this parietal component lasted, whereas the duration of the vertex negative component did not vary according to RT (Figure 7.11).

These results suggest that the negative parietal component of the visual omission response, which is also a "modality-specific" component, reflects,

Figure 7.9. (*opposite page*) Grand means (across subjects and situations of experiment 1) of the various types of visual omission responses obtained after trial by trial detection and triggered on the peak latency of the first positive component. Linked earlobes reference. From one isopotential line to the next, amplitude increases in steps of 2 μV. Components of both polarities peak at the vertex (*upper map*; vertex type) or on the posterior region (*middle map*; parietal type). The mixed type (*lower map*) shows two positive components, the first one on the vertex, the second parietal. On this average single-trial map, the second negative component that usually follows the parietal negativity and peaks on the vertex does not show up. Reproduced with the permission of the publisher from Renault, The visual emitted potentials: Clues for information processing, in A.W.K. Gaillard and W. Ritter, eds., Tutorials in Event-related Potential Research: Endogenous Components. Amsterdam: Elsevier, 1983.

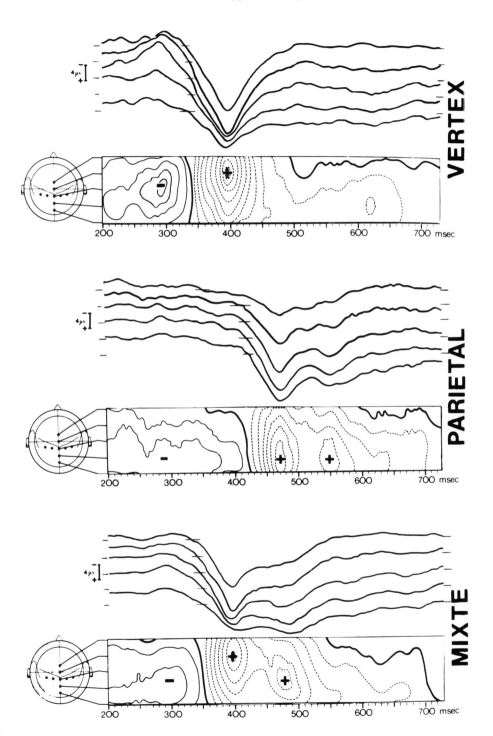

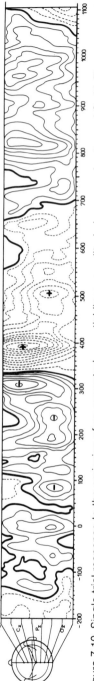

Figure 7.10. Single-trial response to the omission of an expected visual stimulus, obtained from one subject, with a midline longitudinal montage going from Fz to a little lower than Oz (experiment 2). Linked earlobe reference. On the time scale, 0 indicates the moment of the omission. Between two successive isopotential lines, amplitude increases in steps of 2 µV. The response is made up of two distinct negative components peaking successively at Oz and on the vertex, followed by two positive waves, one peaking at the vertex, the second at Pz.

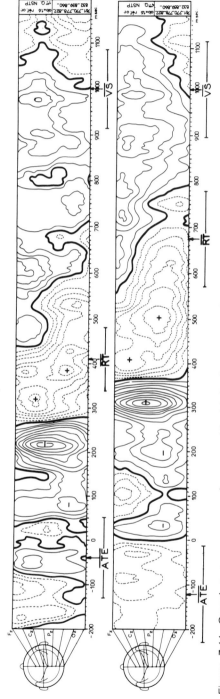

Figure 7.11. Grand mean responses (across subjects) to the omission of an expected visual stimulus grouped according to reaction times (experiment 2,: see text). The responses are triggered by the negative vertex peak for the first RT quartile (responses corresponding to quick RTs, *upper map*) and for the 4th RT quartile (responses corresponding to slow RTs, *lower map*). Linked earlobe reference. Reproduced with the permission of the publisher from Renault and Lesèvre, A trial by trial study of the visual omission response in reaction time situations. In D. Lehmann and E. Callaway, eds., Evoked potentials. New York: Plenum Publishing Corp., 1979.

on-line, certain aspects of perceptual processes. In contrast, the short duration negative component, peaking at the vertex, is probably related to orientation reactions rather than to proper sensory information processing. However, after calculation of the product moment correlations between the onset and offset of each component, the finding that the onset of the vertex negative wave depended upon the ending of the parietal negative wave supports a cognitive interpretation of the orienting reaction, as if orienting could only take place when the stimulus evaluation stage is over [26,27].

The existence of these various foci of activity, whatever their underlying generators, seems to be an important issue in the field of ERP potentials related to cognitive processes. The study of their time relations to behavioral responses might indeed shed some light in the domain of mental chronometry and thus help in the formulation of psychological models of human information processing.

It seems that different topographic approaches and brain mapping displays should be chosen according to the type of problem under study. As for the problem of the location of ERP generators, the spatiotemporal mapping display evidently has the disadvantage of presenting space in only one dimension, although, as we have seen, the use of two or more lines of electrodes related to one another by a common electrode, as on our "cross montage," might help to reconstruct the spatiotemporal organization of the potential field on a given limited region of the scalp, and therefore give clues regarding the most probable underlying sources.

However, whole-brain maps derived from a two-dimensional array of electrodes covering the scalp evidently permit a better representation of potential distribution on the scalp and are thus theoretically better suited for the study of ERP generators. In any case, this problem can only be faced by the use of various approaches providing complementary information, including comparisons of deep and surface recordings in primates, studies of lesion effects on surface ERP components, and topographic analyses of human magnetic evoked fields.

On the other hand, spatiotemporal maps have a distinct advantage over instantaneous whole-brain maps in that they represent amplitude, topography, and time variables on the same chart, making it possible to study these three variables in relation to one another. For this reason spatiotemporal maps are particularly well suited for the study of mental chronometry and information processing stages.

Finally we would like to raise a crucial question concerning analysis of ERP spatiotemporal maps. Indeed, such maps are simply intended to show the EEG data in the best possible way (and to sometimes discover some otherwise hidden aspect of the data), but by themselves they do not perform any proper analysis of the data. What are the useful measures to be taken on such maps? What are the relevant parameters to be picked up among these complex images? Peaks (interpolated or not), averaged "plateaux," onsets and offsets of waveforms (related to which baseline?), slopes, waveform surfaces, or volumes? How can two (or several) maps be statistically compared without reducing these images to a few of their time and space points, as is usually done? It seems that no fully satisfactory answers to such crucial questions have yet been given. But these questions open another chapter of another story.

ACKNOWLEDGMENTS

The authors wish to thank the researchers, engineers, and technicians of the LENA Group, who all have largely contributed to these topographic studies. The authors are, in particular, grateful to Bernard Renault, Ph.D., who has worked on the missing stimulus response and mental chronometry illustrated in the second part of this chapter.

REFERENCES

1. Rémond, A. Orientations et tendances des méthodes topographiques dans l'étude de l'activité électrique du cerveau. Rev. Neurol. 1955; 93:399–432.
2. Rémond, A. An integrating topograph. Electroenceph. Clin. Neurophysiol. 1956; 8:719–720.
3. Rémond, A. Integrated and topographical analysis of the EEG. Electroenceph. Clin. Neurophysiol. 1961; suppl. 20:64–67.
4. Rémond, A. Level of organization of evoked responses in man. Ann. N.Y. Acad. Sci. 1964; 112:143–159.
5. Rémond, A. The importance of topographic data in EEG phenomena and an electric model to reproduce them. Electroenceph. Clin. Neurophysiol. 1968; suppl. 27:29–49.
6. Lesèvre, N. et Rémond, A. Etude du champ visuel par les potentiels évoqués moyens. Rev. Neurol. 1968; 118(6):419–430.
7. Rémond, A., and Lesèvre, N. Etude de la fonction du regard par l'analyse des potentiels évoqués visuels. In A. Dubois-Poulsen, G.C. Lairy, and A. Rémond, eds. La fonction du regard. Paris: INSERM, 1971; 127–175.
8. Lesèvre, N., and Rémond, A. Potentiels évoqués par l'apparition de patterns : effets de la dimension du pattern et de la densité des contrastes. Electroenceph. Clin. Neurophysiol. 1972; 32:593–607.
9. Lesèvre, N. Potentiels évoqués par des patterns chez l'homme: Influence de variables caractérisant le stimulus et sa position dans le champ visuel. In G. Lelord, ed. Activites évoqués et leur conditionnement chez l'homme normal et en pathologie mentale. Paris: INSERM, 1973; 1–22.
10. Lesèvre, N. Topographical Analysis of the pattern evoked response (PER): Its application to the study of macular and peripheral vision in normal people and in some pathological cases. In R. Alfieri and P. Solé, eds., Documenta Ophthalmologica Proceeding Series, The Hague: W. Junk, 1976; 10:87–102.
11. Lesèvre, N., and Joseph, J.P. Modifications of the pattern evoked potential related

to the part of the visual field stimulated (clues for the most probable origin of its various components recorded on the scalp). Electroenceph. Clin. Neurophysiol. 1979; 47:183–203.

12. Lesèvre, N., and Joseph, J.P. Hypothesis concerning the most probable sites of origin of the various components of the pattern evoked potential. In C. Barber, ed., Evoked Potentials. Lancaster, England: MTP Press Limited, 1980; 159–166.

13. Lesèvre, N. Chronotopographical analysis of the visual evoked potential in relation to the visual field (data from normal and pathological cases). Ann. N.Y. Acad. Sci. 1982; 388:156–183.

14. Donchin, E. Use of scalp distribution as a dependant variable in event-related potential studies. In D.A. Otto, ed., Multidisciplinary Perspectives in Event Related Brain Potential Research. Washington D.C.: U. S. Government Printing Office, 1978; 526–532.

15. Vaughan, H.G. The relationship of brain activity to scalp recordings of event related potentials. In E. Donchin and D.B. Lindsley, eds., Averaged Evoked Potentials: Methods, Results, Evaluations. Washington: NASA, 1969; SP 191:45–94.

16. Halliday, A.M., and Michael, W.F. Changes in pattern evoked responses in man associated with the vertical and horizontal meridians of the visual field. J. Physiol. (Lond.) 1970; 208:499–513.

17. Michael, W.F., and Halliday, A.M. Differences between the occipital distribution of upper and lower field pattern-evoked responses. Brain Res. 1971; 32:311–324.

18. Ristanovic, D. The human visual cortex as a system of four generators. Acta Med. Jug. 1971; 2:379–395.

19. Jeffreys, D.A., and Axford J.C. Source location of pattern-specific components of human visual evoked potentials, I, II. Exp. Brain Res. 1972; 16:1–40.

20. Biersdorf, A. Cortical evoked responses from stimulation of various regions of the visual field. Doc. Ophthalmol. (Den Haag) 1974; 4:249–259.

21. Donchin, E., Ritter, W., and McCallum, C. Cognitive psychophysiology: The endogenous components of the ERP. In E. Callaway, P. Tueting, and S.H. Koslow, eds., Event-Related Brain Potentials in Man. New York: Academic Press, 1978; 349–509.

22. Renault, B., and Lesèvre, N. Topographical study of the emitted potential obtained after the omission of an expected visual stimulus. In D.A. Otto, ed., Multidisciplinary Perspectives in Event-Related Potential Research. Washington, D.C.: U.S. Government Printing Office, 1978; 202–209.

23. Renault, B., and Lesèvre, N. A trial by trial study of the visual omission response in reaction time situations. In E. Callaway and D. Lehmann, eds., Event-Related Potential in Man: Application and Problems. NATO Conferences Series III. Human Factors vol. 9. New York: Plenum Press, 1979; 317–329.

24. Renault, B. Ragot, R., and Lesèvre, N. Etude des relation entre le potentiel émis et les mécanismes de préparation perceptivo-motrice. In J. Requin, ed. Anticipation et comportement. Paris: Editions du CNRS, 1980; 167–182.

25. Renault, B. Ragot, R. and Lesèvre, N. Correct and incorrect responses in a choice reaction time task and the endogenous components of the evoked potential. Prog. Brain Res. 1980; 54:647–654.

26. Renault, B., Ragot, R., Lesèvre, N., and Rémond, A. Brain events: their onset and offset as indices of mental chronometry. Science 1982; 216:1413–1415.

27. Renault, B. The visual emitted potentials: Clues for information processing. In

A.W.K. Gaillard and W. Ritter, eds., Tutorials in Event Related Potential research: Endogenous components. Amsterdam: North Holland, 1983; 159–175.

28. Brazier, M.A.B. The electrical fields at the surface of the head during sleep. Electroenceph. Clin. Neurophysiol. 1949; 1:195–204.

29. Brazier, M.A.B. The electrical fields at the surface of the head. Electroenceph. Clin. Neurophysiol. 1951; suppl. 2:38–52.

30. Lilly, J.C. Forms and figures in the electrical activity seen in the surface of the cerebral cortex. The Biology of Mental Health and Disease. New York: Harper, 1952; 206–219.

31. Lehmann, D. Multichannel topography of human alpha EEG fields. Electroenceph. Clin. Neuropysiol. 1971; 31:439–449.

32. Lehmann, D., Kavanagh R.N., and Fender, D.H. Field studies of averaged visually evoked potentials in a patient with a split chiasm. Electroenceph. Clin. Neurophysiol. 1969; 26:193–199.

33. Petsche, H., and Marko, A. Toposkopische Untersuchungen zur Ausbreitung des Alpharhythmus. Wien Z. Nervenheilk. 1955; 12:87–100.

34. Petsche, H., and Stumpf, C.H. Topographic and toposcopic study of origin and spread of the regular synchronized arousal pattern in the rabbit. Electroenceph. Clin. Neurophysiol. 1960; 12:589–600.

35. Petsche, H., Rappelsberger, P., and Trappl, R. Properties of cortical seizure potentials fields. Electroenceph. Clin. Neurophysiol. 1970; 29:567–578.

36. Shaw, J.C., and Roth, M. Potential distribution analysis. II. A theoretical consideration of its significance in terms of electrical field theory. Electroenceph. Clin. Neurophysiol. 1955; 7:285–292.

37. Rémond, A., Ragot, R., and Cecchini, A. Possibilités de la saisie topographique des signaux EEG. Rev. EEG. Neurophysiol. 1976; 6(2):178–184.

38. Ragot, R., and Rémond, A. EEG field mapping. Electroenceph. Clin. Neurophysiol. 1978; 45:417–421.

39. Duffy, F.H. Topographic Display of Evoked Potentials: Clinical applications of brain electrical activity mapping (BEAM). Ann. N.Y. Acad. Sci. 1982; 388: 183–196.

40. Jeffreys, D.A., and Smith, A.T. The polarity inversion of scalp potentials evoked by upper and lower half-field stimulus patterns: Latency or surface distribution differences. Electroenceph. Clin. Neurophysiol. 1979; 46:409–416.

41. Lehmann, D.D., and Skrandies, W. Multichannel evoked potential fields show different properties of human upper and lower hemiretina systems. Exp. Brain Res. 1979; 35:151–159.

42. Cobb, W.A., and Morton, H. Evoked potentials from the human scalp to visual half-field stimulations. J. Physiol. 1970; 208:39–40.

43. Shagass, C., Amadeo, M., and Roemer, A. Spatial distribution of potentials evoked by half-field pattern onset stimuli. Electroenceph. Clin. Neurophysiol. 1976; 41:609–622.

44. Harding, G.F., Smith, A.G.F., and Smith, P.A. The effect of various stimulus parameters on the lateralization of the VEP. In C. Barber ed., Evoked Potentials. Lancaster: MTP Press, 1980; 213–218.

45. Blumhardt, L.D., Barret, G., and Halliday, A.M. The asymmetrical visual evoked potential to pattern reversal in one half-field and its significance for the analysis of visual field defects. Br. J. Ophthalmol. 1977; 61:454–461.

46. Jeffreys, D.A. Cortical source-locations of pattern-related VEPs (visual evoked potentials) recorded from the human scalp. J. Physiol. (Lond.). 1971; 229:502–504.

47. Renault, B., and Lesèvre, N. Variations des PE par des patterns chez l'homme dans une situation de temps de réaction : influence de la vigilance et de la motricité. Rev. EEG Neurophysiol. 1975; 5(4):360–366.

48. Klinke, R., Fruhstorfer, H., and Finkenzeller, P. Evoked responses as a function of external and stored information. Electroenceph. Clin. Neurophysiol. 1968; 25:119–122.

49. Picton, T.W., Hillyard, S.A., and Galambos, R. Evoked responses to omitted stimuli. In M.N. Livanov, ed., Major Problems in Brain Electrophysiology. Acad. Sci. USSR 1974; 302–311.

50. Simson, R., Vaughan, H.G., and Ritter, W. The scalp topography of potentials associated with missing visual or auditory stimuli. Electroenceph. Clin. Neurophysiol. 1976; 40:33–42.

51. McCallum, W.C. Brain slow potential changes elicited by missing stimulus and by externally paced voluntary responses. Biol. Psychol. 1980; 11:7–20.

52. Simson, R., Vaughan, H.G., and Ritter, W. The scalp topography of potentials in auditory and visual discrimination tasks. Electroenceph. Clin. Neurophysiol. 1977; 42:528–535.

53. Ruchkin, D.S., Sutton, S., Munson, R., Silver, K., and Macar, F. P300 and feed back provided by absence of the stimulus. Psychophysiology 1981; 18:271–282.

8

EEG Modifications during Visual and Motor Reactions Observed by Beta, Alpha, and Theta Quantification and Topographic Mapping

D. Samson-Dollfus, Z. Tsouria, I. Bertoldi, E. Dreano, and J. Y. Doris

It is well known both that the alpha rhythm disappears when the subject opens his eyes and that a comparable reactivity to motor function exists in the sensory area. Although it has been reported that the alpha rhythm reacts to eyes open, almost no studies have been done on beta and theta visual reactivity.

During motor reactivity, spectral electroencephalograph (EEG) differences have been observed in the alpha and beta rhythm on the scalp region corresponding to the motor area. In his research, Giannitrapani [1] located electrodes strictly over this motor area. Pfurtscheller [2] and Pfurtscheller and Aranibar [3,4] recorded the central and occipital regions of the scalp; they reported that beta activities decreased and that the alpha band was also modified by movement.

The purpose of the research reported here was to examine whether visual and motor reactivities could be represented by topographic mapping. However, our results had to first be statistically validated in the manner recommended by Etevenon [5].

MATERIAL AND METHODS

The EEGs of 20 right-handed normal subjects (20–40 years old) were recorded on paper and magnetic tape for subsequent data analysis. Twelve electrodes were applied on the scalp, according to a slightly modified 10–20 system (F2, C4, P2, O2, T2, T4, F1, C3, P1, O1, T1, T3). The common reference was linked ears.

The EEG was filtered above 30 Hz to eliminate the aliasing effect of muscle activity. The sampling rate was 100 Hz. Spectral analysis of the 12 data channels was performed off-line, on artifact-free portions of the EEG, and carefully screened by visual analysis. Drowsy periods were excluded from analysis.

Four different behavioral states were recorded: eyes closed, resting (ECL); eyes open, resting (EOP); right-hand voluntary movement (RVM); and left-hand voluntary movement (LVM). Each state was recorded for a 3-minute period, but only 10 spectra of 512 msec were computed and averaged for each condition. In order to verify the repeatability of our measures, the ECL condition was recorded twice, at the beginning and at the end of the session. The five spectral bands computed were delta (1–3.8 Hz), theta (4–7.8), alpha (8–12.8), beta-1 (13–18), and beta-2 (18.2–25). We studied only the theta, alpha, and beta-1 bands, and for each of these bands, an index of reactivity was computed as follows: (EOP-ECL)/ECL or (VM-ECL)/ECL.

Topographic displays of the absolute value of the theta, alpha, and beta power spectra, and of the indexes of reactivity were performed on a machine devised by Sebban and Debouzy [6]. This EEG mapping was not as sophisticated as the topographic analysis given by the methodology described by Duffy et al. [7] but has provided informative pictures.

The absolute values of the activating conditions (EOP, RVM, and LVM) were compared to ECL. Moreover, the first ECL (ECL1) was compared to the second ECL (ECL2). The different indexes (EOP-ECL1)/ECL1 and (VM-ECL1)/ECL1 were compared to (ECL2-ECL1)/ECL1 to differentiate the normal intraindividual fluctuations of the brain electrical activity differences associated with different tasks. We used the nonparametric paired Wilcoxon test with a threshold of 0.05 to test the significance of the differences between results. We also looked at individual data and counted the subjects who were reacting for each different condition.

RESULTS

In the ECL conditions no statistical differences appeared between right and left hemispheres for beta-1, alpha, and theta power spectra.

Visual Reaction

Alpha decreased significantly ($p \leq 0.01$) on all 12 leads upon the subjects' opening their eyes (Figure 8.1B). Beta-1 also decreased significantly ($p \leq 0.01$) in the centro-parieto-occipital area (Figure 8.1A) but exhibited no change in the fronto-temporal regions. Indexes of reactivity were higher for alpha and beta rhythm on the occipital regions and reached the threshold of 0.01 on all the scalp. All subjects demonstrated this large reactivity to opening the eyes.

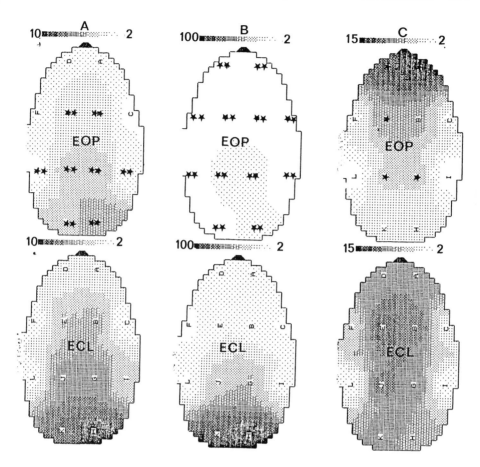

Figure 8.1. *A*. Beta-1 ; *B*. Alpha. *C*. Theta. The differences between ECL and EOP are much more evident for alpha and beta than for the theta bands. $*p \leq 0.05$; $**p \leq 0.01$. Asterisks in figures represent areas of significant differences, where figures depict scalp from above, nose at top, left ear to left.

Theta decreased on the left fronto-centro-parieto-occipital lead, and the right parietal lead ($p \leq 0.05$), but increased significantly ($p \leq 0.05$) on the right frontal lead (Figure 8.1*C*).

Motor Reaction

In this sample of normal subjects, the theta, alpha, and beta-1 bands decreased at each electrode and in each subject for the RVM and LVM, but the significant threshold of $p \leq 0.05$ was not reached for all situations; the differences were significant for the theta band on the left central lead for the right-hand movements and on both central ($p \leq 0.01$) and parietal ($p \leq 0.05$) leads for the left-hand movement (Figure 8.2*A*). For the beta-1 power spectrum, the index of reactivity was significantly higher ($p \leq 0.05$) on the parieto-controlateral leads, but the absolute values of the beta power spectra did not reach the threshold of 0.05 (Figure 8.2*B*).

In spite of the tendency of alpha to decrease during RVM and LVM, no significant difference was observed for the alpha band in our sample of normal subjects, except on T1 for RVM. Surprisingly, the alpha power spectrum increased ($p \leq 0.05$) on T4 and 02 for RVM.

DISCUSSION

Results concerning the resting eyes closed condition did not show a significant difference in the alpha power spectra between right and left occipital regions [8]. It is possible that the condition in which we recorded our subjects (quiet room) was one of the reasons for this result.

The topographic displays have shown that the visual reaction is diffuse for alpha and beta-1 but predominates in the posterior region, an observation well known for the alpha rhythm, but not commonly accepted for beta. It is possible that these beta rhythms were different from the anterior beta rhythms related to the activation of the brain. The visual reaction was not so important for theta, and curiously, theta increased on the right frontal region when the eyes were opened. This did not appear related to eye movements, because we chose artifact-free portions of EEG for subsequent spectral analysis.

Regarding motor reactivity, our results on beta-1 are consistent with those of Giannitrapani [1] and Pfurtscheller [2], who mentioned a bilateral beta reactivity, which we also observed. But the significance threshold was reached only for a limited region of the brain in our sample of normal subjects.

We failed to observe a significant motor reaction on the alpha power spectrum. Ackerman et al. [9] reported that only four of their 11 subjects showed significant changes in the alpha band. R. Harner (personal communication, 1984) thought that alpha rhythm reacted quite well to the motor tasks when bipolar transversal montages were used. Pfurtscheller [2] also used transversal short distance montages. Since we used referential montages, this may explain the differences between their data and ours. Another possible explanation is in the fluctuation of the samples. Pfurtscheller had restricted his study to samples of 2 seconds of RVM and LVM. In our protocol, the tests may have lasted too long. This may allow time for a local reactivity to spread to both hemispheres. Studies on this point are in progress in our laboratory. We still have some methodological problems to solve, especially concerning the best recording time protocols but we wish to emphasize that topographic mapping, even in black and white, will prove to be a valuable method of demonstrating

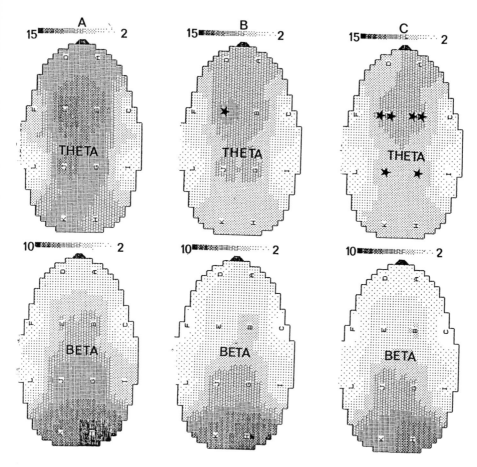

Figure 8.2. Motor reaction. *A*. Rest eyes closed. *B*. Right hand voluntary movement. *C*. Left-hand voluntary movement. Theta: Some significant differences were observed. Beta: In spite of a trend to decrease, no significant threshold was observed on the absolute spectral values of the beta-1 band.

the results of EEG quantification, when statistical studies have shown their validity on pretreated data relative to normal subjects.

REFERENCES

1. Giannitrapani, D. Spectral analysis of the EEG. In G. Dolce and H. Künkel, eds. Computerized EEG Analysis. Stuttgart: Gustav Fischer Verlag, 1975; 384–402.
2. Pfurtscheller, G. Central beta rhythm during sensori-motor activities in man. Electroenceph. Clin. Neurophysiol. 1981; 51:253–264.
3. Pfurtscheller, G., and Aranibar, A. Occipital rhythmic activity within the alpha

band during conditioned externally paced movement. Electroenceph. Clin. Neurophysiol. 1978; 45:226–235.

4. Pfurtscheller, G., and Aranibar, A. Evaluation of event-related desynchronization (ERD) preceding and following voluntary self-paced movement. Electroenceph. Clin. Neurophysiol. 1979; 46:138–146.

5. Etevenon, P., Trotrat, T., Guillou, F., Benkelfat, C. EEG cartography by means of statistical group studies, activation by visual attention. Neuropsychology 1985; in press.

6. Sebban, C., Debouzy, C., and Berthaux, P. EEG quantifié et cartographie numérisée. In N.A. Lassen, and J. Cahn, eds., Drugs and Diseases. Paris: John Libbey, 1984; 176–181.

7. Duffy, F.H., Burchfiel, F.L., and Lombroso, C.T. Brain electrical activity mapping (BEAM): A method for extending the clinical utility of EEG and evoked potential data. Ann. Neurol. 1979; 5:309–321.

8. Butler, S.R., and Glass, A. Asymmetries in the electroencephalogram associated with cerebral dominance. Electroenceph. Clin. Neurophysiol. 1974; 36:481–491.

9. Ackerman, R.H., Baron, J.C., Correia, J.A., Chiappa, K.H., Wolpow, E.R., Nelson, C., Young, R.R., Taveras, J.M. Comparison of two methods for monitoring cerebral activity: 133 xenon inhalation blood flow studies and compressed spectral analysis of EEG. In J.S. Meyer and H. Lechner, eds., Cerebrovascular Diseases 1979. Amsterdam: Excerpta Medica, 1979; 1:11–12.

9

Physical Aspects of EEG Data as a Basis for Topographic Mapping

Bo Hjorth

Pictures showing anatomical structures have obvious diagnostic value, whether produced as geometrical projections or as the result of more sophisticated processing. The classical x-ray image displays a pattern based on selective absorption, i.e., on a passive property of the investigated structure, whereas an electroencephalograph (EEG) topogram depicting EEG background activity displays a pattern formed by active neuroelectrical events generated within the structure. However, no clear distinction can be made between active and passive features from a physical point of view. Recorded EEG data may be regarded as being determined by both active events and features of passive systems that propagate these events. In this chapter, EEG measures that relate to this hypothetical model are described and topographically mapped.

The EEG represents variations in an electrical potential that, as a physical quantity, is governed by certain basic laws of physical systems. Although the actual systems may be complex, some of their properties can be expected to characterize or limit the dynamics of the observed EEG potentials. The occurrence of an event in a physical system means that an amount of energy is suddenly made available to, or released in, the system. The energy is then dissipated by the system in a process that is defined by the type of system and its determinative constants. This process, that is, the system response to an event, is available for observation through the related physical response manifestations. Thus, analysis of the dynamic features of EEG tracings should make it possible to detect changes in the basic states of underlying neural systems.

CHOICE OF COMPUTED VARIABLES

EEG background activity appears to be a mixture of more or less rhythmic components that may represent sequential organizations of events. Therefore,

175

quantitative measures intended for identification of dynamic system features should possess minimum sensitivity to sequential order and maximum sensitivity to dynamic features of the measured quantity. This can be achieved by computing the variances of derivatives during the EEG epoch. Variances accumulate during the epoch regardless of sequential order in the derived values, whereas the ratios between variances relating to different order derivatives reflect dynamic properties of the observed quantity. When the variances are computed from sampled data, each derivative can be represented by the difference of corresponding order. The variance of amplitude, formerly equal to the derivative of order zero, is required for completeness. The derivatives of orders zero, one, and two consistently convey basic information on fundamental physical systems. Their variances, denoted $s_0{}^2$, $s_1{}^2$ and $s_2{}^2$, can be computed on-line from the consecutive samples a_v. The consecutive differences $a_v - a_v - 1$ are denoted d_v.

$$s_0{}^2 = (a_1{}^2 + a_2{}^2 + \ldots + a_n{}^2)/n$$
$$s_1{}^2 = (d_1{}^2 + d_2{}^2 + \ldots + d_n{}^2)/n$$
$$s_2{}^2 = ((d_1 - d_0)^2 + (d_2 - d_1)^2 + \ldots + (d_n - d_{n-1})^2)/n.$$

With a view to the dynamic properties of physical systems, the variances should be rearranged into three new variables, activity (*a*), mobility (*m*), and complexity (*c*):

$$a = sqrt(s_0{}^2)$$
$$m = sqrt(s_1{}^2/s_0{}^2)$$
$$c = sqrt(s_2{}^2/s_1{}^2 - s_1{}^2/s_0{}^2).$$

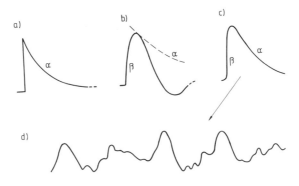

Figure 9.1. *a*. A first-order physical system response. *b*. A second-order physical system response. *c*. A fourth-order bioelectrical system response. *d*. A random superposition of 2000 bioelectrical responses. The horizontal scale is identical to that of the single response in *c*, but the amplitude has been scaled to appropriate size.

These variables are also designated normalized slope descriptors (NSD) because of their meaning with reference to graphic features of the tracing:

where a is the root mean square (*rms*) value, or standard deviation, of the EEG tracing with respect to the static mean (normally "zero").

m expresses the mean (*rms*) slope (actually, the *rms* value with respect to zero mean) as a number of standard deviations (*rms*) of the tracing per unit of time (normalization to a). If the time unit is made equal to $1/2\pi$ seconds, m will express the frequency of a pure sine wave in Hz. When the tracing is not a pure sine wave, m expresses the mean (*rms*) frequency of the power spectrum.

c expresses the complexity (e.g., average "sharpness") of the tracing and can be regarded as a measure of frequency spread; a pure sine wave yields $c = 0$.

BASIC PHYSICAL SYSTEMS

The simplest possible system, a first-order system, is defined by one system constant (α) and displays the exponential system response shown in Figure 9.1a, mathematically described as $\exp(-\alpha t)$. Computing the variables defined above for this response yields $m = c = \alpha$, the system constant.

A second-order system, of a type which is fundamental in physics, displays a system response as shown in Figure 9.1b; $\exp(-\alpha t) \cdot \sin(\beta t)$. Computation of mobility and complexity yields:

$$m = sqrt(\alpha^2 + \beta^2)$$
$$c = 2\alpha$$

Thus, the computed variables directly reflect the two constants which govern the behavior of the system.

Another type of system, more common in chemical or biological contexts, has a system response equal to the difference between two exponentials; $\exp(-\alpha t) - \exp(-\beta t)$. Computation of m and c yields:

$$m = sqrt(\alpha \cdot \beta)$$
$$c = \beta - \alpha$$

In fact, this third system type constitutes the basis for a suggested model describing the generation of postsynaptic potentials [1]. While this model requires four exponentials, the number of independent system constants can be reduced to two by making certain assumptions. The system response (Figure 9.1c) is then described as $\exp(-\alpha t) + \exp(-\beta t) - 2\exp(-(\alpha+\beta)/2)$. Computation of m and c yields:

$$m = sqrt(\alpha \cdot \beta/3)$$
$$c = sqrt((3\alpha + \beta) \cdot (\alpha + 3\beta)/6)$$

This type of response has a finite second derivative everywhere. Therefore the variance ratios can also be computed from superimposed, randomly distributed responses. The variances of the superposition are then equal to the results obtained by linear addition of the variances of the single responses, thus making the variance ratios equal for the random superposition and the single response.

Computer simulations [2] confirm that system constants defining a single response can be determined from the variance ratios of the superposition, the latter bearing apparent resemblance to an EEG tracing. Figure 9.1*d* shows a superposition obtained by iterated addition of the system response shown in Figure 9.1*c* with randomly distributed horizontal displacement and amplitude projection (multiplied by the cosine of a randomly distributed angle between 0 and 180 degrees). The computed values of *m* and *c* relating to Figures 9.1*c* and 9.1*d* are identical.

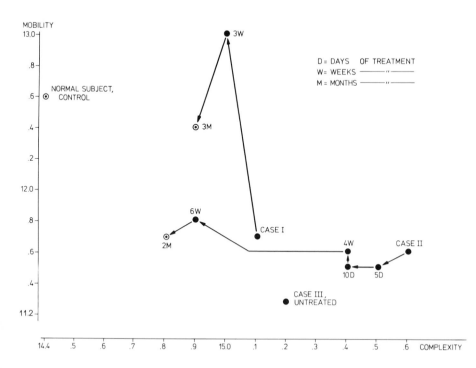

Figure 9.2. Mobility (*m*) and complexity (*c*) values derived from published spectra in two cases of hypothyroidism. Differential values as a result of treatment are plotted over time.

SYSTEM CONSTANTS AND PHYSIOLOGY

This discussion does not imply that the EEG necessarily represents a superposition of field components generated by fluctuating membrane potentials. The EEG could also reflect variations in ion density, i.e., in the energy state obtained as a balance between energy-dissipating cell discharges and energy-restoring metabolic activity. Such a model for EEG generation describes a physical system with, for example, one system constant defining the rate of locally available energy inflow.

The proposed variables m for mobility and c for complexity consistently reflect determinative parameters in the physical systems described in the introductory examples (Figure 9.1). In an unknown system, the dependence of m and c upon a given parameter can be determined from empirical data, or at least approximated as a linear combination of m and c.

Metabolic activity constitutes a fundamental parameter in the EEG generating process. In an effort to study the sensitivity of m and c to metabolic changes, a tentative evaluation was made [3], based on published spectral data relating to treatment of hypothyroidism [4]. Conversion of spectral data to m and c was based on the fact that variance s_n^2 of the derivative of order n is equal to the even spectral moment μ_{2n} of order $2n$. The variances were derived from the power spectrum $S(\omega)$ as:

$$ s_n^2 = \mu_{2n} = \int \omega^{2n} \cdot S(\omega) d\omega $$

Figure 9.2 shows how m and c changed during the treatment of the two published cases of hypothyroidism, as computed from the spectra. These changes were less conspicuous in the original spectral data. The sensitivity to metabolic activity indicates that m and c reflect the functional state of the physiological systems involved.

A report on applications of a, m, and c in psychotropic drug research [5] concludes that "The NSD procedure proved to be sufficiently sensitive to objectify the time course of action of psychoactive drugs, to monitor changes in vigilance, and to quantify drug effects on the sleep-wakefulness cycle." Another report [6], dealing with the application of currently available EEG quantifying methods in cardiac surgery, noted that use of the NSD method yielded the best classification performance. High figures of merit were obtained in feature ranking relative to the different EEG states during cardiac surgery.

These examples from drug research and cardiac surgery, as well as a number of reports from related areas [7–12] support the observation that a, m, and c respond to physiological changes in the central nervous system.

THE TOPOGRAPHIC PATTERN

The useful information provided by a picture displaying, for example, x-ray absorption, ultrasound reflectivity, or neurophysiological data is mainly contained in the density pattern formed by spatial variations in the measured quantity. Isometric contours formed by these variations can often be evaluated qualitatively in terms of displacement, asymmetry, etc., even when normality or abnormality cannot be quantitatively assigned to the individual value. In this instance there is little point in displaying a value which is topologically invariant, since only the occurrence of differences in the data contribute to the topographic pattern. Subtracting from the data any topologically constant component, such as the value by which a generalized abnormality affects the topological average, enables display of the pattern formed by the remaining distribution of differences within a more limited dynamic range. Thus, topographic pictures essentially provide a means of attaining spatial differentiation. Generalized changes, as reflected in the topological average, can be given a separate, quantitative presentation. The topographic pictures included in the following discussion have a dynamic range comprising only seven density grades centered at a level representing the average of the displayed quantity.

Which Quantity Should Be Displayed?

In order to assign a meaning to the topographic pattern, intermediate stages of the computation process must be determined on the basis of empirical data. The variables a, m, and c were shown to be closely linked to the generating physical and therefore probably physiological systems.

In accordance with the statement that topographic pictures essentially provide a means of attaining spatial differentiation, variables a, m, and c are used to form the ratios a/a_0, m/m_0, and c/c_0 in which a_0, m_0, and c_0 are computed from the totals of the variances s_0^2, s_1^2, and s_2^2 for all electrode positions. The ratios express relative topological variations within a recording, regardless of absolute values. Since the ratios vary around unity with zero as an asymptotic minimum, they must be "linearized" by logarithmic conversion before being entered into linear operations:

$$A = \ln(a/a_0)$$
$$M = \ln(m/m_0)$$
$$C = \ln(c/c_0).$$

While the values of the ratios are asymmetrically distributed with unity means, the new variables, A, M, and C, have more symmetric distributions with means of approximately zero and equal deviations for equal relative changes in the intrinsic variables.

The variation in A, M, and C between affected regions and unaffected regions was studied in individual cases with localized lesions. Virtually 100% negative correlation was found for A and M in each case, whereas C displayed no systematic behavior with respect to the lesion. The connection between A and M confirms the well-known fact that a lesion is associated with an increase in amplitude and a decrease in mean frequency, the only new finding being that the relative changes are quantitatively equal. An abnormality feature based on linear combination of the quantities $+A$ and $-M$ must also include the component $+0.75C$ in order to counterbalance the effect of local alpha activity, the latter causing a combined increase in A and decrease in C.

Representing the abnormality feature by density in the topographic image requires an asymptotic minimum equal to zero. This is achieved by means of the antilogarithmic conversion:

$$f = \exp(A - M + 0.75C).$$

Finally, computation of f_0 as the average of f for all electrode positions and forming the ratio f/f_0 yields a quantity suitable for display. Assigning the average of the ratio f/f_0, i.e., unity, to the intermediate density grade centers density variations in the picture with respect to the average of the abnormality feature.

Sensitivity of the Derived Abnormality Feature

Detecting changes in the structure of composite signals normally requires objective, quantitative methods. The procedure for computing the abnormality feature, described in the preceding section, constitutes one such method. The fact that the abnormality feature is based on the variables a, m, and c is likely to make response to a change in the EEG nonspecific with respect to the cause of the change. The interpretation of a, m, and c in relation to physical systems suggests that these variables reflect fundamental features of generating systems, rather than more intricate processes. This is the reason for adapting the abnormality feature to changes caused by local lesions, since lesions can be expected to affect physiological conditions basic to the EEG generating process.

Low specificity of the response to changes necessitates a well-defined reference state in relation to which deviations can be quantitatively determined. This is also the reason why research methods based on activity, mobility, and complexity have proved useful in such research as drug and sleep studies in which well-controlled reference states can be established.

In order to obtain a corresponding reference state from which topologically conditioned deviations can be quantified by means of the abnormality feature, the values for a_0, m_0, and c_0 are considered representative of all positions on the scalp and chosen as references for a, m, and c relative to each individual electrode position. This makes the abnormality feature only sensitive to differences in the topological pattern, regardless of the topological average.

The differential patterns formed by changes in EEG, shown as topographic pictures of the abnormality feature, can be visually compared to other diagnostic displays, such as computed topography (CT) scans. This type of topogram, produced on-line as part of the EEG examination procedure, can greatly enhance the information conveyed from the neurophysiologist to the clinician.

A simple example of the practical utility of topographic map sequences for diagnosis can be taken from our laboratory experience [13]. A patient with a cerebrovascular lesion had an EEG from which we developed a sequence of topographic maps. These mappings clearly demonstrated abnormalities over one hemisphere, with a constant maximum in the temporoparietal region. The distribution of the abnormalities was not readily discernible from the original EEG record.

SPATIAL RESOLUTION

The resolution in local features in the electrical field of the scalp surface is limited by the spatial sampling density, i.e., by the number of electrodes applied over the area of interest. The electrode positions defined by the internationally established 10–20 system for electrode placement is used in the research presented here so as to make the method clinically applicable.

Limits for the spatial resolution are set by the electrical transfer function from neuroelectrically active regions to the measuring channel for each electrode position. An essential part of this transfer function defines the relationship of the potential distributions at the cerebral convexity and the scalp surface. The potential field at the scalp surface is generated by the potential distribution on the cerebral convexity, which can be represented by a dipole layer. The transfer function is considered equal to a superposition of all the dipole fields. According to this model, shown in Figure 9.3, potential variations at a particular point on the cerebral convexity will generate contributions to the surface field equivalent to those generated by a dipole at this point. This means that a recording of an electrode potential is not selective with respect to source location. Thus, optimization of spatial resolution requires careful choice of derivation technique.

The relevance of referential derivation using a common reference electrode is doubtful, since spatially distributed sources have no physical reference to any common position. No common reference can be neutral with respect to sources having different locations and different orientations. Attempts to use centrally placed (nasopharyngeal) or remote (noncephalic) reference electrodes do not eliminate the inclusion of field components from sources in neighboring regions. Using the common average potential as a reference incurs additional disadvantages through the entry of interfering higher amplitude activity, originating in some other region, into the local channel via the reference. The two effects cancel out in a given zone, due to equal magnitudes and opposing polarities, creating the erroneous impression that the channel for a local position

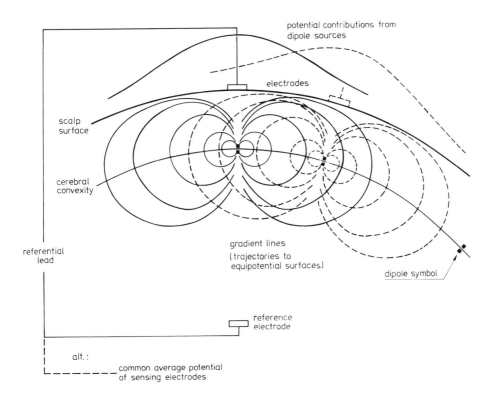

potential contributions from
dipole sources

electrodes

scalp
surface

cerebral
convexity

referential
lead

gradient lines
(trajectories to
equipotential surfaces)

dipole symbol

reference
electrode

alt.:

common average potential
of sensing electrodes

Figure 9.3. The distribution of potential on the cerebral convexity, as seen from the scalp surface, can be represented by an equivalent dipole layer. The effect of a local source in this distribution on the potential field of the scalp surface can be studied as the field contribution generated by a dipole in the dipole layer. A referential lead responds to a local source (solid lines) as well as to sources in other regions (dashed lines). The potentials build up as integrals along the gradient lines.

cannot be affected by interfering activity originating beyond this zone. However, based on certain mathematical principles, reference to the common average potential may be of some advantage in subsequent processing [14].

Bipolar derivation from adjacent electrodes basically records the local potential gradient (field strength), which decreases more rapidly with the distance from its source than does potential, the latter representing the spatially integrated gradient. The disadvantage of bipolar derivation is the fact that its spatial sensitivity distribution, basically that of a dipole sensor parallel to the surface (Figure 9.4a,b), cannot be directed at a single, well-defined, enclosed area. However, spatial selectivity can be obtained by systematic combination of bipolar leads. The resulting sensitivity distributions for the arithmetic means of opposing bipolar leads are shown in Figure 9.4c,d. These distributions can also be combined into the spatially selective sensitivity distribution

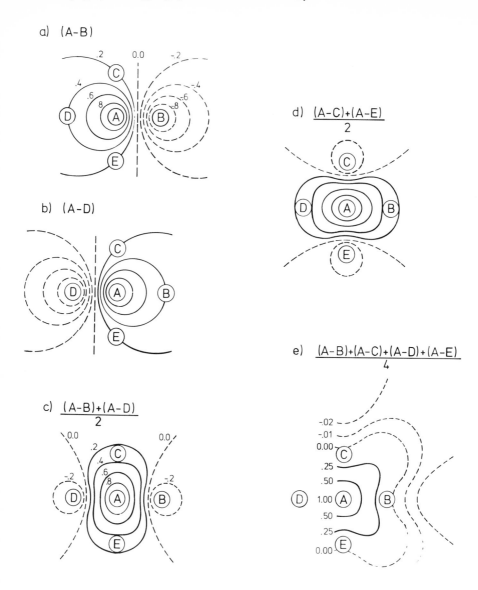

Figure 9.4. The sensitivity of a potential measurement to a source below the surface can be plotted as a function of the location of the source in relation to the electrodes involved. *a.* The sensitivity distribution obtained when measuring the potential difference between electrodes *A* and *B*, i.e., from the bipolar derivation *A-B*. *b.* The sensitivity distribution of the bipolar derivation *A-D*. *c.* The combined sensitivity distribution obtained by adding the potential differences obtained from *A* to *B* and *A* to *D*, followed by division by two, i.e., forming the arithmetic mean. *d.* The sensitivity distribution of the arithmetic mean of the derived values from *A* to *C* and *A* to *E*. *e.* The sensitivity distribution of the arithmetic mean of all four potential differences in two perpendicular directions.

of the arithmetic mean of four bipolar leads directed at the central electrode. The resulting sensitivity distribution is shown in Figure 9.4*e*.

The combination of the potential differences into an arithmetic mean, as shown in Figure 9.4*e*, is mathematically equivalent to forming the Laplacean source operator. This operator constitutes a general tool for derivation of the local source component in a field and can be implemented for finite sample distances in a two-dimensional field by deriving the total of the second-order differences in two perpendicular directions [15,16]. The total of second-order differences in the electrode configuration shown in Figure 9.4 is proportional to the arithmetic mean of the potentials recorded by the four bipolar leads directed at electrode A. Using the arithmetic mean instead of the Laplacean operator provides approximations for the Laplacean operator in the 10–20 systems's positions where available directions are not perpendicular. Compensations can be made for variations in the interelectrode distances by dividing each potential difference by the corresponding interelectrode distance before forming the mean.

The derivation technique thus outlined is referred to as "source derivation." The improvement in spatial resolution of source derivation, as compared to referential and bipolar derivation, was confirmed in a tentative investigation [15] that demonstrated reduced correlations by factors of 0.5 to 0.25 between signals from adjacent electrode positions. Application in routine clinical EEGs [17–20] has confirmed the value of the improved spatial resolution provided by source derivation in detecting and observing localized abnormalities.

The various approaches to derivation technique can be generalized by introducing the concepts of matrix algebra [16,21]. Any type of derivation technique can be expressed as a matrix of coefficients that defines the relationship between the potential at each electrode and the resulting tracing obtained from each electrode position. An adaptive computer algorithm has been devised [14] to adjust the coefficients of the derivation matrix to minimize the average of all off-diagonal elements of the correlation matrix related to the resulting tracings. These tracings have been found to be virtually identical to those obtained from source derivation and display a minor improvement over source derivation only in a few cases. Therefore, we have chosen source derivation, as a basis for topographic mapping, keeping in mind the possibility of on-line implementation using an inexpensive analog network.

GENERATING A TOPOGRAPHIC PICTURE

The mapping of an approximately spherical surface into a two-dimensional picture necessarily entails an inaccurate representation of distances. However, locations on the head surface can be well defined in the picture by means of predefined points representing the electrode positions. Partition of the head

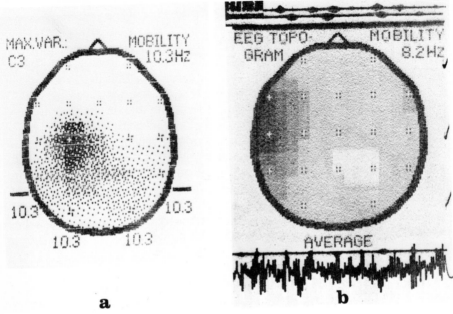

Figure 9.5. Examples of topographic pictures composed with 128-x-128 pixels. *a.* A picture produced by a dot matrix printer using squares comprising 7-x-7 pixels surface elements within the head contour to produce varying density grades. *b.* A picture produced by modulating the vertical scanning velocity of an ink jet printer.

contour area of the representation into approximately 200 surface elements is adequate for the limited resolution in the derivation technique. The density value assigned to each surface element is obtained by adding contributions from the computed values for surrounding electrode positions. The contribution from each electrode position is obtained by multiplying each computed value by the factor $1/(1 + R^2)$, in which R represents the distance from the electrode position to the surface element, and is normalized to two-thirds of the interelectrode distance. This procedure represents an interpolating spatial filter.

A picture comprising 128-x-128 pixels (picture elements) permits allotment of 7-x-7 pixels to each surface element. Figure 9.5*a* shows how these 49 pixels can produce different density grades through variations in the number of pixels assigned black, while remaining pixels in the surface element are assigned white. The picture in Figure 9.5*b* is generated by an ink jet EEG recorder producing different density grades by modulating the vertical scanning velocity of the ink jet. This picture can be printed on the EEG paper with the tracings from which it is computed.

MICROPROCESSOR IMPLEMENTATION

A microprocessor-based system was designed to implement the topographic mapping principles described in this discussion. Such a system is small enough to be built into or closely attached to the individual EEG recorder. The integration of a topography device and an EEG recorder thereby makes the printing of topograms part of the recording routine.

Each 1-second long EEG interval is contiguously processed into three variance values for each of the 19 electrode positions, so that a set of 57 values is derived each second. Data from the last 13 seconds are stored in memory and updated each second through replacement of the oldest data set by the newest. Pressing a button starts final processing of the data for the first 8 of the most recent 13 seconds. This leaves the operator 5 seconds of decision time to prevent the inclusion of unanticipated artifacts in the data from which the topogram is derived. When the recording is considered representative and free from artifact, the operator can initiate the printing of a topogram by simply pressing a button.

Due to the averaging effect, the mapping of an abnormality feature associated with a full 8-second EEG section would yield reduced sensitivity to episodic abnormalities of brief duration. We eliminate this effect by generating a second, optional topogram using the abnormality feature in each second. The electrode position displaying the widest abnormality variation in the 8 seconds is selected for determination of the second in which abnormality was at maximum. The data for this second are used in computing the optional topogram. Figure 9.6 shows how an episodic abnormality affects the two types of topogram; one representing the 8-second average and the other representing the 1-second subepoch containing the episodic abnormality.

Since the topograms only display differential patterns formed by topologically conditioned variations in the EEG, the average state of the EEG must be separately assessed by the neurophysiologist. Support for this assessment is provided by the average value for mobility (designated m_0 here) which is printed numerically in the topographic picture. The mobility values obtained from some posterior electrodes are also printed in the picture. As mentioned, mobility is identical to mean (*rms*) frequency and, unlike the relative quality of the abnormality feature, constitutes an absolute quantity.

EXAMPLES FROM CLINICAL PRACTICE

The EEG segment shown in Figure 9.6 is for a 52-year-old man who, periodically during the preceding two months, had felt weakness in his right arm and leg. Clinical status indicated slightly decreased reflex on the right side. Our diagnosis was left-sided cerebral dysfunction due to vascular disease. Figure 9.7

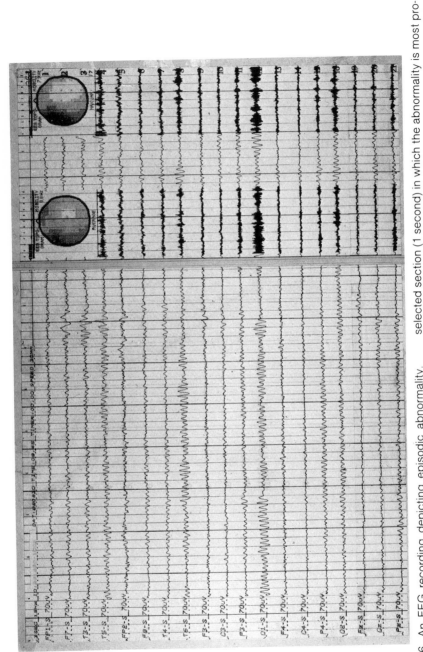

Figure 9.6. An EEG recording depicting episodic abnormality. The method shown in Figure 9.5*b* is used for printing the topograms. The first topogram represents the average during 8 seconds, while the second topogram represents the automatically selected section (1 second) in which the abnormality is most pronounced. A section immediately preceding the topograms, providing the operator with 5 seconds of decision time, has been deleted from the picture.

shows an interictal EEG segment and topogram for a 27-year-old man with occasional grand mal attacks. Neither anamnesis nor clinical status was indicative of a focus. An EEG derived by means of the Laplacean source derivation technique showed, more conspicuously than bipolar tracings, a localized left-sided abnormality (theta waves) as depicted in the topogram. Asymmetry was also visible in the mobility values relating to positions T5 and T6. Figure 9.8

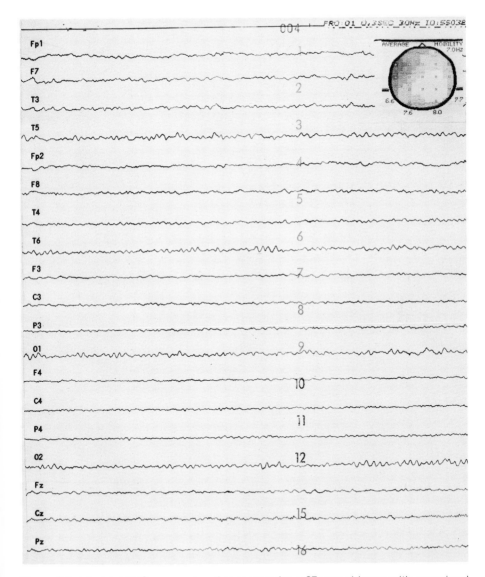

Figure 9.7. Interictal EEG segment and topogram for a 27-year-old man with occasional grand mal attacks. Theta waves occur over the left frontotemporal region.

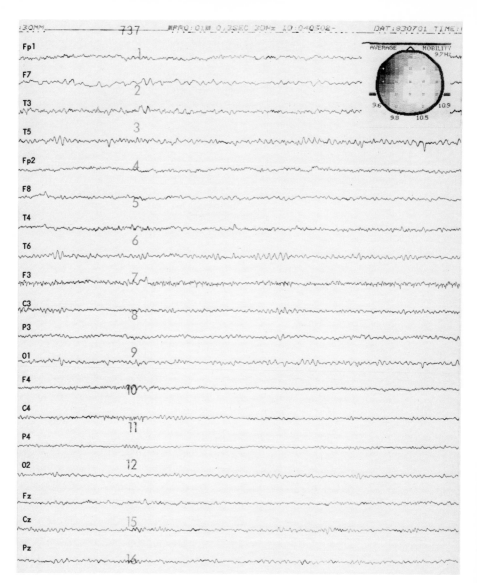

Figure 9.8. EEG segment and topogram for a 79-year-old man with short, repeated absence attacks. A left-sided focal abnormality is seen both in the EEG and in the topogram.

shows the EEG segment and topogram for a 79-year-old man with recent onset of short, repeated attacks of absence. A left-sided, fronto-temporal focal abnormality in the EEG is prominent in the topogram. Figure 9.9 shows the EEG segment, topogram, and CT scan for a 62-year-old woman whose acute illness was characterized by difficulty in controlling her left hand, followed by generalized convulsion one hour later. The EEG topogram displayed severe abnormality in the posterior right temporal region. The CT scan showed decreased density in the same region, indicating cerebral infarct.

SUMMARY

A physically oriented method of signal analysis has proved to be sensitive to EEG changes associated with local lesions when the analysis is applied to EEG

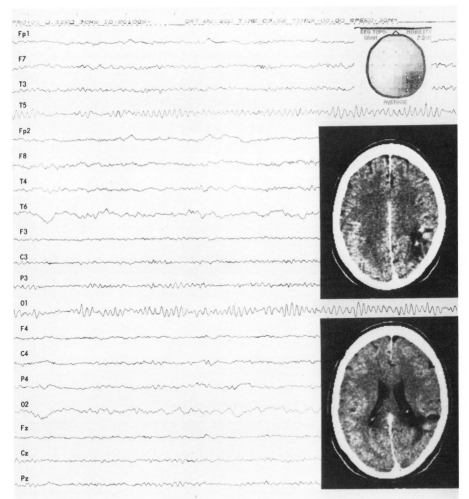

Figure 9.9. EEG segment, topogram, and CT scan for a 62-year-old woman. The CT scan shows decreased density in the posterior right temporal region, indicating cerebral infarct.

background activity. Therefore, the method has been chosen as a basis for topographic mapping of EEG changes of this type.

This chapter provides brief presentation of the method of analysis, describing its on-line implementation and the relationship between derived quantities and properties of possible generating systems. An example was given to illustrate how the derived quantities reflect metabolic changes.

Special emphasis is placed on derivation technique, since spatial selectivity is a prerequisite for topographic mapping. A physical approach to potential distribution in the scalp surface leads to "source derivation," a practical use of the Laplacean source operator. Further attempts to improve spatial resolution within the established 10–20 system for electrode placement, based on measured spatial correlation of the EEG signals, have yielded only minor improvement over source derivation but considerable increase in equipment complexity.

Output data from the analysis for each electrode position consists of three values. These data are combined into a single quantity termed "abnormality feature" with optimum sensitivity to EEG changes of the type associated with localized lesions. The 19 resulting values, one for each electrode position, are interpolated into a printed gray-scale array forming the final EEG topogram.

The principles outlined have been implemented in a microprocessor-based system that can be attached to an EEG recorder. Pressing a button initiates printing of a topogram comprising an 8-second section of the most recent 13 seconds of the EEG, leaving 5 seconds of decision time for the technician. The primary aim of these EEG topograms is to convey information complementary to the written EEG report sent by the neurophysiologist to the referring clinician. But experience has shown that the neurophysiologist can also derive additional information from the topograms.

ACKNOWLEDGMENTS

The author thanks Dr. A. Persson, head of Department of Clinical Neurophysiology at Huddinge University Hospital (Stockholm), for supporting the development of this method by applying it to EEG data during routine recording, and evaluating the clinical relevance of the results obtained.

REFERENCES

1. Lopes da Silva, F.H., Hoeks, A., and Smits, H. Model of brain activity. Progress report 3, 1972, Utrecht: Inst. Med. Phys. TNO 1972; 97–104.
2. Hjorth, B. Time domain descriptors and their relation to a particular model for generation of EEG activity. In: G. Dolce and H. Künkel, eds., CEAN Computerized EEG Analyses, Stuttgart: Fisher, 1975; 3–8.

3. Hjorth, B. Time domain descriptors quantify EEG changes related to hypothyroidism (abstract). Electroenceph. Clin. Neurophysiol. 1975; 38:208P.

4. Lenard, H.G., and Bell, E.F. Bioelectric brain development in hypothyroidism. A quantitative analysis with EEG power spectra. Electroenceph. Clin. Neurophysiol. 1973; 35:545–549.

5. Matejcek, M., and Devos, J.E. Selected methods of quantitive EEG analysis and their applications in psychotropic drug research. In P. Kellaway and I. Petersen, eds., Quantitative Studies in Epilepsy, New York: Raven Press, 1976; 183–205.

6. Pronk, R.A.F. EEG Processing in cardiac surgery. Dissertation, Free University, Amsterdam. Inst. Med. Physics TNO, Report R-1982-1, 1982.

7. Devos, J.E., and Carruthers-Jones, I. Drug induced modifications in the circadian rhythm and EEG of rats. In: Sleep 1976, 3rd Europ. Congr. Sleep Res., Montpellier 1976, Basel: Karger, 1977; 355–357.

8. Kanno, O. Clarenbach H., Kapp, H., and Cramer, H. Normalized slope descriptors in the evaluation of sleep profile and drug effects (abstract). Electroenceph. Clin. Neurophysiol. 1980; 50:125P.

9. Kayed, K., and Godtlibsen, O.B. Central effects of the beta-adrenergic blocking agent acebutolol. Eur. J. Clin. Pharmacol. 1977; 12:327–331.

10. Marciano, F., Monod, N., and Nolfe, G. Computer classification of newborn sleep states (abstract). Electroenceph. Clin. Neurophysiol. 1977; 43:475P.

11. Matejcek, M., Tjeerdsma, H., and Neff, G. Normalized slope descriptors (NSD) applied to sleep research. In Sleep 1978, 4th Europ. Congr. Sleep Res., Tirgu-Mures, 1978. Basel: Karger, 1980; 403–406.

12. Spehr, W., and Stemmler, G. Postalcoholic diseases: Diagnostic relevance of computerized EEG. Electroenceph. Clin. Neurophysiol. 1985; 60:106–114.

13. Persson, A., and Hjorth, B. EEG topogram: An aid in describing EEG to the clinician. Electroenceph. Clin. Neurophysiol. 1983; 56:399–405.

14. Hjorth, B. An adaptive EEG derivation technique. Electroenceph. Clin. Neurophysiol. 1982; 54:654–661.

15. Hjorth, B. An on-line transformation of EEG scalp potentials into orthogonal source derivations. Electroenceph. Clin. Neurophysiol. 1975; 39:526–530.

16. Katznelson, R.D. EEG recording, electrode placement, and aspects of generator localization. In P.L. Nunez, ed., Electric Fields of the Brain. New York: Oxford University Press, 1981; 176–213.

17. Grass, H., and Gottschaldt, M. Improvement of the visual estimation of EEG tracings by source recording (abstract). Electroenceph. Clin. Neurophysiol. 1980; 48:21P.

18. Lütcke, A., Gabel, U., and Mertins, M. Comparison of Hjorth's source derivation and conventional methods in focus detection (abstract). Electroenceph. Clin. Neurophysiol. 1981; 52:39P.

19. Sitzer, G., Matz, D., and Brune, G.G. Toposelective derivations as a new EEG method for better localization of organic cerebral processes (abstract). Electroenceph. Clin. Neurophysiol. 1981; 52:S60.

20. Wallin, G., and Stålberg, E. Source derivation in clinical routine EEG. Electroenceph. Clin. Neurophysiol. 1980; 50:282–292.

21. Hjorth, B. Multichannel EEG preprocessing: Analogue matrix operations in the study of local effects. Pharmakopsychiat. Neuro-Psychopharmakol. 1979; 12:111–118.

10

EEG Topography: Experience and Comments

Anders Persson

Topographic presentation of the electroencephalogram (EEG) has been described and used by several researchers over the last 30 years. Grey Walter and Shipton's toposcopic display systems of 1951 [1] were among the first published. Our method for EEG topography [2], technically described in Chapter 9, was primarily designed for clinical use as a complement to the EEG record and the ordinary clinical report. Our approach to EEG topography was founded on a wish to improve the information to the clinician about signs of functional disturbance visible in the EEG record. A topographic picture might facilitate the understanding of an EEG abnormality, its localization, and intensity. It adds information to the clinical report, which for many reasons must be quite short. The possibility of developing topograms on-line was a further advantage. This is provided by the graphic output capacity of the ordinary Mingograph EEG writing system of Siemens-Elema.

METHODS

The basis of the EEG topograms was a mathematical analysis of the EEG, according to the methods described by Hjorth [3] using the normalized slope descriptors activity, mobility, and complexity. Schematically, these can be said to carry information about mean amplitude, mean frequency of the power spectrum, and frequency spread.

EEG abnormalities usually consist of increased amounts of slow waves. The degree of abnormality is related to the degree of cerebral dysfunction and is inversely proportional to frequency and directly proportional to amplitude. Based on examinations of EEG records with pronounced local EEG abnormalities, we constructed an abnormality feature (f), that is proportional to activity and inversely proportional to mobility. The average f_0 was formed as an average recording of f from 16 electrodes, with the three frontal electrodes (Fp 1,

Fp 2, Fz) excluded to diminish the effect of artifacts from eye movements. After filtering, the ratio f/f_0 determined the ink intensity for a particular electrode. The dynamic range was chosen such that minimum and maximum ink densities represented 0.5 and 1.5 times the scalp average f_0. (For further technical description refer to Chapter 9.) Thus the topogram displays local deviations from the scalp average, regardless of its absolute value.

The EEG was recorded on a 21-channel polygraph (Siemens-Elema) into which a microprocessor-based system for the EEG analysis was built. The electrodes were applied according to the 10–20 system, and the source derivation technique was used [4]. The recording procedure followed the ordinary clinical routine. Special care was taken to reduce artifacts, particularly slow waves, which influence the abnormality feature. To obtain a topographic display in our lab, a topogram is printed by simply pressing a button. The topogram is computed from data stored in the memory from the last few seconds. We have primarily used topograms of 4 or 8 second periods. Slight abnormalities were better shown by the longer periods, but were also more susceptible to artifacts.

RESULTS

Our method was primarily designed to indicate local EEG abnormalities, particularly slow-wave activity. Figure 10.1 shows the EEG and topogram from a 41-year-old patient with a vascular lesion in the left hemisphere. The topogram corresponds to the first 4 seconds of the EEG recording, leaving 2.5 seconds to exclude artifacts before printing starts. During printing of the topogram, the paper speed is reduced but EEG recording continues. When the printing is finished the data from which the topogram is computed are removed from the memory. The marked slow-wave activity on the left side in the EEG is clearly shown in the topogram.

The tendency for slight EEG abnormalities to be more pronounced in the topogram than in the EEG record is because the topogram shows a relative rather than an absolute abnormality feature. Based on our experience this may sometimes provide support for the interpretation of the EEG. This is illustrated in Figure 10.2 which provides a recording from an 18-year-old man suspected of having partial epilepsy. The EEG shows a slight abnormality at the T6 electrode. From the topogram it is obvious that the abnormality is more pronounced and abnormal readings also appear in adjacent electrodes. The diagnostic accuracy of the topogram was supported by further examination, which revealed a local organic lesion in the right posterior temporal region.

Figure 10.3 is a recording from a 30-year-old man with partial epilepsy due to a left-sided traumatic lesion. The focal EEG abnormality is well shown in the topogram. The diffuse EEG changes, on the other hand, are not visible due to the design of the method to show local changes relative to scalp average. The average mobility is, however, written out on the topographic picture. In

this 4-second period the reading for mobility was 6.2 Hz, which is well below
the normal limit for healthy adults. With eyes closed, average mobility in patients with normal EEG (in the 20–60 year range) was 9.81 ± 1.0 Hz (mean ±
standard deviation). The calculation was based on the mean of at least ten 4-
second epochs in 30 healthy subjects with a normal EEG.

Another effect of showing relative values of the abnormality feature is
shown in Figure 10.4. Recording with eyes closed and eyes open did not show
significantly different topograms. The mean mobility, however, decreased

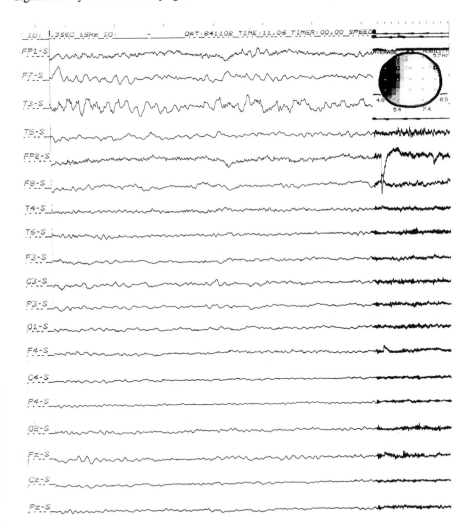

Figure 10.1. EEG and topogram recorded in a 41-year-old patient with a left-sided vascular lesion. The topogram was based on data from the first 4 seconds of the recording between the markings at the bottom of the picture.

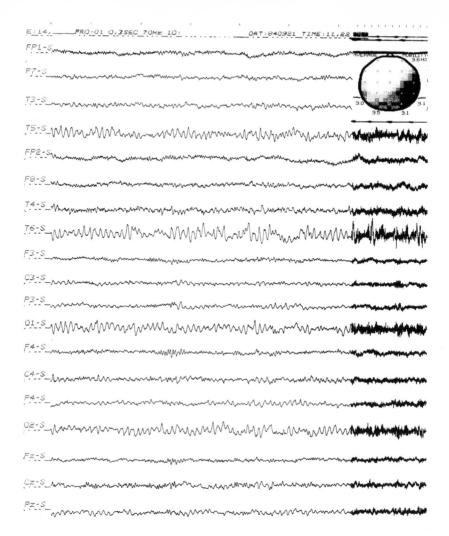

Figure 10.2. EEG and topogram from a 18-year-old man suspected of having partial epilepsy.

about 2 Hz at eyes open compared to eyes closed. The mobility values shown in the picture are the mean of ten 4-second epochs at each state.

Disturbance of cerebral function may appear as increased frequency and reduced amplitude of the EEG activity. In our computation of the EEG data, this gives rise to decreased abnormality features, shown in the topogram as light areas.

Listening to music is known to activate the right posterior temporal region [5]. Figure 10.5 shows five consecutive topograms from a normal subject at rest and then listening to music (*Eine kleine Nachtmusik* by Mozart). The region around the electrode T6 remained light, indicating a small relative abnormality feature. As the absolute mobility values of this electrode were written out on the topogram picture, it was possible to see that the mobility in this electrode increased while listening to music compared to rest. In this subject, the mean of 10 epochs was 11.44 ± 0.46 Hz while listening to music and 10.76 ± 0.30 Hz at rest. If a symmetry coefficient is constructed to compare left and right temporal electrodes [$100 \times (T5-T6/T5+T6)$], the difference between acti-

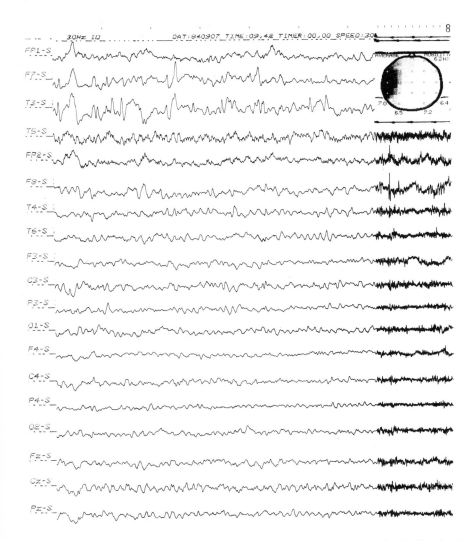

Figure 10.3. EEG and topogram from a 30-year-old patient with partial epileptic fits due to a left-sided traumatic lesion.

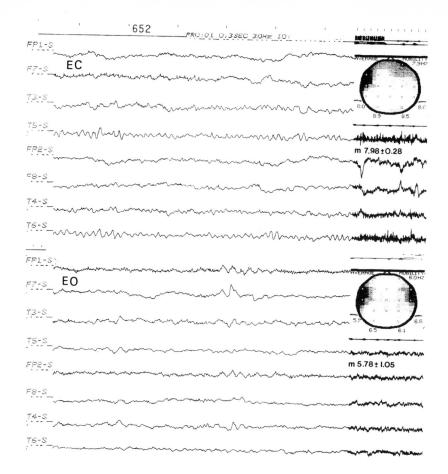

Figure 10.4. Topograms and part of their corresponding EEG with eyes closed (EC) and eyes open (EO). The EEG was recorded on a 14-year-old girl.

vation and rest was more pronounced and statistically significant ($P<0.005$). The means for this coefficient were -9.050 while listening to music and 0.545 at rest.

In summary we believe that this method for on-line EEG topography facilitates communication between the neurophysiologist and the clinician. Furthermore, it can be used to decide if a slight EEG abnormality is significant.

The chapters in this volume convincingly demonstrate that various methods of topographic mapping of EEG and evoked potential data can be used, all giving information about the relation between spatial distribution and time. Several problems with the techniques have been presented—artifact, type of reference electrode, scaling, etc.

Topography is thus an elegant method of presenting local abnormalities.

REST   **MUSIC**

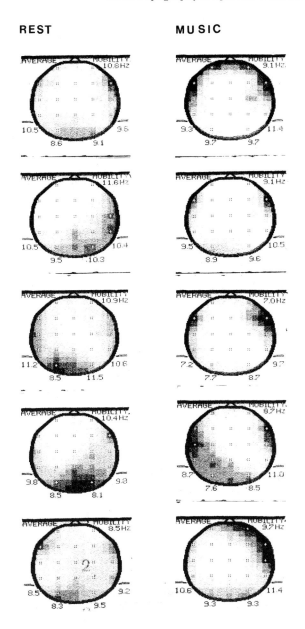

Figure 10.5. Topograms from a healthy subject during rest (*left*) and while listening to music (*right*). A constant appearance of a light area at the T6 electrode while listening to music is a probable sign of local cerebral activation.

It is also capable of yielding useful data on normal distribution of various frequency components. In combination with statistical methods, topography shows differences between groups of patients and normal controls in such pathologies as schizophrenia and Alzheimer's disease.

Topography obviously adds valuable information as compared to the ordinary visual analysis of EEG and evoked potentials, but is that information of clinical importance for the individual patient? For a clinical neurophysiologist, that is a very important question. We cannot afford to make examinations that add data which, although statistically significant, are not clinically significant. This volume gives promise for the future in this respect. However, more studies about the clinical utility of topography are necessary. Such research should be given highest priority. We must define those situations where topographic mapping on clinical grounds is a justified complement to the ordinary EEG and evoked potential examination.

ACKNOWLEDGMENTS

The studies presented in this chapter were performed in collaboration with Mr. B. Hjorth, engineer at the Research and Development Laboratory of Siemens-Elema. Technical support from Siemens-Elema AB, Solna, is gratefully acknowledged.

REFERENCES

1. Walter, W.G., and Shipton, H.W. A new toposcopic display system. Electroenceph. Clin. Neurophysiol. 1951; 3:281–292.
2. Persson, A., and Hjorth, B. EEG-topogram: An aid to describe the EEG to the clinician. Electroenceph. Clin. Neurophysiol. 1982; 54:35.
3. Hjorth, B. The physical significance of time domain descriptors in EEG analysis. Electroenceph. Clin. Neurophysiol. 1973, 34:321–325.
4. Hjorth, B. An adaptive EEG derivation technique. Electroenceph. Clin. Neurophysiol. 1982; 54:654–661.
5. Duffy, F., Bartels, P.H., and Burchfiel, J.L. Significance probability mapping: An aid in the topographic analysis of brain electrical activity. Electroenceph. Clin. Neurophysiol. 1981; 51:455–462.

11

A Simple Add-on Personal Computer Procedure for Color Displays of Electrophysiological Data: Advantages and Pitfalls

Reginald G. Bickford and Barry Allen

Many areas of science are now displaying data processing results in color. Although color displays are visually attractive, in many intances they show virtually the same data as black-and-white displays. This raises the question of perceptual and psychological bias attached to results presented in color. It would be remiss not to discuss some of the problems and illustrate some of the pitfalls by review of examples. Thus, for instance, a skeptic might argue that there are disadvantages in presenting data in color if the point to be displayed can be clearly seen in noncolor presentations. If color is used, its persuasive qualities might bias the observer toward the colored result as against a black-and-white rendition. In fact color displays have been tried in virtually all the imaging techniques and have been mostly discontinued in computed tomography (CT), magnetic resonance (MR), and sonographic imaging. The use of color, however, has many advantages over noncolor presentation in specified circumstances, particularly where a large number of variables have to be displayed simultaneously. Thus color processing seems to have become standard in positron emission tomography (PET).

METHODS

History

Electroencephalographers have been vitally concerned with localization of varied waves since the inception of the technique; it is therefore natural that in the past a good deal of attention has been given to the problem of toposcopic displays. The first attempt at contouring electrophysiological data generated by the cortex was by Lilly [1,2] in 1949. Lilly used various ingenious methods, including a rubber membrane peg display for field visualization, after which a movie camera was used to make a total moving sequence. He named the display images that appear under these circumstances "icons" and discussed the perceptual problems that these techniques might be prone to produce. In 1948 Goldman [3] showed an interesting display of human alpha rhythm in which a curious rotatory movement could be perceived. Before the inception of digital methods, Shipton and Grey Walter [4] provided a multioscilloscope analog display with rotating time base. With the development of digital methods, Harris [5,6] contoured both EEG and evoked potential onto head maps. Recently there has been a rapid development of black-and-white and color displays from commercial enterprises and physiological laboratories whose aim is to represent processed brain electrical activity on some kind of simulated head manikin. With the advent of color display systems, Duffy [7] demonstrated a convincing use of evoked potential field displays in color of EEG and evoked potentials on clinical cases at the American EEG Society meeting in 1977. This was the inception of the more recent BEAM System that has now been given a significant statistical background. Extensive work on many of the problems raised in this report have been covered by Lehmann and his collaborators [8,9].

This chapter presents the following: (1) a simple interpolation and color display system for a personal type computer (Zenith 100); (2) the conversion of static displays into movie presentation of evoked potential wave invasion of the cortex; (3) a scheme for testing topographic accuracy of interpolation and display procedures (tank experiments); (4) a "field injection" technique for testing accuracy of these methods in human subjects; (5) some examples of advantages and pitfalls of color processing of EEG spectra and evoked potentials.

Data Generation

Data came from several sources (Figure 11.1). There were saline tank experiments in which potential fields were injected from (1) a sine wave generator for spectral studies, and (2) a special damped sine wave generator (designed by Dr. Peter Fortescue), the onset of which could be triggered by an appropriate stimulus pulse. This allowed the injection of simulated evoked potential waveforms into the tank or subject's scalp for the generation of simulated evoked potential maps. Similarly, coutour plots were made using the spectral fast Fourier transform (FFT) program to provide binned data of the appropriate waveform (delta, theta, alpha, beta).

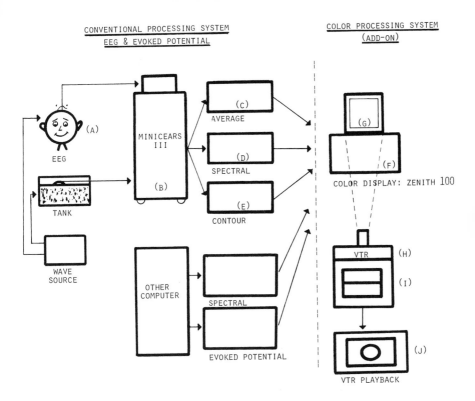

CONVENTIONAL PROCESSING SYSTEM
EEG & EVOKED POTENTIAL

COLOR PROCESSING SYSTEM
(ADD-ON)

(A) EEG

TANK

WAVE SOURCE

MINICEARS III

(B)

OTHER COMPUTER

(c) AVERAGE

(D) SPECTRAL

(E) CONTOUR

SPECTRAL

EVOKED POTENTIAL

(G)

(F)

COLOR DISPLAY: ZENITH 100

VTR (H)

(I)

(J)

VTR PLAYBACK

Figure 11.1. Diagram of a basic computer (Minicears III) and computer add-on (Zenith 100) system: Patient (*A*) connected to Minicears III (*B*) which undertakes averaging and spectral analysis on 16 channels. This system produces a 16-channel average (*C*) together with voltage numerical data indicating the voltage on the scalp at appropriate times following the stimulus. Spectral analysis numerical results (*D*) with numbers referable to wave frequencies (delta, theta, alpha, and beta) and locations (10–20 system) and black-and-white contour (*E*) of evoked potential or spectral data. The numbers generated by the Minicears III program are then transferred to the Zenith 100 microprocessor (*F*), the software of which converts the numbers, following interpolation, to color displays appearing on the terminal face (*G*). This computer generates three different graphics, a vertical perspective, and right and left lateral perspectives (see Figure 11.2). Multiple images representing a sequence can be printed on a smaller scale to indicate changes with different spectral frequencies or with sequential EP latencies. A VHS video system (*H*) recording onto videotape is available for documenting the movie displays appearing on the color terminal. These can be viewed subsequently as a videotape movie (*J*). Reference electrode consists of a continuous heavy-duty copper wire located on the bottom of the tank 5–6 inches from the electrode pickup grid. This achieves an adequate indifferent electrode arrangement.

Tank Experiments

A rectangular 10-gallon saline tank was used for injection of the waveforms by means of an appropriately located pair of electrodes (copper plates) into the saline medium (Figure 11.1). Pickup of the generated field was by means of a 10–20 electrode grid (16 channels) placed on the fluid surface. This arrangement allowed the pickup of sinusoidal or evoked potential waveforms that had been injected in appropriate directions and locations by stimulus electrodes in the tank.

Human Scalp Field Injection Experiments

Three normal subjects were used to provide an "experimental head" into which simulated waveforms, generated as in the tank experiments, were injected into the human scalp. After an appropriate location had been chosen for the injection electrodes and they had been sealed to the scalp with electrode paste, a standard conventional Electrocap with 16 electrodes was pulled over the head and adjusted appropriately. The Electrocap electrodes were then filled as in a conventional recording. This provided a human experimental setup in which sine wave or evoked potential fields could be injected with known relationship to the 10–20 electrode array (by feeling through the Electrocap material and marking the location of injection electrodes in relation to the 10–20 arrangement of the Electrocap). No sensation was produced by the injected fields, which ranged in voltage from 100 to 1000 mV.

Patient Observations

A small number of patients from the clinical lab provided data on artifact and selected pathologies (Plate 4).

Computer Techniques

Basic Processing

Sixteen-channel spectral bin data and the 16-channel evoked potential voltages were obtained by use of the Minicears III computer system [10]. As shown in Figure 11.1, data collected from either the patient or by techniques described earlier resulted in the generation of black-and-white contour plots of chosen spectra (delta, theta, alpha, beta) or evoked potential distribution voltage maps at a chosen interval following the stimulus.

Further Processing of This or Other Data

For this purpose, data was transferred to a Zenith 100 microcomputer with color terminal and color printer. The color display software was written by Allen [11]. While the usual procedure was to transfer data from the Minicears III computer (via the keyboard or cable interface), the 16 data values representing the voltages necessary for production of color contours (after interpolation) can be taken from other 16-channel average plotted data after the latency line has been inserted and the appropriate 16 voltages from the traces. Likewise, the 16 integrated voltage number required for the spectral programs can be taken from another computer or other spectral processing system (or from a table of random numbers for system tests).

Movie Display of Evoked Potentials

A convenient way to form the sequenced color images appearing on the terminal face consisted of using a Quasar VHS taperecorder and camera. Images were programmed to appear on the terminal at 0.25–1.0-second intervals. A complete sequence of 150 images contained in the sweep was then filmed as a color movie lasting 1 to 2 minutes and showing the detail of evoked potential wave invasion of the cortex. Such a videotape gives details of distortions of wave spread that may be encountered in clinical conditions.

RESULTS

Saline Tank Experiments

Good correspondence was demonstrated between the location of artificial fields and the placement of injection electrodes, indicating that the processing and the interpolation procedures have an acceptable accuracy (about 5%).

Activity on the Reference Electrode

One of the advantages of contour plots for the electroencephalographer is that they provide an easily recognized location of some abnormality such as the tumor (if it produces delta waves or other abnormal discharges) free from interference by activity appearing on the reference electrode. This contention is generally accepted on the intuitive basis that activity on a reference electrode would have the effect of moving a display in a vertical plane, affecting all electrodes equally and therefore not changing the differences exhibited between lines in a contour plot. In these experiments we had the opportunity of placing artificial wave forms on the reference electrode (Figure 11.1), which were close in frequency to those produced by the evoked potential simulator. This experiment confirmed the contention that reference activity can be eliminated from the contour graphics by this technique. While this is true for black-and-white line plots, interference can be severe from the reference electrode if color plots of the same data are made because activity that causes changes in the average level of the plot also changes the detail of the color display, including the color at zero cross. Unless special precautions are taken, the use of a color display under these circumstances is disadvantageous.

Field Injection of Normal Subjects

An example of this technique is shown in Figure 11.2 for injection of a sinusoidal theta wave located in the right lateral temporal area. The distribution of the impressed theta plot is evident since in this normal awake subject, theta activity was minimal before the injection process. These lo-

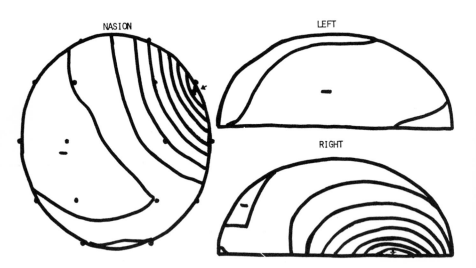

Figure 11.2. An example of a sine wave rhythm field injection into the scalp of a normal subject in the right temporal area from two electrodes, one of which is indicated by an arrow. The other (reference) is approximately 6 inches further down on the neck. Note that the injected field is accurately portrayed in relation to one end of the injection site and that there is adequate correspondence between anterior-posterior and lateral views, bearing in mind the difficulties of transfer between polar coordinates of the 10–20 system and the flat field of the vertical and lateral contour views.

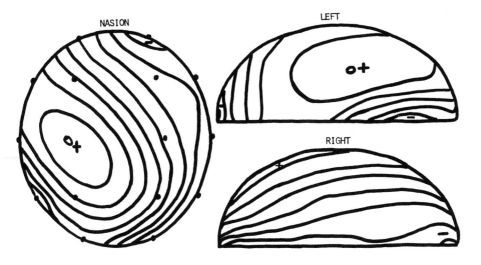

Figure 11.3. An artifact seen when there is unilateral eye movement with the appearance of artifactual delta frequency and theta activity in the right frontal region. Eye blinks, which may appear intermittently and unexpectedly, both unilateral and bilateral, can easily contaminate the primary data, and unless this is inspected continuously during the processing, serious errors may occur.

cal field injection techniques also give a visual check on the reliability of interpolation procedures and the method used for the vertical and lateral displays. These displays showed acceptable spatial accuracy (about 5%).

Artifact

The reason for illustrating some of the varied types of artifact is related to concerns about the reliability of area displays when they are used in isolation of the accompanying data-processing stages, including the processing of primary EEG data. Figure 11.3 gives an example of the apparent localized slow-wave activity that can occur in a patient with unilateral eye blink. This can occur clinically for a variety of reasons (ocular palsy, artificial eye) and produces localized changes. Likewise the more common intrusion of eye blink artifact is as a bilateral phenomenon that can cause problems by its possible confusion with genuine delta activity in the frontal regions. These difficulties are not, in fact, confined to processed displays and present considerable difficulty in the routine clinical interpretation of the EEG by conventional methods. Another common artifact due to muscle activity contamination on the electromyogram (EMG) is illustrated in Figure 11.4. Many patients are in an agitated, uncomfortable, or restless state when they have an EEG recording. Thus when con-

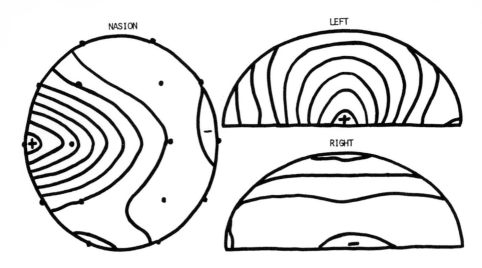

Figure 11.4. EMG artifact as it appears in a spectral display (13–18 Hz). These lower frequencies are contained in the EMG envelope. In this subject, while EMG was evident in the primary, it is not always appreciated that this may produce the kind of spectral change shown in this illustration. Since minor degrees of EMG contamination can easily occur in experimental situations and in patients who are tense, this is a viable artifact and has to be carefully guarded against.

toured data are reviewed, lateralized effects may have come from EMG contamination in the alpha, theta, or beta ranges. This is because EMG spectra commonly show small amounts of these frequencies. Unless primary EEG data is viewed, this problem may be overlooked.

Perhaps one of the most difficult artifacts encountered in spectral analysis, and therefore in topographic displays related to such data, is that due to shifts of alertness in the subject or patient. Such changes are a particular hazard in drug test experiments or in patients taking medication. The onset of drowsiness is accompanied by profound changes in the EEG, with shifts to the left of most frequency components (sometimes associated with conspicuous left-right asymmetries) in the spectral display and forward shifts of the alpha process. In a drug study of a particular agent that is apt to produce drowsiness, there may be conspicuous differences in the spectral contour of the patient before and after taking the drug, but these differences may merely reflect the fact that the patient was not in a comparable state of alertness in the two situations.

Another biological artifact that can generate considerable error is that produced by intrusions of the electrocardiogram (ECG) in a patient who has a rather constant heart rate. Because of the sensitivity of spectral programs to repetitive events (such as ECG) that can appear quite small and inconspicuous in the primary EEG trace, this source of error is often unrecognized. It is promoted by the presently popular ear reference technique used in computer displays. Change in heart rate is a common accompaniment of a drug study (from anxiety or from direct effects on the cardiovascular system). Consequently this artifact can be a problem in drug studies, particularly if the drug produces changes in heart rate and consequent shifts in spectral components.

Those who use contouring algorithms for the production of black-and-white and color displays need to be aware of the propensity of these mathematical devices to produce the appearance of an electrical focus when the input data is entirely random. An example is shown in Figure 11.5.

DISCUSSION

A topogram of EEG and evoked potential is a simple, convenient, and efficient way to communicate electrophysiological information to a neurologist or other clinician, and it is particularly helpful when it yields a clear localization of disturbed function. However, this ease of communication in localized lesions tends to obscure a number of difficulties of this electrical imaging method when compared to those presently in use in clinical neurology such as the CT, PET, and MR. Data on localization may depend on spectral localization of slow waves (the conventional delta focus). Localization may also be argued from asymmetries occurring in spontaneous rhythms such as the alpha rhythm or in distortions of the amplitude or invasion pattern of the evoked potential, e.g., as a result of a pattern shift or other stimulus. Problems may arise when the results of spontaneous activity distortion are not entirely coherent with those of other measures. On the other hand, the asymmetries of evoked potential development seen in learning disorders are sometimes considerable and naturally invite comparison with other imaging methods.

Considerable difficulties may be encountered with electrical imaging when characteristic displays are sought for special types of diseases such as schizophrenia. In these cases there is a tendency for investigators to produce area displays of a colored and impelling type in the absence of backup data so that the observer has very little clue as to whether these are really unbiased choices of display pattern. Because of the complexity and lack of sequential data in topographic techniques, it is easy for the experimenter to be unaware that artifact is making its appearance in the final display data. The difficulty is increased by the fact that many artifacts are intermittent in appearance and may not, for instance, have been present when a routine artifact check was made. It is for this reason that the examples given in this chapter illustrate the far-reaching changes that such artifactual intrusion can produce. In order to reduce this type of error, it is recommended that some effort be made to include at least a portion of primary data along with (or even on top of) the contour plots.

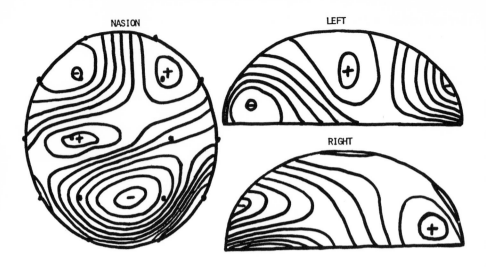

Figure 11.5. A random-number display with the plotting values chosen from a table of random numbers. It illustrates the powerful nature of interpolation algorithms that, because of their tendency to make contours from numbers, may mislead the investigator. In this instance it points to contoured activity (let us suppose in the delta range) that might be interpreted as two lesions located at left frontal and posterior midline. Lateral displays correspond. This kind of error can easily occur if the data numbers from a low amplitude display, which is presumably close to random because of predominant noise (amplifier or electrode), are processed by spectral or evoked potential display after having been brought up (amplified) beyond appropriate limits.

FUTURE STUDIES

Will electrical images hold their own among the competitors (CT, PET, MR) in the imaging field? It is often said that electrical events represent function and therefore will always have an edge on the competitors. This statement should be modified to say that electrical events are related to function but often in a complex way. Experienced electroencephalographers recognize many of the paradoxes related to function such as (1) the inverse relationship of alpha amplitude to brain activity such as is seen in alpha blocking, and (2) the low amplitude of the EEG in the REM (rapid eye movement) stage of sleep when metabolic data indicate a high state of brain activity. While these anomalies can be accounted for by subsidiary hypotheses, they do in fact cause difficulty in clinical interpretation. For instance, during resuscitation of a patient who has suffered some kind of cerebral insult, it is noted that EEG amplitude (presently much higher than normal due to slow waves) is progressively decreasing in voltage. Is this a good or bad prognostic sign? There is no easy answer.

The other problem with electrical recordings is that in general we do not know from what structure the pattern or wave is arising. For example, we know that activity recorded at the vertex and left ear when the patient is stimulated by clicks comes from the brain stem and the diencephalic area and not from the region of the recording electrodes. However, in the brain stem average evoked response (BAER), it is not known whether the origin of the waves is from axon fibers or from synaptic activity. Electroencephalographers know about these problems, but the associated paradoxes coupled with our basic ignorance concerning the structures involved in generation of electrical waves makes clinical interpretation difficult.

COORDINATION

The answer to some of these problems could come from comparison of data with that from other imaging systems that produce anatomical, metabolic, or other information from the production of EEG patterns or waveforms. Thus, for instance, if a CT scan shows a subcortical lesion in a circumscribed area, we should know what effect such as deafferentation has on EEG activity and its spectrum from an overlying area. In its historical evolution, the EEG has unfortunately not had the advantage of such correlative information and has had to depend on notoriously inaccurate clinical lesion localization. There is now an opportunity to reassess this area, a reassessment that could provide a major reevaluation of electroencephalography. Toposcopy and imaging methods present a ready procedure to complete these important tasks. Similar comparisons could be made where metabolic information is available and is likely to be important in elucidating such complex syndromes as schizophrenia, where abnormalities in both the metabolic and EEG fields have been reported but their relationships and topography are virtually unknown.

Initially such comparisons should be made within the field of EEG and evoked potentials because such knowledge might be expected to yield both functional and diagnostic information. It was this kind of expectation that led Bickford [10] to emphasize the ACE (automated clinical electrogram) test for clinical use. In our limited exploration of an older population (relatively symptom-free), we discovered surprising anomalies with, for instance, a slowed and low-voltage alpha rhythm associated with a large occipital evoked response to pattern shift. A simple interpretation would be that the alpha mechanism is suppressed, and the evoked potential mechanism arising from the same general region is enhanced. The clinical question is: How do such ambiguities predict the future for this patient? In other words, what is the prognostic meaning of such a discordant finding? Note that the approach suggested here is somewhat different from an equally valid approach taken by Duffy and his group of using comparative statistics applicable to topographic displays. The problem encountered with statistical estimates of likelihood of differences from a normative group is that the answer is often not sufficiently definitive (i.e., probabilities are not high enough) to speak with the certainty demanded of a clinical situation. Here the patient demands to know if he has the disease. The causal approach emphasized here, together with statistical approaches in other imaging methods, might in the long run be expected to clarify the field of diagnostic and research toposcopy and improve diagnosis in the field.

ANATOMICAL PROBLEMS IN IMAGING COMPARISONS

The suggestion of relating topographic maps emerging from CT, PET, and MR scans overlooks a considerable problem, namely, that they do in fact have different spatial projection parameters. These problems became evident when an attempt was made to produce a lateral view of the topograms normally viewed in a vertical projection. The 10–20 system is essentially a polar coordinate projection; thus, there are difficult transformations to transfer the data with any accuracy onto a flat surface. In the data section, we indicated that this can be done with present projective techniques within an acceptable degree of error. However, complex problems (possibly insoluble) arise when maps comparable to the slice techniques of the CT, PET, and MR scanners are attempted. This requires some kind of projective transfer algorithm that tells us what electrical activity might look like along a defined and flat slice-like display. We know so little about the EEG and its origin that such a venture is little short of guesswork and in fact may not be appropriate. In the meantime, relationships can be established using anatomical concepts such as identification of the fiber tract that is involved, or designation of the neuronal population. Some of these problems can be solved by probe techniques of the depth electrogram since these can access and in fact be implanted on coordinates that match those in use by the more modern imaging methods.

Another technique of interest is that of magnetic electroencephalography (with both the spontaneous and the evoked potential maps). The topographic maps in these instances are thought to represent current paths that are simpler than those involved in more classical resistive "network" problems of the EEG. Thus, for instance, brain slices illustrative of current flows within the slice might become available which would be more relevant to other slice techniques (CT, PET, and MR).

The most important aspect of topographic projection techniques might turn out to be their ability to spatially interrelate information from diverse technical areas. These may be the constellations that define the diseases of the future.

Some of the advantages and pitfalls attending color as contrasted with black-and-white in area displays are discussed. The methods in use are tested by means of saline tank experiments and field injection techniques used in normal subjects.

Because of the difficulty involved in artifact recognition when only the final process of contoured display is used, care has to be taken in the interpretation of clinical toposcopic results. When feasible, it is recommended that at least a small sample of primary EEG data be included with the final display to assure no untoward contamination of the data.

The commercial availability of color display microcomputers at a relatively low cost (home computers) and the ability of simple video recording techniques to form a movie presentation of wave-front invasion of the cortex by evoked potentials bring these techniques into the realm of feasibility for those with low budgets.

Future progress in the field will come from interrelating the independent information from anatomical, metabolic, and magnetic measures for which the toposcopic display would form an incisive technology with many clinical and diagnostic advantages.

ACKNOWLEDGMENTS

Supported in part by Alzheimer's Disease Research Center Grant #AGO5131-01.

REFERENCES

1. Lilly, J.C. A method of recording the moving electrical potential gradients in the brain: The 25-channel Bavatron and electroconograms. Paper presented at Conference on Electronic Instrumentation in Nucleonics and Medicine, New York, N.Y., 1949.
2. Lilly, J.C. Instantaneous relations between the activities of closely spaced zones on the cerebral cortex: Electrical figures during responses and spontaneous activity. Am. J. Physiol. 1954; 176(3):493–504.
3. Goldman, S., Vivian, W.E., Chien, C.K., and Bowes, H.N. Electronic mapping of the activity of the heart and brain. Science 1948; 108:720.
4. Walter, W.G., and Shipton, H.W. A new toposcopic display system. Electroenceph. Clin. Neurophysiol 1951; 3:281.
5. Harris, J.A. A spatial interpolation procedure for electroencephalography. Thesis, University of Minnesota, 1967.
6. Harris, J.A., Melby, G.M., and Bickford, R.G. Computer-controlled multidimensional display device for the investigation and modelling of physiologic systems. Comput. Biomed. Res. 1969; 2:519–536.
7. Duffy, F.H., Burchfiel, J.L., and Lombroso, C.T. Brain electrical activity mapping (BEAM): A method for extending the clinical utility of EEG and evoked potential data. Ann. Neurol. 1979; 5:309–321.
8. Lehmann, D., and Brown, W.S. The EEG as scalp field distribution. In A. Rémond, ed., EEG Informatics. Amsterdam: Elsevier/North Holland, 1977; 365–384.

9. Lehmann, D., and Skrandies, W. Reference-free identification of components of checkerboard-evoked multichannel potential fields. Electroenceph. Clin. Neurophysiol. 1980; 48:609–621.
10. Bickford, R.G. A combined EEG and evoked potential procedure in clinical EEG (automated cerebral electrogram: ACE test). In N. Yamaguchi and K. Fujisawa, eds., Recent Advances in EEG and EMG Data Processing. New York: Elsevier, 1981; 217–235.
11. Allen, B.A., Bickford, R.G., and Hajdukovic, R. Area display of EEG and EPs: Mathematical considerations. Electroenceph. Clin. Neurophysiol. 1984; 58:13P (abstr.).

12

From Entertainment to Education, from Education to Enlightenment

Harold W. Shipton

This chapter is intended to serve both as a commentary on some parts of the Boston conference and also as an introduction to topographic methods for those who have not followed their development. Because an excellent history of these methods and applications from their inception until 1970 has been produced [1], early technologies are only briefly discussed. There is also some reference to recent developments in my own approach to toposcopic technology.

The chapter title refers to a comment by Grey Walter [2] that the introduction of some degree of frequency sensitivity turned toposcopes from devices with a high entertainment value (the flickering images of early systems were seductively suggestive of Sherrington's description of the brain as an "enchanted loom") to educational tools. For the first time, useful data could be obtained about the variations of the electroencephalogram (EEG) simultaneously in terms of space and time. Educational these systems undoubtedly were, and in the hands of their proponents, they served as "hunch generators" about the nature of the mysterious quasi-rhythmic activity that we call the EEG. Most of the systems were complex, and few, if any, were exported from their innovator's laboratory. In part the purpose of this volume is to determine whether the information-processing capability of inexpensive digital computers will move us from education to enlightenment.

It must be conceded that the EEG is essentially a low data rate signal. The electrical generators, whatever they may be, are usually protected from the electroencephalographers's probes by skin, scalp, cerebral spinal fluid (CSF), and the conductive soup in which the cells in aggregate are immersed. If we accept that in the spontaneous EEG there are no useful signals above 100 Hz and, if we assume that 20 channels are independently connected to surface electrodes, then we have a signal which, according to the Nyquist theorem, can be completely described by 4000 samples per second. This is about the rate required to specify good-quality speech in a telephone system. Even when evoked potentials are considered, the data rate is not much more than 10 times better than the conditions for the raw EEG signal. If one then adds to these rather modest data rates the constraint that one cannot repeat an experiment an indefinite number of times since the biological preparation is always changing—certainly because of its nature, and perhaps because of the stimulation that we are applying—it should not surprise us that the information so far obtained from the EEG has yielded few of the secrets of sophisticated brain function.

An early justification for toposcopic techniques [3] was that the classical technique of measuring a few isolated variables against time was neither practical nor justified. It was also recognized [1] that a complete representation of EEG brain electrical activity requires a minimum of five dimensions: the classical x, y, z spatial dimensions, at least one electrical parameter, and time. These constraints, when combined with the fact that n electrodes can present information to $(n^2 - n)/2$ channels, indicated to early workers the magnitude of the task with which they were confronted. We may reasonably speak of the early toposcopes (with the exception of a few that did not operate in real time) as only existing in the 10 years B.C. (before computers). In the earliest types, accuracy was only obtained in the x and y dimensions. There was generally no ability to measure amplitude, and the only useful indication of frequency was the ability that these devices had to draw attention to a phase reversal focus. The only survivor of these early devices appears to be the dot-density topogram [4] of Barlow, which makes use of computer technology. These simplistic systems became useful only when time was reintroduced as a parameter by making recordings on moving film [5,6]. Because of the need to present the data aligned along a vertical axis in order to see time shifts, the topological relationships in these devices were confined generally to a single line of electrodes placed along the head. Typical of the next development in topographic techniques were the "chronotopograms" of Rémond. Here again the output was either a snapshot of the activity at a single instant of time or, in Petsche's system, a plot of activity as a function of time in a limited linear space. These systems all pointed out the essential difficulty of contour maps either in terms of time or voltage. They are an ideal way of indicating on two-dimensional paper the height of mountains or depth of valleys, and they are useful to indicate slowly changing data such as the isobars on a weather map. If, however, the brain electrical activity is changing rapidly, and by this I mean changing at EEG rates, either the number of maps must be increased dramatically, with a consequent difficulty in interpretation, or the interval between contours must be rather coarse. Attempts to improve contour presentation by color or by computer symbols have not overcome this fundamental problem. If, however, contouring is combined with one of the other methods of signal analysis, such as frequency analysis, then the average activity over an integration period of a few seconds can be described by using various degrees of shading if the system is monochromatic or by the attribution of color to particular frequencies if a suitable presentation is available. A number of such systems have been made and represent a useful addition to the electroencephalographer's armamentarium. They suffer, however, from the weakness of all transforms between the time domain and frequency domain, that is, that somewhere in the process, integration over a time period occurs and, because the octave range of an EEG is high (although its bandwidth is low), it is difficult to choose an appropriate interval. If 4 seconds (which is a commonly used time value) is chosen, only four samples are available at 1 Hz, and the well-known difficulties of splice effect can significantly reduce the confidence which one may have in these transforms of signals at very low frequencies. Nonetheless, toposcopic systems using this type of transform represent a substantial improvement over those where instantaneous data are presented, if only because they reduce the large mass of data to manageable proportions.

One class of systems that was developed in the B.C. era and which has been resurrected is the spiral scan toposcope of Walter and Shipton. These have been described in an early form [3] and also in a greatly simplified modern version [7]. These are powerful instruments for studying the complexities of the normal EEG because they preserve frequency and phase information and do not depend on conventional frequency transforms. The early version was very complex and had all the problems of reliability and stability associated with vacuum tube and analog systems. The original machine used 22 channels, the outputs of each of these brilliance modulated a cathode ray tube. The 22 tubes were so placed as to represent a plan view of the head, and electrode positions were indicated on an edge-lit transparent screen. Frequency and phase were indicated by means of a radial time base common to all tubes which was rotated by means of an electromechanical servo mechanism. In these devices, if speed of rotation coincides with any multiple of the signal frequency, a stationary pattern results. Frequency is determined from a knowledge of the rotational speed of the servo, and means are provided for indicating this rate. The time relations between signals in different channels can be directly observed. The display is photographed with an exposure time of several sweeps of the time base. An apparent improvement in signal-to-noise ratio results from the fact that signals not integrally related to sweep speed do not appear at the time bearing in successive traces. The appearance of a typical trace is shown in Figure 12.1*A*. Means were provided to fire a stimulus generator when the sweep passed a fiduciary mark, usually "12 o'clock." This version of the toposcope was well suited to the observation of evoked potentials since locking to the stimulus in all channels was automatic.

In the second version of this toposcope the radial time base was replaced by a circular sweep that increased in diameter during the camera exposure (the display was mistakenly called helical and the misnomer appears to have stuck). In the first version there were 24 lines per exposure, irrespective of sweep speed, this being controlled in the same manner as the early equipment. Signals

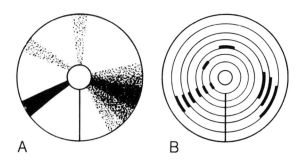

Figure 12.1. *A.* The display features of the original Walter/Shipton toposcope. As can be seen, the radial scan produces ambiguities when presented with short duration signals. *B.* The ability of the helical scan system to discriminate between signals of slightly different frequency is easily observed.

which have an integral relationship to the rotation speed would appear at the same angular bearing on successive sweeps but with changing radius. If the relationship was not integral but departed by even a small amount from a whole number, a spiral would result, and very accurate estimations of relative frequencies could be made. Another major problem of this system was that the camera exposure could not always be related to the signal, and thus some of the features obtained by this technique were fortuitous. In 1981, a revised version of this device was designed and built using a combination of analog and digital technology. An outline of the system is presented in Figure 12.2. This system had a number of advantages compared to the earlier device. First, a sample of 12.5 seconds of data could be accumulated and studied at will so that photography was only required when the operator was satisfied that the desired features were under observation. A further advantage was that the system was extremely simple and a 9- or 16- channel version required only a standard oscilloscope as the display. The operation of this system is shown in Figure 12.3. The method has probably little value in clinical medicine but has elucidated a number of features of the normal human alpha rhythm. It does of course have disadvantages. It is relatively ambiguous in its measurements of amplitude and it is not possible to interpolate between the electrodes; thus the resolution in terms of space is limited. Further spatial accuracy is probably unjustified in studies with surface electrodes because of the "smearing" that occurs as a result of the electrolytic nature of the pathway between signal source and electrode. This system is inexpensive, reliable, and simple to operate. The version currently in use is being extended to permit easier time measurements and to increase the period in which data can be collected without interruption.

A criticism leveled at the early toposcopes is that they present data in a form unsuited to quantification. In fact, until the advent of Duffy's significance probability mapping [8], statistical analysis of the EEG depended largely on computer storage of raw data and subsequent (usually off-line) processing. The analyses ranged from simple tables of significance to complex multivariate analyses. Many procedures were typically hampered by the small population available, by the lack of normative data, and by the imprecision of many of the measures. In any event, the end product was often a plethora of numbers that approached or surpassed the complexity of the raw record.

The helical scan toposcope frequently presented startlingly clear evidence

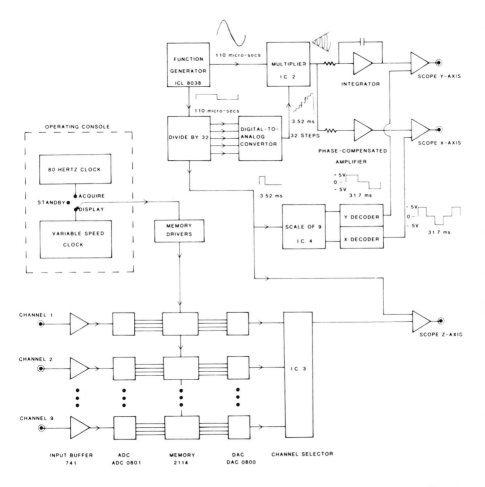

Figure 12.2. A block diagram of the new version of the helical scan toposcope. Signals from nine EEG channels are digitized and stored in a memory which is clocked at low frequency (80 Hz). For display purposes, the memory is read at speeds determined by a variable high-speed clock. The sweeps are produced by a function generator running at 9K Hz. These are modulated as a function of sweep number by the multiplier. Position information is indicated by a pair of decoders in the *x* and *y* planes. From "A Modern Frequency and Phase Indicating Toposcope" published EEG Journal 1981: Vol. 52/Issue 6:659–662.

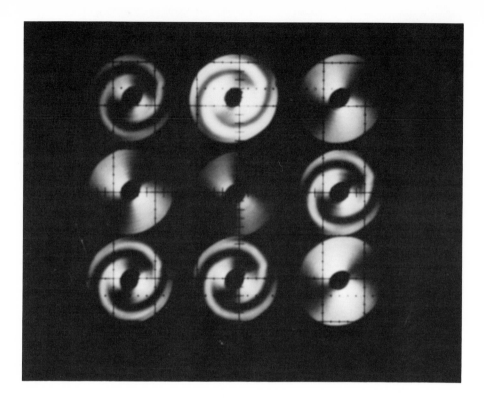

Figure 12.3. The appearance of the helical scan toposcope when fed with a series of simulated alpha waves. At the beginning of the scan (spot nearest the center) all channels were fed with a 9.0 Hz sine wave signal. At approximately halfway through the traces, the frequency in four channels was reduced. The resulting spirals clearly indicate this. Frequency is approximately 9 Hz, equivalent to 7 seconds of data. The top center trace is fed with signal at one-fifth the amplitude of all other traces.

of interaction between the cerebral hemispheres, a subject of interest both to the clinician and to the researcher. It is probably only the lack of appropriate statistical method that has prevented its wide use. It may be that statistical verification of data has become an end in itself. Numbers are not (Lord Kelvin notwithstanding) the only route to knowledge. An analogy can be found in the analysis of handwriting. It is exceedingly difficult to represent a signature by a polynomial; a bank clerk can quickly recognize a valid or invalid signature even in the presence of considerable artifact.

The introduction of significance probability mapping and related techniques has greatly changed the outlook for toposcopic methods in clinical and experimental medicine because it is now possible to make useful statistical statements about EEGs. The method is described by Duffy [9]. Its application depends on computer technology, since a point-by-point statistical comparison between a population data base and an individual record is computed and then displayed in spatial coordinates with color used to indicate the statistically significant differences. The use of this and closely related techniques is the major subject of this book, and it would be repetitious to do more than emphasize the range of clinical conditions in which they have given promising results. Schizophrenia, lead poisoning, and dyslexia, although widely different in their neurological manifestations, seem to be identifiable by the method.

This is not to say, nor have its proponents claimed, that topographic mapping is free from difficulties. The use of color, because it is so dramatic, may influence the electroencephalographer in subtle ways, and shading between one hue and another is hard to quantify. Prosaically, too, the use of color inhibits publication by increasing page and reprint costs.

There is also the problem of independence between points obtained by interpolation. The brain does not have a smooth surface, and the orientation of signal sources near the surface presents a classical physiological dilemma. However, the use of many points may be esthetically pleasing and the images may suggest comparison with x-ray-based displays. Whether such comparisons between methods that show structure and methods that show function are valid (or useful) is unclear. Nor has the problem of artifact rejection been solved. Computers cannot yet discriminate with any degree of confidence between brain and extracerebral potentials. Advanced display and measurement techniques must be fed with data that have been censored by the electroencephalographer. Too often we hear that "60 seconds of artifact free EEG were fed into. . ." The treatment of the EEG as a more-or-less stationary time series may in part be due to the engineer's ability to handle such signals with facility.

This survey has only touched on the implications of these new statistical and computer-based toposcopes. I have not considered their use in evoked potential studies, and though many of the advances in EEG technology have in the past few years come from the study of these events, EEG itself has been relatively static. There has been, it is true, renewed interest in spectra (often displayed topographically) but, by and large, "eyeballing" has remained the technique of choice. This book gives us a view of the future where the combined efforts of many workers in many disciplines promise to refine the study of the mysterious potentials that intrigue us so much. Will we go from education to enlightenment? The question was well posed by Grey Walter [3] when, at the conclusion of the description of the first large-scale toposcope, he wrote: "the warp and the woof of cerebral function may have different hues. Enlightenment in one field may be balanced by bewilderment in another, but it would be foolish to expect the enchanted loom to weave a fustian fabric."

REFERENCES

1. Petsche, H. EEG Topography. In Rémond A., ed., Handbook of EEG & Clinical Neurophysiology. Amsterdam: Elsevier, 1972; 5:5–54.

2. Walter, W.G. The Living Brain. New York: WW Norton, 1953.
3. Walter, W.G. and Shipton, H.W. A new toposcopic display system. EEG Clin. Neurophysiol. 1951; 3:281–292.
4. Dubinsky, J., and Barlow, J.S. A simple dot-density topogram for EEG. EEG Clin. Neurophysiol. 1980; 48:473–477.
5. Petsche, H. Die erfassung von form und verhalten der potentialfelder an der hernoberfloche durch eine kombinierte EEG-toposkopische methode. Wien Z. Nervenheilk, 1967; 25:373–387.
6. Bekkering, D.H. The EEG-magnetograph and the EEG spectrograph: Apparatus for fast poly-analysis. EEG Clin. Neurophysiol, 1956; 8:721.
7. Shipton, H.W. and Armstrong, G. A modern frequency and phase indicating toposcope. EEG Clin. Neurophysiol, 1981; 52:659–662.
8. Duffy, F.H., Burchfiel, J.L. and Lombroso, C.T. Brain electrical activity mapping (BEAM): A new method for extending the clinical utility of EEG and evoked potential data. Ann. Neurol. 1979; 5:309–321.
9. Duffy, F.H., Bartels, P.H., and Burchfiel, J.L. Significance probability mapping: An aid in the topographic analysis of brain electrical activity. EEG Clin. Neurophysiol. 1981; 51:455–462.

13

Classification Strategies for Topographic Mapping Data

Peter H. Bartels and Hubert G. Bartels

Electroencephalograph (EEG) recordings provide an extraordinarily rich source of information. It is difficult even for an experienced encephalographer to extract by visual inspection of the multiple waveforms all the diagnostically relevant information. When presented in pictorial form and as a time sequence of two-dimensional images, the perception of underlying patterns is made easier; this accounts for the interest in topographic mappings of EEG recordings. It should be understood that in interpolated maps a much better pictorial presentation is achieved, but that no additional information over that provided by the individual points sampled by the electrodes is gained. However, the maps lend themselves ideally to the recognition of discriminating features, and thus aid in the full and effective use of diagnostic clues.

The human eye/brain complex is excellent at detecting themes underlying such topographic maps in patients with different diagnoses. Even when these themes are very subtle, and constitute "poor patterns," an encephalographer will, after exposure to many instances of such maps, almost instantly recognize the identifying feature complex and arrive at a diagnosis. It is only poorly understood exactly how an experienced encephalographer might do this. As a rule, even the successful diagnostician is hard put to it to verbalize the discriminating criteria. It is possible that the recognition of such subtle pattern differences eventually emerges as a skill, rather than as an analytical process. There is no doubt though that human diagnosticians do very well in this task, and that they are doing better by viewing topographic maps than routine EEG recordings.

Yet, the diagnostic skill is tied to individuals, who may find it hard to transmit their skill to others. There is a high degree of subjectivity left in the diagnostic assessment. The uniformity of assessment in different diagnostic centers may not be as controlled as one might like. These considerations support efforts to assist encephalographic diagnosis by computer-based expert systems. It is the purpose of this chapter to survey some of the considerations that enter into the design of computer-based classification programs, evaluation of diagnostic clues and features, and of automated classification procedures.

Topographic mapping of brain electrical activity is based on data descriptive of the spatial distribution of evoked potentials, of the temporal distribution, of the spectral distribution, and of the multiple dependencies among all these. The primary measurements in brain electrical activity mapping are voltage values recorded as a function of location, time, and frequency. There are numerous efficient schemes for a reduction of this massive volume of data to a manageable size. One such approach is to define "features," quantities descriptive of specific properties of the dynamic process that is being mapped. An example for such a feature is the symmetry of brain wave propagation, expressed by a single value. Such a feature fulfills a very useful purpose. It summarizes by its single value a great many individual voltage readings, and thus accomplishes a valuable data reduction. At the same time the feature provides a descriptive entity that can be directly related to a diagnostic interpretation.

One may define a great many features, each descriptive of and summarizing certain aspects of the recorded process. Not all these features can be expected to contribute useful, diagnostically discriminating information. Therefore, the next data reduction step involves a selection of a small subset of features useful for a given diagnostic problem. Only this set of features is used to represent a patient. The different features are kept in an arbitrary, but consistent, ordering. The selected set of values p-tuple in number, is also referred to as a "feature vector." In the following, patients are always considered as represented by a feature vector.

The feature vector actually represents a point in a p-dimensional feature space; but the terms "patient," "feature vector," and "point in the p-dimensional feature space" are often used as synonyms.

This chapter surveys the methodology of classification, i.e., how those features may be used to assign a given patient to a certain diagnostic category. The practice of classification encompasses an extremely wide range of both human, and scientific-technological activities. We are specifically concerned with objective classification procedures, i.e., with procedures where decision rules and object assignments are derived in an objective, automated manner [1–4]. Such procedures are based on measurements, allow reproducible results, and permit an assessment of the performance of the classification rule.

In any event, each brain electrical activity map [5,6] is condensed from thousands of measurements to maybe two hundred features, and even though effective feature selection methods may allow one to find a small subset of features that offers adequate discrimination for diagnostic classification, one is still dealing with multivariate data. A brief introduction to multivariate data is therefore given, to introduce some terms and concepts.

MULTIVARIATE DATA: GEOMETRIC REPRESENTATION

Feature vectors are used to describe brain maps. They are multivariate data. Most everyone is familiar with univariate data: every observation is expressed by just one single number. In multivariate data every observation is expressed by a set of numbers, arranged in an arbitrary but consistent order. A patient could, for instance, be described by a four-tuple of values, such as age, weight, height, blood pressure. The decisive difference between univariate analysis and multivariate analysis is that in the multivariate case one considers the mutual dependence of all the variable values.

In univariate statistics a sample is described by two "descriptive statistics," the sample mean and the sample variance. When one goes to the simplest multivariate situation, the observation of two variables on each object, the sample is described by five descriptive statistics: the sample mean for the first variable (or the first component in the bivariate feature vector), the variance for the first variable, the sample mean for the second variable, the variance for the second variable, and the covariance between the two variables.

The transition from one-dimensional to two-dimensional to p-dimensional data is strictly formal. One must not think of "dimensions" in the sense of "extension in physical space." Rather, each dimension, variable, or feature merely represents a different property of the object that is being described. One can of course easily think of p different, relevant properties of an object. The object is thus represented in a p-dimensional feature space. For a mathematical treatment it really does not make much difference how many properties one is considering. For example, one may readily compute a distance between two points in a multivariate space. In a bivariate case everybody remembers Pythagoras: the distance d is given by the square root over the difference in coordinate values for the two points for the first variable $(a_1 - a_2)$, squared, plus the difference in value of the second variable $(b_1 - b_2)$, squared. It is known as the "Euclidean distance."

$$d = \sqrt{(a_1 - a_2)^2 + (b_1 - b_2)^2}$$

In going to a trivariate case we merely have under the square root three differences, squared. And, in going to a p-dimensional case, the distance is computed as the square root taken over the sum of p squared differences in coordinate values for the two points:

$$d = \sqrt{(a_1 - a_2)^2 + (b_1 - b_2)^2 + \ldots (p_1 - p_2)^2}$$

There are two ways to represent multivariate data. One may write down arithmetic expressions, or one may prefer a geometric/graphic representation.

Clearly, when one wants to compute numerical results one has to use arithmetic representations.

To write down the full algebraic equations for a probability distribution is practical only for the univariate and maybe the bivariate case. For situations involving more variables one has to use matrix notation. In matrix notation the dispersion of the multivariate data set is expressed in a variance-covariance matrix. Matrix notation allows one to write down and do computations on multivariate distributions with great simplicity. But, in many situations a conceptualization of multivariate data in geometric/graphic terms is extremely helpful [7]. In introducing such a geometric/graphic representation, it is best to start with some concepts from univariate statistics and extend them to the bivariate case. All the basic concepts can then still be visualized on paper. From the bivariate case the extension to the p-variate case is simple.

In the univariate case, the distribution of observed values is often represented by a bell-shaped curve, the gaussian distribution. The peak of that curve indicates the mean value, and the spread of the curve indicates the variance. One may define an interval on the abscissa, extending symmetrically from the mean value, such that 95% of all observations can be expected to fall within its range. This interval is known as the "tolerance region," an expression originating from applications in quality control.

In the bivariate case the tolerance region is an ellipse. Three situations are of interest: noncorrelation, positive correlation, and negative correlation. When the two variables are not correlated the covariance is zero, and the axes of the ellipse are parallel to the ordinate and abscissa, i.e., the variable axes. The shape of the ellipse is determined by the variances of the two variables: if the variance of the variable plotted along the abscissa is larger, then the larger axis of the ellipse is horizontally oriented.

If there is a covariance, the axes of the tolerance ellipse are tilted, with a positive slope for the larger axis in case of positive covariance, and a negative slope in case of negative covariance. The bivariate case lends itself to the introduction of some concepts and terms commonly used in multivariate analysis. The axes of the ellipse are also called the "eigenvectors," and the variances in direction of the eigenvectors are also called the "eigenvalues." A bivariate distribution thus has two eigenvectors and two eigenvalues.

The area of the ellipse expresses the total variability in the bivariate data set; it is given by a single number, the "determinant." When the dependence between the values of the two variables is very strong, the ellipse becomes increasingly slender, until in the extreme case of perfect correlation it degenerates into a sloped line. The second eigenvalue then goes to zero.

To extend the bivariate representation to p dimensions is straightforward. The elliptical tolerance region becomes an ellipsoid—in the three-dimensional case an ellipsoid with three different axes, in the p-dimensional case a hyperellipsoid with p different axes. The position of the ellipsoid's center marks the multivariate mean vector. The ellipsoid's shape expresses the covariance structure of the feature vector's components: it is determined by the eigenvalues of the multivariate distribution. The ellipsoid's orientation is determined by the eigenvectors of the multivariate distribution, which also reflect the covariance structure. The volume of the ellipsoid expresses the overall dispersion of the p-variate data. It is expressed by the determinant of the variance-covariance matrix.

Whether one considers a multivariate distribution as a p-dimensional point cloud, as a p-dimensional balloon, or as a hyper-ellipsoid is all quite immaterial. What is of value is that one has a way of thinking about the relationship between different distributions in a high-dimensional space. It aids greatly in understanding the rationale in many of the multivariate analytical approaches, for instance, discrimination and classification. One can imagine two multivariate distributions as two balloons, and one can imagine surfaces separating them—surfaces that could represent decision boundaries for classification. One can imagine directions along which two distributions are maximally separated, directions which would make good discriminant functions. One can see how different variance-covariance matrices in two distributions would be represented by two "balloons" of different shape, size, and orientation, which would affect the tilt one would want to give a separating plane in the feature space. Also, the geometric/graphic representation allows one to think about effective ways of reducing the dimensionality. For instance, one could imagine a number of clouds in the sky, and the sun casting their shadows onto the earth. There could well be a direction for the sun such that all the shadows are clearly separated on the ground: for our multivariate data this means that a reduction in dimensionality from three-space to two-space is possible, without loss of discrimination quality.

CLASSIFICATION

Classification means that an entity is being assigned to one of two or more possible categories. The procedure presumes that (1) categories have been established, and (2) a prescription has been developed to accomplish the classification into one of these categories. The establishment of categories may be based on either "external truth" or the "data structure." In the first case it is unequivocally known from other sources into which diagnostic category the object should be placed. What remains to be done is the finding of features that will distinguish between patients from different diagnostic categories. The procedures for this are known as "supervised learning" [8]. In the second case the observed patients are a priori all members of the same category. What one would like to know is whether the observed group is indeed homogeneous, or whether it contains subgroups. This determination is made by observing the data structure. For example, if the value distribution for one or more features shows a pronounced bimodality one might draw the conclusion that the patients falling into different modes might indeed be considered to represent different subcategories. They certainly are different. The situations underlying supervised learning, and unsupervised learning applications are schematically shown in Figure 13.1. In the first case one has two distributions, known to represent different categories, and one is looking for the best discriminating features. In the second case one has only one distribution, and one is searching for an indication of inhomogeneity, or different modes, to define subsets of data to be used as categories.

For a few features one can, find such inhomogeneities by visual inspection of plotted data. When the bimodality is expressed as only a slight shift in a higher dimensional feature space, computer algorithms known as unsupervised learning algorithms [9–12] may be used for the search. However, these algorithms are designed to find inhomogeneities; whether the detected subclasses are statistically significant is another matter. One should not accept a subcategorization unless it passes a multivariate significance test [13]. Once a group is found to consist of subclasses, the identified members can be treated as belonging to different groups, and may then be entered into the supervised learning procedures.

SUPERVISED LEARNING

In supervised learning procedures, representative samples from each category are identified and assembled into training, or learning, sets. Development of classification procedure requires at least two such sets. For classification algorithms that can handle multiple categories, there have to be as many training sets as there are categories. For every member of a training set the full complement of features, which can be substantial, is computed. It is easy to imagine that topographic mapping data might have several hundred different features. It is of course totally impractical to use all these in a classification rule. The next step in supervised learning, therefore, is usually a reduction of the number of features to those that show potential for discrimination [14–17]. This begins

A 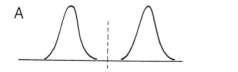   B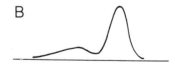

Figure 13.1. *A.* Supervised learning methods apply when two data sets known to belong to different categories are given. The task is to find a set of features which separate the two data sets so that the tolerance limits of their feature distributions have as little overlap as possible. Misclassifications can then be avoided. *B.* Unsupervised learning methods must be applied when there is no prior information available about the homogeneity of a data set. One searches for features that reveal a modality, or inhomogeneity that would indicate the presence of subsets of data.

with a search for features whose value distributions in the training sets show statistically significant differences. Significant differences are a necessary but not a sufficient condition for selection. Such differences merely identify good candidates for discriminating features. Statistical differences indicate that the confidence regions for the mean values in the different training sets do not overlap. To be useful as a discriminator the feature should have nonoverlapping tolerance regions for the two training sets. This first step in "dimensionality reduction" usually results in 40–50 features with discrimination potential. From these features other algorithms will be used to select a small subset of the best discriminating ones. No more and if possible fewer than 10, discriminating features are best for the derivation of a classification rule.

A classification rule is derived by some algorithm of the form:

If the value of feature X is larger than, or equal to, a threshold T, assign the object to category I.

If the value of feature X is smaller than the threshold T, assign the object to category II.

The selected best features are very often combined into a linear combination, such as:

$$D = w_3 X_3 + w_5 X_5 - w_8 X_8 + w_2 X_2$$

and the classification rule becomes:

If $D \geq T$, assign object to category I.
If $D < T$, assign object to category II.

Other classification rules may take the form:

If the value of $X_3 \geq T_3$ and, if the value of $X_5 < T_5$ and, if the value of $X_{14} \geq T_{14}$, then assign object to category I.
Otherwise, assign object to category II.

All the items in training sets are then classified, and one counts the proportion of correctly and incorrectly classified objects.

In the next step the classification rule is applied to data of known categories, not included in the training sets. These data are often called object, or test, sets. One tests the classification rule for general validity and consistency on new data to ensure that one did not fit the rule to the training sets. There is always a danger that one tailors a classification rule to the training sets. Such a rule might perform badly on new data, which implies that the system has been overtrained. The sequence of steps in supervised learning is summarized in Table 13.1.

Table 13.1   Supervised Learning

Learning Set I and Learning Set II
Compute all features
Evaluate all features
Select best features
Weight features
Derive classification rule
Apply rule to test sets

SAMPLE SIZE/DIMENSIONALITY RATIO

Overtraining is apt to occur when certain precautions are not taken, such as failure to maintain an adequate sample size/dimensionality ratio. Every component in the feature vector describes a certain object property and is in fact a random variable forming a dimension in the feature space. The sample size/dimensionality ratio describes how many observations per variable were recorded. Since for each object the full feature vector is recorded, this assesses how many objects were examined per dimension of the feature space. It should be understood that sample size per object category/dimensionality is actually meant by sample size/dimensionality ratio, the customary term in the literature. Too low a sample size/dimensionality ratio leads to spurious classification rules, as demonstrated by the following extreme example.

It is obvious that if one had only two observations and observed only a single object property, one could always separate the two observations. Using the learning set only, one could claim 100% classification success. This estimate of classifier performance is misleading. The sample size/dimensionality ratio is only 1:1. Or if only two variables form a feature space and there are two objects in each training set, one can nearly always separate the pairs with 100% classification success (Figure 13.2*A,B*).

Guidelines for a choice of appropriate sample size/dimensionality ratio vary in the literature [18,19]. The classic study by Foley [20] suggests a minimum ratio of 3:1. Practical experience in the automated classification of data from medical diagnostic imagery and other fields of pattern recognition suggests sample size/dimensionality ratios of 10:1 as useful, and of 20:1 as providing reliable decision rules. What sample size/dimensionality ratio one should maintain depends on the intended use of the decision rule. If plenty of test set data are available, one could quickly ascertain whether the decision rule had indeed been tailored too closely to the training set data only, and corrective action could be taken. Under such circumstances one may well start a first, iterative development of a decision rule at a sample size/dimensionality ratio of as little as 5:1. If no test set data are available much more stringent requirements for sample size/dimensionality must be met, such as a ratio of 50:1, so that the estimate of the error rate is realistic.

PERFORMANCE OF A CLASSIFIER

The performance of a classifier may be tested in a number of ways. Three widely used methods are as follows:

1. The resubstitution method. Here, the training set data are used to derive the classification rule. The rule is then applied again to the training sets to classify every object. This approach leads to an underestimation of the error rate to be expected in an application of the classification rule to new data. The underestimation gets worse the lower the sample size/dimensionality ratio. If one decides to use the resubstitution method for a performance test one should have a sample size/dimensionality ratio of at least 50:1. Even then error rate estimates are apt to be 10–15% too low.
2. The training set/test set approach. Here the available data are partitioned. Half to two-thirds are used as training set data, and the remainder are held in reserve to test the classification rule. This is a safe procedure and the method of choice, but even here a sample size/dimensionality ratio of at least 5:1, and better of 10:1 or 20:1, should be maintained in the training sets.
3. The hold-one-out method, also known as jack-knifing [21]: Here, training is done using all feature vectors except one. The single withheld feature vector is then classified. This process is now exhaustively repeated for every feature vector. This method is held to provide very good estimates of the performance of a classifier. It is often the only feasible method with very small data sets and under this condition may indeed be the best approach. It has recently come under some criticism, and practical experience confirms that the obtained error rate estimates may not be as reliable as the early users of the technique believed.

CLASSIFICATION PROCEDURES

It is useful in a discussion of classification procedures to distinguish between classification constraints, classification algorithms, and classification strategies. In practice, they increase in importance in that order.

Classification Constraints

Classifier constraints affect the manner in which a threshold is established for discrimination. There is usually some overlap between the distribution functions for the discriminator values from, e.g., two training sets. When a decision threshold is set, a certain proportion (alpha) of objects from category I will erroneously be assigned to category II. And another proportion (beta) of objects

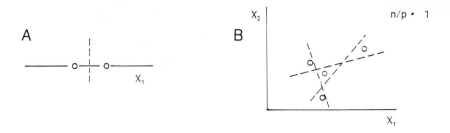

Figure 13.2. In situations where the sample size/dimensionality ratio *n /p* is only unity, one can practically always claim 100% classification success. Yet, the result is meaningless.

really belonging to category II will fall into the region below the threshold and will be erroneously classified as category I. The classifier constraints allow the designer of a decision procedure to control these errors. Three methods are commonly considered. These are the Neyman-Pearson constraint, the Bayes rule, and the minimax method [22].

In the Neyman-Pearson method one concentrates on one category only and determines the greatest error one would be willing to accept for that category. This is where one sets the threshold, whatever proportion of errors this might mean for the other category (Figure 13.3*A*).

In the Bayes approach the risk of error is distributed equally between two categories, and the threshold is set to equalize errors. In Figure 13.3*B* the threshold is set so that an equal proportion of observations from both categories is correctly classified, and likewise, that equal proportions are misclassified. Equal costs for misclassification are assumed.

The minimax method is sometimes used when very little prior information about the relative proportions of objects from either category is available. One adopts a minimax approach as a defense; the worst could always happen. The threshold for category I is set such that under the most unfavorable circumstances a certain error rate will not be exceeded. Assuming the distribution to the left in Figure 13.3*C* represented category I, the worst case would be the highest curve, i.e., highest prior probability for the occurrence of objects from category I. Then one does the same for category II, and between these two limits one minimizes the maximum error that could possibly occur in both categories. It clearly is a damage-limiting posture; if the worst case does not happen one has not taken advantage of this. But, if the worst case does happen, one still classifies with a limited error rate.

Classification Algorithms

A large number of different classification algorithms have been developed, often to satisfy a particular problem. One therefore has the option to select an algorithm that best fits one's own data classification problem.

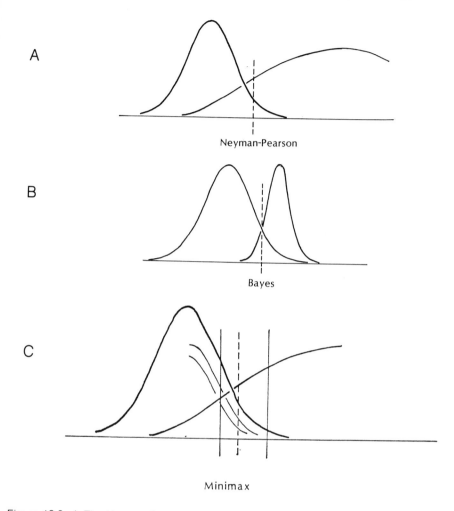

Figure 13.3. *A.* The Neyman-Pearson constraint considers one distribution only. The largest acceptable error has been determined for the distribution on the left, as has the threshold set to that point. This is done regardless of whatever errors for objects from the distribution on the right might now be misclassified. *B.* In the Bayes approach, the proportion of misclassifications is made equal for both categories and the boundary is set accordingly. Equal cost of misclassification has been assumed in the example. *C.* The minimax method is employed when one knows very little about the prior probabilities of objects from both distributions, and when one wishes to take a defensive stand. One sets the threshold so that for each distribution of maximum acceptable error is never exceeded, even when the prior probability for the category should reach its largest possible value. This is indicated by the series of curves for the distribution on the left: the highest curve would constitute the case where the maximum error might occur. Between these two limiting maximum errors for both distributions lies the minimum for the overall classification error.

A classification algorithm uses quantitative measurements taken from objects to map them into a certain region of a feature space. With certain regions being allocated to different categories, the algorithm thus classifies objects into different categories. Some examples of classification algorithms are linear discriminant analysis, quadratic discriminant analysis [21,23], maximum likelihood classifiers [24], the k-nearest neighbor algorithm [25,26] algorithms applying separating hyperplanes, nonparametric partitioning methods, potential function classifiers, and distance classifiers.

Linear Discriminant Analysis

Linear discriminant analysis is one of the oldest and most widely used procedures to assign objects to one or more different categories in an objective manner [27–29]. For each data set the mean vectors and the variance-covariance matrix are computed. Then a projection of all feature vectors from a p-dimensional discriminant space onto a single direction, i.e., into a univariate representation, is made. This direction is chosen so that it provides maximum separation for feature vectors from the different categories. It is formed as a linear combination of the original features, each weighted according to its contribution toward category separation, and it is called a linear discriminant function. For each feature vector a "discriminant score" is computed that reflects onto what location on the discriminant function a given feature vector has been projected. If the discriminant score falls below a certain threshold, the feature vector is assigned to one class; if it has a larger score, it is assigned to another class. A two-dimensional example is shown in Figure 13.4.

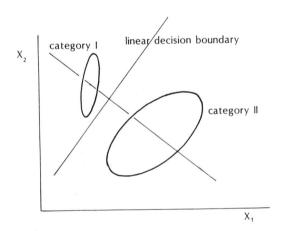

Figure 13.4. In this two-dimensional example, the tolerance regions for two categories are shown. A discriminant function, extending from the upper left to the lower right, has been defined, and a linear decision boundary has now separated the feature space into two regions associated with classification into category I or category II.

The result is that the feature space is divided by plane decision surfaces into regions assigned to different categories. Different discriminant algorithms offer a great many options for the selection of variables, for instance, a stepwise selection and tryout procedure to find the best discriminating variables or criteria for assessment of category separation and the selection of weighting coefficients for the original feature vector components. In linear discriminant analysis it is usually assumed that the variance-covariance matrices of the different categories are equal; this is practically never the case. Fortunately the procedure is rather robust, i.e., results are not too seriously affected when differences in the categories' variance-covariance matrices do exist. When such differences are pronounced and especially when the mean vectors are not well separated in the feature space, one would do well to use a quadratic rather than a linear discriminant procedure.

Maximum Likelihood Classification

In maximum likelihood classification an object is assigned to the category for which its probability density is highest. This offers several advantages. For example, in situations where distributions show substantial overlap, regions can be identified for which membership in one category is more likely than in another. This is shown for a univariate example in Figure 13.5*B*; Figure 13.5*A* demonstrates how a simple discriminant function might set the threshold. The feature space is not simply divided into regions for different categories by plane surfaces. The distance of a feature vector from each category mean vector is actually measured in terms of the variance-covariance of that category. In maximum likelihood classification the feature space is no longer isometric: rather, distances are expressed in terms of each category's variance-covariance. For example, the marked point in Figure 13.6 is linearly much closer to the bivariate distribution to the left. Yet, it is outside that distribution's 90% tolerance region but inside the tolerance region of the more disperse distribution to the

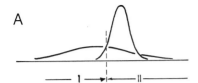 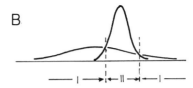

Figure 13.5. *A.* One-dimensional example of the effect on classification of a simple threshold setting, such as a linear discriminant score. All items to the left of the threshold are assigned to category I, all items to the right are assigned to category II, even though the probability density for category I is larger again at high values on the feature axis. *B.* A maximum likelihood classifier assigns objects to categories on the basis of the highest probability density, and thus sets nonlinear decision boundaries.

right. A maximum likelihood classifier assigns this point to the category on the right. The separating decision boundaries are highly nonlinear, as shown in Figure 13.7 for a Bayesian decision boundary.

The kNN Algorithm

The use of the k-nearest neighbor classifier algorithm, also known as the kNN classifier, is a nonparametric procedure; i.e., no assumptions are made about the multivariate distributions in each category. Its behavior is well studied, and kNN algorithms have been extensively used. A point in multivariate feature space is always assigned to the diagnostic category to which the majority of its neighboring points belong. If the feature vector components recorded for a given patient have values that position the patient in a region of the feature space where all neighbors belong to a given diagnostic category, the assignment is obvious and logical. On the other hand, if the feature vector components position the patient in a region where feature vectors representing different diagnostic categories occur, i.e., borderline cases, the kNN algorithm lets simple majority rule (Figure 13.8).

Two problems with the kNN algorithm are as follows: (1) The training sets feature vectors have to be retained in the computer, since each and every one is needed in the future to compute distances to new data points. This can

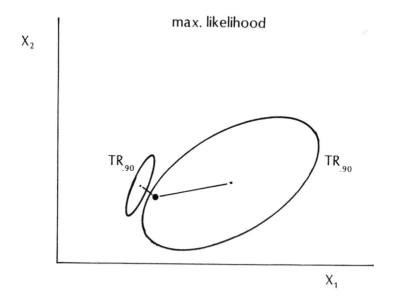

Figure 13.6. The maximum likelihood classifier considers the distortion of the feature space due to the variance-covariance structure of the data sets. Shown is the classification of the marked point into one of two distributions, defined by their 90% tolerance regions. It is assigned to the more disperse distribution to the right.

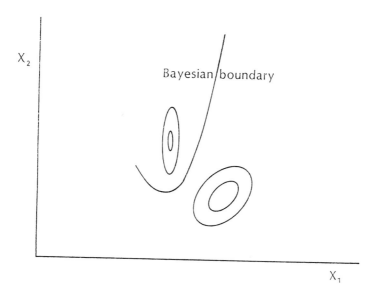

Figure 13.7. The Bayesian boundary provides a nonlinear decision boundary based on likelihood.

be awkward but is not a serious drawback. (2) Even though most textbooks refer to the kNN algorithm as nonparametric, this is not necessarily true. If one uses Euclidean distances to the nearest neighbors, the feature space is assumed to be isometric. One then comes close to a nonparametric procedure, yet the metric may be ill-fitted to the actual data distributions. Most data sets have significant correlations between the components of the feature vectors. This means that the feature space is stretched in accordance to the covariance structure of a training set. Two data points at a distance giving them the same probability density, i.e., at the same Mahalanobis distance [30], could have drastically different Euclidean distances from the group mean, Figure 13.9. Some kNN algorithms therefore offer, as a distance metric, the Mahalanobis distance, making the kNN algorithm a parametric procedure. Also the covariance structure in the feature space is usually quite different for the different training sets. The algorithms work with the "pooled covariance" structure, or the averaged covariance structure over all training sets. In some situations one then has all the disadvantages of a nonparametric procedure and all the problems of a parametric technique. A certain circumspection therefore is advised before one applies such an algorithm.

The DSELECT Algorithm

The DSELECT algorithm [31] was first developed in 1969. A similar algorithm was proposed by Henrichon and Fu, also in 1969 [32]. We have used our version of the DSELECT algorithm almost unchanged since 1969. Voss [33–35] describes a virtually identical algorithm. An identical algorithm is called "recursive partition generation" [36].

The algorithm is a nonparametric procedure, which leads to a binary decision sequence. At each decision node only one feature is utilized—that feature which allows the most profitable unequivocal classification of a subset of objects into a terminal node. All other objects are left in the remainder group, and a search for the best feature for splitting the remainder group is initiated. The DSELECT procedure generates a binary decision tree (Figure 13.10).

The DSELECT algorithm requires two training sets of feature files. Processing starts with the data for the first feature. The files from both training sets are merged. The feature values are ranked, but each feature value retains a tag, identifying it as having come from one or the other training set.

A threshold is moved through this ranked list starting at the lowest value. As long as feature values from only one training set are encountered, the threshold continues to advance. Upon encountering the first value belonging to the second training set, the previous threshold is temporarily stored and an exploratory threshold is advanced. If the encountered value is just an outlier and is followed by many more values from the original set, the single misclassification is accepted, and the process continues. The first stored temporary threshold is moved on, replacing the exploratory threshold. If, however, more values from the second training set continue to be encountered, the temporary thresh-

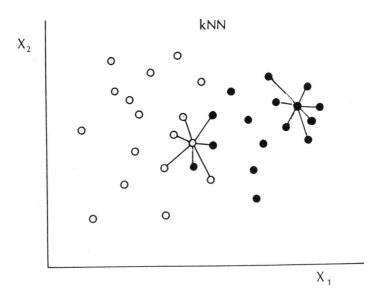

Figure 13.8. Schematic example of new data classification by the kNN rule. The new point at the center of its neighborhood on the right would be assigned to the black category; the new entry to the left would be assigned to the white category, by majority rule.

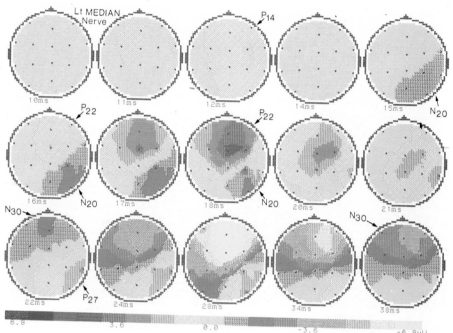

Plate 1. Bit-mapped color imaging of scalp potential fields to upper limb stimulation. Stimulation of left median nerve at wrist in a normal 22-year-old woman. Electrode sites indicated by black pixels. The latency of each map after stimulation is indicated in milliseconds at lower left. The zero baseline $\pm$ 0.4 μV appears in green. Voltage increments of 0.8 μV are represented by red yellow hues for negative and blue purple for positive as shown by the calibration scale. From Desmedt and Bourguet [6] (With permission from Elsevier Biomedical Press, Amsterdam).

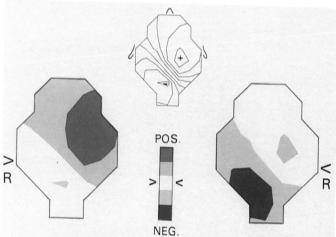

Plate 2. Effects of the choice of a real electrode as the reference for mapping of the instantaneous field of Figure 3.2A (copied as equipotential contour map in inset). The field distribution is displayed as color-coded equipotential area map using the left or the right mastoid as reference (arrowheads). Note how the suggestion of a "positive component, right anterior" is strong when the left mastoid was chosen, and that of a "negative component, left posterior" is strong when the right mastoid was chosen. Although the distribution is identical, the labeling is different in the maps.

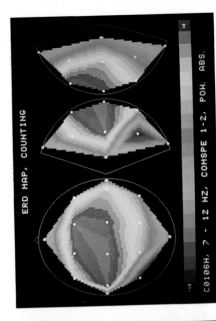

ERD MAP, SPONTANEOUS SPEECH

C0104H, 7 - 12 HZ, COMSPE 1-2, POW. ABS.

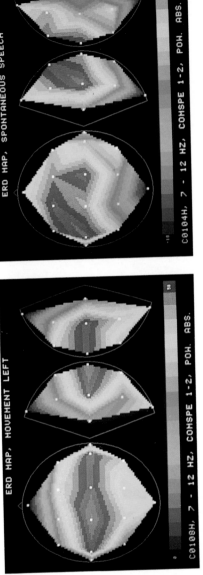

ERD MAP, MOVEMENT LEFT

C0108H, 7 - 12 HZ, COMSPE 1-2, POW. ABS.

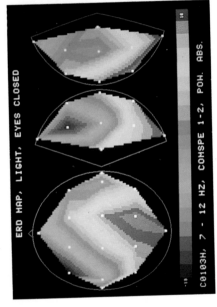

ERD MAP, COUNTING

C0106H, 7 - 12 HZ, COMSPE 1-2, POW. ABS.

ERD MAP, LIGHT, EYES CLOSED

C0103H, 7 - 12 HZ, COMSPE 1-2, POW. ABS.

Plate 3. ERD maps (lateral and top views) calculated in a healthy volunteer during voluntary, self-paced movement of the left hand (*upper left*), spontaneous speech (*upper right*), 1-sec light stimulation (*lower left*), and spontaneous counting (*lower right*). ERD scale in percentage. Dark blue minimal values; red, maximal values. Each map is scaled according to extreme values. Bipolar electrode positions. The interelectrode positions are marked.

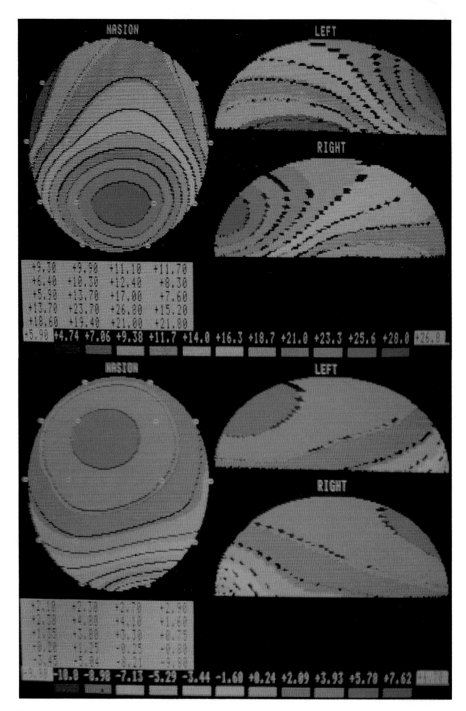

Plate 4. Examples of color display for spectra (*upper*) and for evoked potential voltage distribution (*lower*). The area displays include lateral right and left head views for spectra and evoked potentials. The displays come from a 15-year-old patient with a learning disorder. Note (*upper illustration*) slight asymmetry of alpha (8–12 Hz) spectral distribution with maximal intensity of voltage on the right. The evoked potential display (*lower illustration*) to binocular pattern shift (L.E.D.) shows a marked asymmetry of voltage distribution with maximum intensity in the right occipital-parietal region.

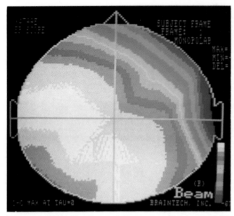

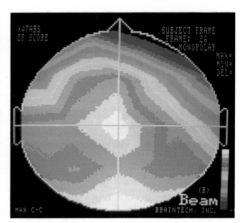

Plate 5. Distribution of the correlation coefficient between the AER of a reference population and a subject with a tumor in the right anterior quadrant.

Plate 6. Distribution of the maximum value of the correlation coefficient computed for the first 100 msec of the AER of the same subject of Figure 15.11.

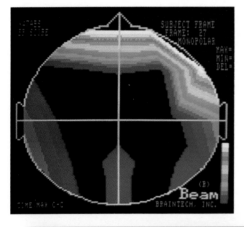

Plate 7. Distribution of the latencies where the maximum value of the correlation coefficient was measured in the first 100 msec of the EP. High values of this parameter indicate an increased latency of the EP.

Plate 8. Topographic distribution of alpha activity for one minute of EEG averaged across 20 subjects, shown for lateral view as depicted in Figure 16.1. Left-hand map is for alpha in the band 7 to 10 cps and right-hand map for band 10 to 13 cps. Color scale shows increasing magnitude of activity (square root of the power spectrum).

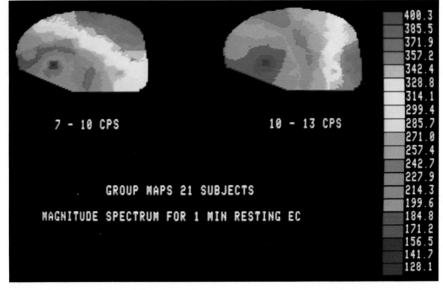

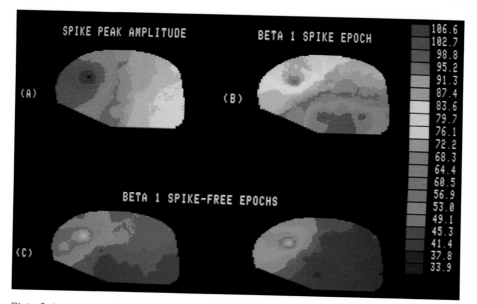

Plate 9. Interictal activity from a patient with complex partial epilepsy. *A.* The topography of the raw EEG at the peak of an interictal spike. *A* uses a bipolar scale such that negative microvolts are represented by blues and positive potentials by reds (same scale as shown on the right except for different values). *B.* The topography for beta activity (13–20 cps) from the magnitude spectrum for a 2.56-second epoch centered on the spike. *C.* The topography with same spectrum parameters except for epochs that were spike-free.

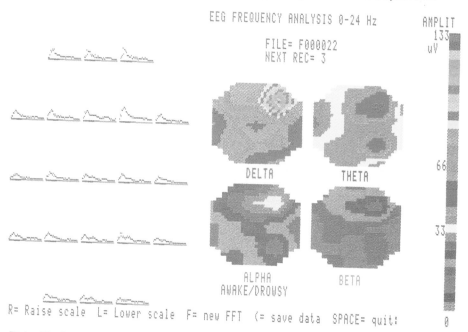

Plate 10. CET of a spike focus at Fp2, adolescent male. Note broad-band increase in power in the right frontal region. Power spectra from 21 channels (1–20 system) shown at left, using sec. epoch, 1–24 Hz. CETs of delta, theta, alpha, and beta bands at right; color scaled in square root of power.

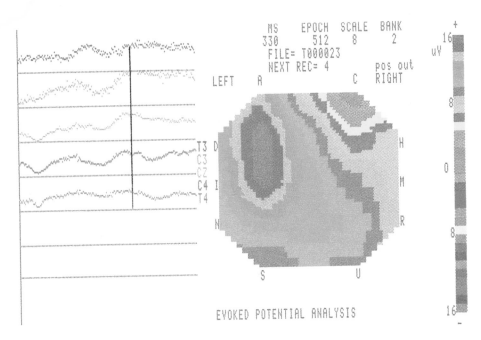

Plate 11. Same patient as Figure 18.3. CET of flash evoked potential (FEP), 21 channels, average of 100 trials, 512 msec epoch. Five channels shown at left (T3, C3, Cz, C4, T4). CET of FEP, latency 330 msec, at right. Color scale in microvolts.

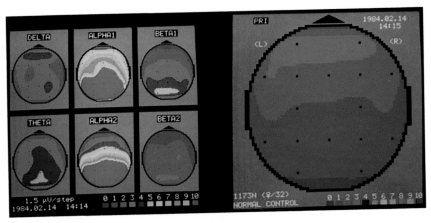

Plate 12. Six frequency domain equipotential maps (*left*) and PRI maps (*right*) from a healthy volunteer.

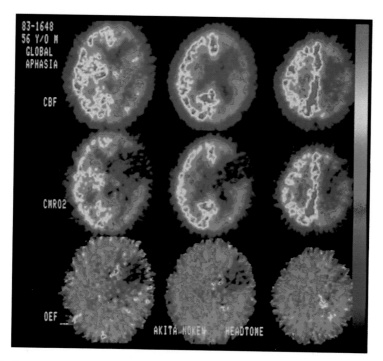

Plate 13. CBF (*top*), CMRO2 (*middle*), and OEF (*bottom*) images from case 1 exhibiting motor aphasia. The right-hand side is the left and the left-hand side is the right on PET images.

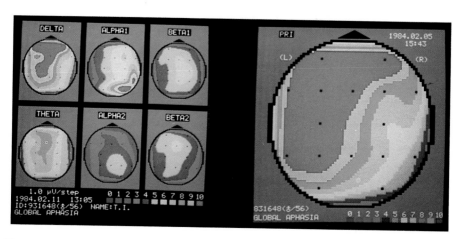

Plate 14. Six frequency domain equipotential maps (*left*) and a PRI map (*right*) from case 1.

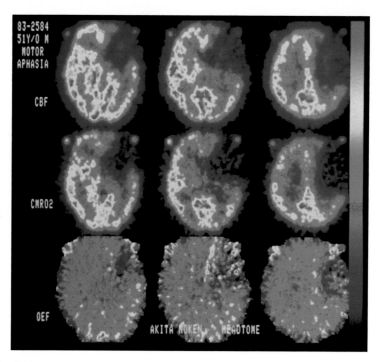

Plate 15. CBF (*top*), CMRO2 (*middle*), and OEF (*bottom*) images from case 2 exhibiting motor aphasia.

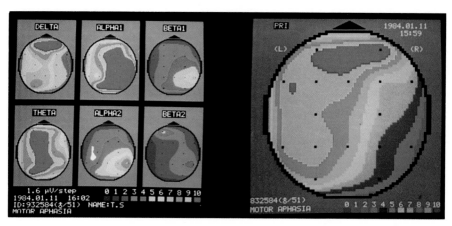

Plate 16. Six frequency domain equipotential maps (*left*) and a PRI map (*right*) from case 2.

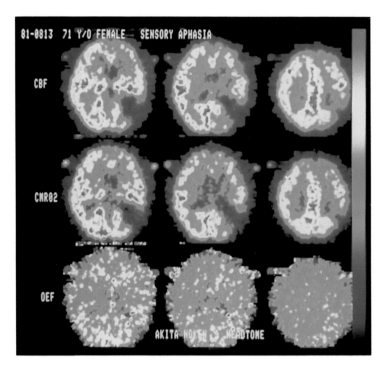

Plate 17. CBF (*top*), CMRO2 (*middle*), and OEF (*bottom*) images from case 3 exhibiting sensory aphasia.

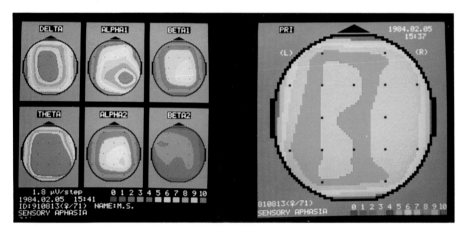

Plate 18. Six frequency domain equipotential maps (*left*) and a PRI map (*right*) from case 3.

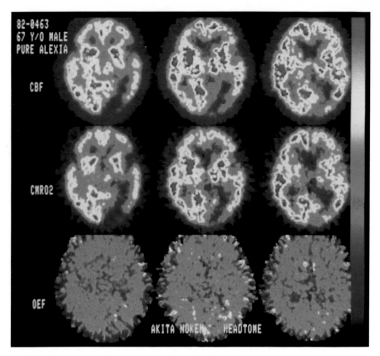

Plate 19. CBF (*top*), CMRO2 (*middle*), and OEF (*bottom*) images from case 4 exhibiting pure alexia.

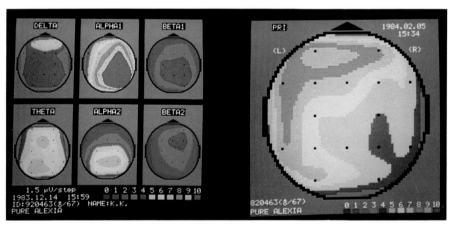

Plate 20. Six frequency domain equipotential maps (*left*) and a PRI map (*right*) from case 4.

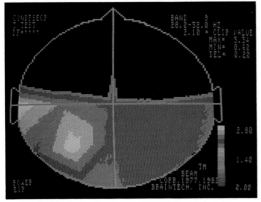

Plate 21. BEAM image: Significance probability map (SPM) exhibiting regional EEG difference between schizophrenic patients and a control group for increased beta activity in the left posterior quadrant during eyes open alert but resting state. Reprinted by permission of Archives of General Psychiatry, July 1983, 40: 719–728. Copyright 1983, American Medical Association.

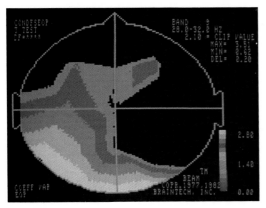

Plate 22. BEAM image: SPM exhibiting coefficient of variaton for the increased beta activity shown in Plate 20. Reprinted by permission of Archives of General Psychiatry, July 1983, 40: 719–728. Copyright 1983, American Medical Association.

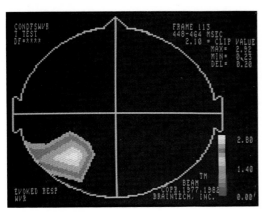

Plate 23. BEAM image: SPM exhibiting between-group difference for schizophrenic patients and a control group based on visual evoked potential, from 448 to 468 msec after onset. Reprinted by permission of Archives of General Psychiatry, July 1983, 40: 719–728. Copyright 1983, American Medical Association.

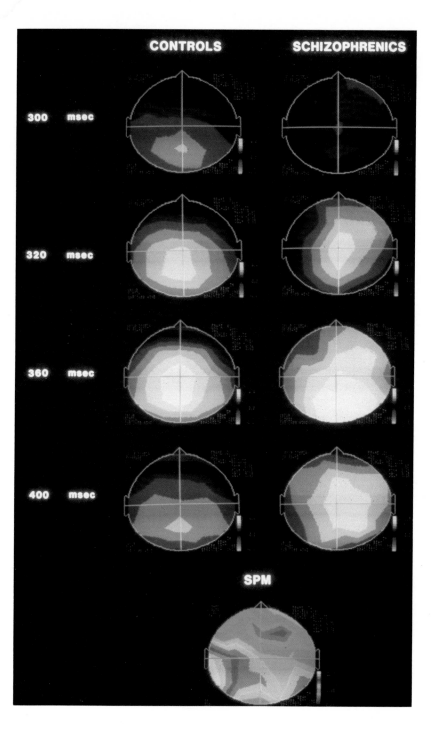

Plate 24. *Top*. Topographic distribution of P300 activity at 300, 320, 360, and 400 msec after stimulus. Scaling of colors was adjusted to allow topography in lower amplitude schizophrenic group to be clearly visible; color scale ranges from −5 to +5µV in controls and −2 to +2µV in schizophrenics. Lowest (negative) values are represented by blues; larger (positive) values by reds, yellows, and white, in that order. Compared with controls, P300 development in schizophrenics shows maxima that are displaced anteriorly and to right and deficiency of activity in left temporal region. *Bottom*. Significance probability map (see text) shows regions of maximal separation between schizophrenic and control groups. Lowest *t* values are shown by blues, with larger values indicated by yellows, reds, and white, in that order. White codes region containing *t* values greater than 2.10. Maximal separation occurred at left middle and posterior temporal electrode sites.

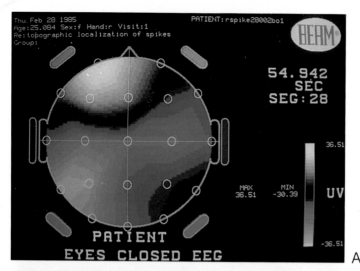

A

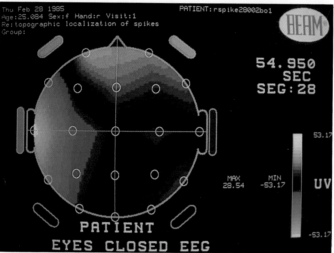

B

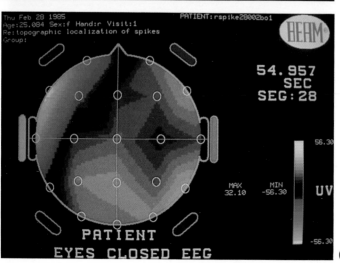

C

Plate 27. (Case 1) Unusual abnormalities in a "schizophrenic" patient. Four sets of three images are shown. Within each set of three, the top left image shows topographic data for the subject, the top right image corresponding data from age-matched controls, and the bottom image the statistical deviation (SPM) of the subject's data from the control group. The top two sets of three images (A,B) show the topographic distribution of spectral-analyzed EEG data utilizing rainbow-colored gray scale for spectral data and red (above normal) and blue (below normal) colored gray scale for the SPM. EEG theta (4–7.5 Hz) is shown in A and beta 1 (12–15.5 Hz) is shown in B. The bottom two image sets (C,D) show the topographic distribution of visual evoked response (VER) data. The red (positive) and blue (negative) scale is used for both the subject's data (*top left*) and control group data (*top right*). The SPM data (*bottom*) is also shown in red and blue scale. The VER from 148 to 184 msec is shown in C and 352 to 388 msec in D. For all four image sets, the color scale to the lower right is for the SPM. Maximum deviations of the patient from control group values are shown in units of standard deviation (Z scores) next to the scale.

Data are derived from Case 1 (see text), a 21-year-old man who developed constant auditory hallucinations and a "schizophrenia-like" syndrome following a minor head injury. Note in A the tremendous increase of bilateral theta, over 7 standard deviations (SD) from control group mean value. This was slightly more marked on the left anteriorly. In the left anterior quadrant, beta 1 was increased by 2.59 SD (B). The VER demonstrated broad negative activity, excessive by over 450 in one epoch, in the left posterior quadrant (D) as well as abnormal negativity in the right posterior temporal during another epoch (C). This was region/interpreted as consistent with organic abnormality. The previous EEGs had been unremarkable and the CT scan normal. The patient responded rapidly to carbamazepine.

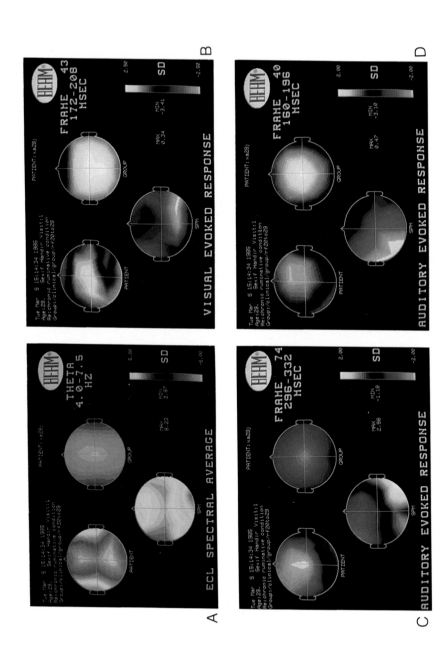

Plate 28. (Case 2) Unusual abnormalities in a depressed patient. Display convention is as for Plate 27. In *A*, spectral-analyzed theta is displayed. *B, C,* and *D* represent evoked potential data. *B* is the VER from 172–208 msec. *C* is the auditory evoked response (AER) from 160–196 msec and *D* the AER from 296–332 msec.

Data are derived from Case 2 (see text), a 29-year-old woman with depression, extreme seriousness, hyperlexia, hypergraphia, hyperphasia, and extreme swings of sexual behavior. In *A*, theta is seen to be greatly increased, by over 8 SD, maximal in the right posterior quadrant (RPQ). In *B*, a regional negativity aberrant by 3.4 SD is seen in the RPQ during the VER. In *D*, the RPQ is abnormal by 2.56 SD during the VER. In *C* the AER is abnormal by 3.1 SD in the left posterior quadrant. Previous EEGs had been considered normal and subsequent CT scans were read as normal. On the basis of BEAM findings, a more diligent historical search uncovered symptoms commensurate with partial complex seizures. The patient has improved slowly on anticonvulsant therapy.

Euclidean distance

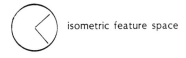

isometric feature space

Mahalanobis distance

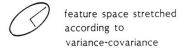

feature space stretched
according to
variance-covariance

Figure 13.9. Schematic representation of the distortion of the feature space by the variance-covariance structure. Use of a Euclidean distance metric ignores this distortion.

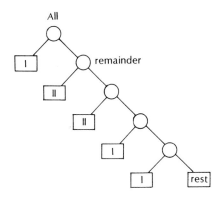

Figure 13.10. Schematic representation of the classification sequence followed by the DSELECT algorithm. At each node, only a single feature is considered in the decision rule, and only terminal descendent nodes are formed in one branch of the binary decision sequence.

old is fixed. The proportion of values unequivocally classified by this threshold setting is stored, as a figure of merit.

This process is now repeated for the same ranked list, but starting from the highest value and moving the threshold downward. Again, a figure of merit is calculated. After the classification potential of the first feature is established, the second feature is examined in a like manner. This procedure continues until a figure of merit for each feature in the files is determined and each threshold is found. Then the feature and the threshold that provides the highest figure of merit is chosen as the first decision element. The classifiable items are assigned to a terminal node, the node is given its proper label, and all other items are assigned to the remainder group.

The algorithm begins again, searching for the best feature to reduce the number of items in the remainder set. The second-best feature from the first decision node is not necessarily the best feature for the second decision node. A two-dimensional example is shown in Figure 13.11.

The user can specify the number of features to be selected, i.e., how many decision nodes the classifier should set. However, the algorithm will terminate on its own if a new feature and decision threshold cannot classify at least a minimum number or proportion of the remainder set. This precludes the algorithm from establishing spurious thresholds in a region of the feature space where two training sets overlap. Values falling into that region are declared as unclassifiable.

It is not unusual for the same feature to be selected repeatedly. Even though the algorithm as implemented, is set up for processing two categories only, a hierarchic sequencing allows multiple categories to be processed. In principle, even a multiple-category, single-stage classifier could be implemented on this basis. This algorithm has been in use for many years and has proved stable, reliable, and insensitive to particular aspects of data distributions.

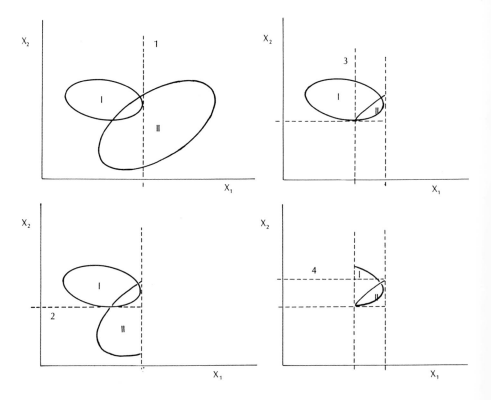

Figure 13.11. Setting of sequential decision boundaries by the DSELECT algorithm.

Classification Strategies

It is useful to distinguish between classification algorithms and classification strategies. A classification strategy defines the manner in which one or several classification algorithms are employed to achieve a final assignment of objects to a category. Examples for classification strategies are single-stage classification procedures and multiple-stage hierarchic classification procedures [37–43]. The principle of the structure of a single and a multiple stage hierarchic classifier is shown in Figure 13.12. A choice has to be made only when more than two categories have to be discriminated. However, even in a two-category situation, hierarchic multiple-stage classification may be useful.

A single-stage classifier will classify an object into one of a predetermined number of categories in one step. Single-stage classifiers are widely used and offer many advantages. However, they also have significant disadvantages. The classification is done for any object from all different categories on the basis of the same features. And each object is tested against all categories for possible assignment. This leads to inefficiency. Features that are very efficient in discriminating objects from one category from those of one or two other categories are often not chosen because they may not be effective in separating other categories. The overall best features, in the sense of minimizing classification error, may not be the best features for the discrimination between particular pairs of categories. This problem becomes especially serious when one faces a classification problem with numerous categories. Theoretically one could combine all features useful in discriminating between all possible pairs of categories and employ all of them in a single-stage classifier. Given this approach, however, one faces the restrictions imposed by the sample size/dimen-

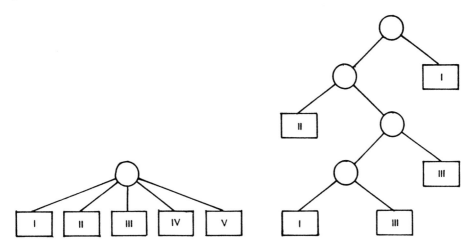

Figure 13.12. Single-stage classification strategy and hierarchic multiple-stage classification strategy.

sionality ratio. These problems are remedied by the use of a hierarchic classifier.

Hierarchic classifiers have a dendritic structure, and have therefore also become known as "tree classifiers." The field has recently received comprehensive treatment in a volume on classification and regression trees by Breiman et al. [36]. A decision hierarchy consists of a starting node, a number of nonterminal nodes, and a number of terminal nodes (Figure 13.12). The nonterminal nodes are indicated as rectangles, terminal nodes as circles.

Literature on hierarchic classifiers often uses terminology derived from tree graph theory. Thus, the starting node becomes the root node; graph edges become branches. It is customary to denote nodes closer to the root node as lower level nodes and nodes more distant from the root node as higher level nodes. A terminal node has only an ascendent node, and no descendent nodes. A nonterminal node has both—an ascendent and a descendent node. At the starting node the entire set of categories are entered. A nonterminal node provides intermediate decisions, the outcome of which results in routing an object to a descendent node. A terminal node corresponds to a final assignment to a category—the decision sequence terminates there for that object.

The construction of a decision tree involves three major considerations: the selection of partitions at each nonterminal node; decisions whether to declare a node a terminal node, or to continue the partitioning; and the assignment of a category label to a terminal node. A hierarchic classifier starts an unknown object at the starting node and has it traverse a path through the graph. At each nonterminal node a decision concerning the routing to the next descendent node is made until the unknown object arrives at a terminal node. It is then assigned to the category represented by that terminal node. The subsets routed to the terminal nodes form a partition of the complete data set entered at the starting node. Each terminal subset represents a distinct category, although there may well be several terminal nodes for the same category.

A hierarchic classifier has several advantages. At any given stage the features offering best separation may be selected. This helps in attaining a high rate of correct assignments. Since the number of features can be kept small, it allows a favorable sample size dimensionality ratio. This in turn leads to decision rules performing well on test set data.

It is generally accepted that a hierarchic classifier may not perform better than a single-stage classifier, but it cannot give a poorer performance. Therefore, in adopting a hierarchic classification strategy one may gain without having to give up anything as far as error rates are concerned. A hierarchic decision structure allows recovery of misclassified objects on the basis of additional features at a more descendent node. In some hierarchic decision schemes it may not be necessary to compute all the features for all objects. Rather, feature values are only computed as needed. There may be a reduction in computational effort.

A binary decision hierarchy allows each nonterminal node to be split into only two descendent nodes. A binary decision tree has the greatest chance of attaining a high rate of correct assignments since at each nonterminal node the "best" features are used to separate the pair of subsets into descendent nodes. A binary decision structure also avoids the problem of unclassifiable objects, which arises when discriminant functions are used to separate objects into more than two descendent nodes. In such a case a cyclic sequence of assignments may result, such as:

Object is category: B rather than category A

C rather than category B

A rather than category C

There are, however, disadvantages associated with hierarchic classification strategies. They share with single-stage classifiers the problem of optimum design as far as feature selection is concerned. Optimum selection would demand exhaustive evaluation of all possible subsets of features, and the number of possible combinations is very high even for a modest number of features. For the same reason, even for a moderate number of categories, the number of possible hierarchic structures is extremely high. Thus one cannot guarantee that an optimum hierarchic structure has been attained. Finally, evaluation of classifier performance of a hierarchic structure is difficult.

Problems of Classification Strategies

Single-stage classifers, such as stepwise linear discriminant algorithms or maximum likelihood classifiers, often rely on some parametric model and are adversely affected in their performance by several circumstances. Among these is the fact that in real-world data, there rarely are equal variance-covariance matrices in all categories. Classification into categories with unequal covariance matrices has received considerable attention [44], especially with respect to the effect on classification procedures when the dimensionality of the feature space increases [45]. The robustness of Fisher's discriminant function to unequal covariance matrices has been investigated [46–49], and the performance of generalized linear and quadratic discriminant functions, using robust estimates, has been examined [50]. Parametric rank-order approaches to discriminant analysis have been used, precisely because parametric models can present serious problems [51].

It has been shown that discriminant analysis is a fairly robust procedure, and that differences in the mean vectors of different categories can be correctly demonstrated to be statistically significant, even when rather substantial differences in the dispersion and dependence structure exist among the categories. However, this robustness breaks down when group centroid distances are of the same order of magnitude as the extension of the confidence regions about the means. Under such conditions deviations from the assumptions of the parametric model are not well tolerated. For the purpose of the correct classification of individual objects from different categories, overlap of the tolerance regions is decisively detrimental. The tolerance regions specify what proportion of the individual feature vectors they enclose. Much of the robustness of statistical inference applies only to the demonstration of mean differences, not to the overlap of tolerance regions. Procedures have been developed to minimize errors in classification due to overlap in tolerance regions [50], but these problems become increasingly intractable as the number of categories to be discriminated increases.

When a classification problem involves multiple categories, the ratio of sample size to dimensionality soon becomes a serious constraint for single-stage classification [18,20], and this has in fact been why the hierarchic classification schemes have been so widely adopted. This has been the case even though it is true that classification of medical diagnostic data rarely demand more than 6–10 features to distinguish objects from two different categories. Unfortunately, these are not the same 6–10 features for all pairs of categories. Thus, it may be necessary to use as many as 25 different features for an overall discrimination.

In a hierarchic binary decision sequence, a small and effective subset of features can be selected at each decision node, so that a high reliability of feature selection and computational economy is attained. However, even in hierarchic classifiers, and especially in complex hierarchic structures, a serious problem arises from the paucity of objects routed to given higher order nodes. To train a decision procedure at such a node on the basis of so few samples may lead to unpredictable results on test set data. It is difficult to maintain an adequate sample size/dimensionality ratio for ensuring reliable feature selection.

In the past designers of decision structures often found that only very few objects of a given category had been routed to a given node. Yet, more feature vectors for objects of this category were needed to maintain an adequate sample size/dimensionality ratio, so that a realistic decision rule would ensue. In such instances the problem was usually resolved simply by going back to a disc file and retrieving more feature vectors from the category in question. However, experience has shown that such data are unrepresentative, unless the objects are routed to the decision node through the entire preceding decision sequence. Routing through a series of decision nodes causes the feature value distributions to be truncated [43]. If data are retrieved from file and entered as they are at any node in the decision structure, they are not representative of the data that are routed to a given node.

Truncation of feature value distributions is a serious problem even for the two-category discrimination at each of the decision nodes distant from the root node. The distributions of feature values for objects routed to these more distant nodes are truncated by decision rules applied at nodes closer to the root node.

Truncation effects even propagate from one feature distribution to another. Consider a feature which is sharply truncated at a node close to the root node. Now consider another feature employed for the first time at a node far distant from the root node. Since this feature had not been used before, one would not expect its distribution to be truncated, but unfortunately this is not so. If the new feature is highly correlated to the first truncated feature, then the distribution of the new feature is truncated even before it was used. In other words, truncation may be introduced to a feature distribution by the truncation of another correlated feature.

Such truncation can and does cause dramatic shifts in the descriptive statistics for location and dispersion. If a distribution function is abruptly cut off by a threshold, and only the segment below threshold is routed to the next decendent node, then the objects of the represented category will have drastically different mean value and less dispersion for that feature. Truncation thus introduces stark deviations from any parametric model distribution to an extent that far exceeds the range of effects that robustness of discriminant analysis algorithms could tolerate.

Truncation of feature value distributions may take many forms. When a classifier sets thresholds for individual features, threshold setting leads to abrupt discontinuity and cutoff at the threshold value. Figure 13.13 shows the distribution functions for a given feature, in category I, indicated by the bell-shaped curve, and another category, for which only the low end of the distribution is shown. The dotted line indicates the threshold set by a classifier. At the two descendent nodes A and B, the feature distributions for category I are now

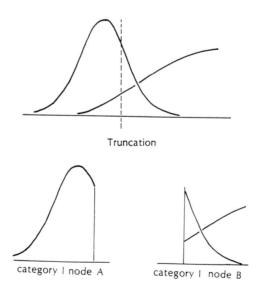

Truncation

category I node A   category I node B

Figure 13.13. Effect of truncation of a feature value distribution by a decision threshold on the distribution of that feature at the descendent nodes.

drastically different in mean value and dispersion, and certainly in the form of the distribution. Yet, both distributions represent category I throughout the descendent nodes in the hierarchic sequence that follows.

Such thresholding need not apply to the feature itself. Consider a case where a feature X_1 is highly correlated with a feature X_3. Now consider the situation where close to the root node a threshold had been set for feature X_3. Much further in the decision sequence, at a node distant from the root node, feature X_1 is called for the first time. The original distribution of X_1 for the considered category has a large dispersion; however, most of the objects contributing to the large variance were cut off when feature X_3 was truncated. X_1, in the subset routed to the descendent node now under consideration, has a rather small variance. The truncation effect here is thus not a sharp cutoff, but a pronounced shift in mean value, a reduction in variance, and in some instances a pronounced asymmetry. Figure 13.14 demonstrates truncation effects as propagated from one feature to another correlated feature.

Quite often a feature enters into a decision rule as a component of a linear combination with a certain weight or coefficient (Figure 13.15). Categories I and II are separated by a linear combination of the two features X_1 and X_2. All feature vectors falling into the region to the lower right are routed to the next descendent node. At that node, the distribution of X_1 becomes asymmetric, due to the effects of the cutoff by the linear discriminant function.

Figure 13.14. Effect of truncation of X_3 at an earlier node on the distribution of X_1 at a higher order decision node, assuming that the two features are highly correlated.

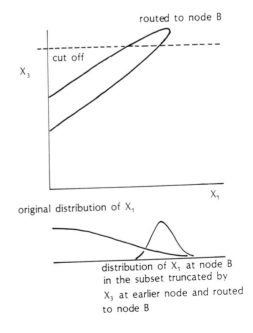

routed to node B

cut off

X_3

X_1

original distribution of X_1

distribution of X_1 at node B in the subset truncated by X_3 at earlier node and routed to node B

Figure 13.15. Truncation of value distribution of feature X_1 by a linear combination of features being subjected to a threshold setting.

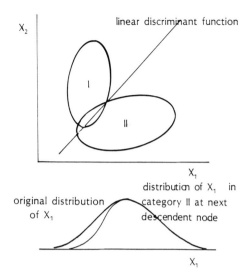

TREND DETECTION

It is true that classification methods are most frequently used to assign an object to a given diagnostic category on the basis of the values observed for some selected features. In the evaluation of diagnostic tests, one should consider using classification methodology to develop early detection capabilities, based on trend analysis. Consider the situation schematized in Figure 13.16. In a bivariate feature space two regions are assigned to two different diagnostic categories, one representing a healthy population, the other a pathologic one. A decision boundary has been established, based on a Bayes maximum likelihood classifier. Let it now be assumed that a patient's values for the two featured variables are found well within the normal range. Let it furthermore be assumed that this patient returns periodically, is evaluated each time, and that each time the bivariate mean of the patient's test results is well within the normal range. However, if one projected the consecutive test results onto an axis connecting the mean of the healthy population to the mean of the diseased population, and if one found that every test showed a progression toward the pathologic condition, one certainly would have to consider the implications.

Whether such a trend is statistically significant can easily be determined by a simple sign test [52]. For five consecutive test results to project progressively closer to the pathology region has a probability of less than 0.04, and thus reaches the confidence levels normally accepted as significant in hypothesis testing (Figure 13.17). Even though all test results clearly fall into the normal region, there is a statistically significant trend observed in this patient, which may be detected by observing very small changes in a number of variables.

Figure 13.16. Detection of a trend in repeated clinical test outcomes.

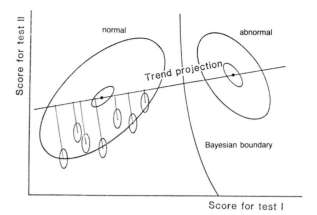

The statistically based classification strategies I have described provide a basis for the reliable identification of features to be utilized in the diagnosis of neuropathologies. These classification paradigms isolate the most powerfully discriminant neurological features for analysis of difference between a given individual and a control group or between two groups under examination. Ultimately, diagnosticians may have available highly sensitive signature sets of features based on topographic imaging which provide extremely reliable results for a wide variety of neurological conditions.

Figure 13.17. Chances for significance of the detected trend as function of number of test repetitions.

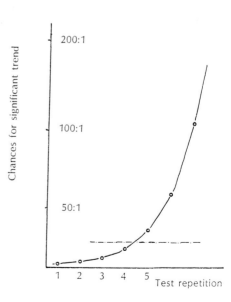

REFERENCES

1. Sokal, R.R., and Sneath, P.H.A. Principles of Numerical Taxonomy. San Francisco: W.H. Freeman, 1963.
2. Duda, R.O., and Hart, P.E. Pattern Classification and Scene Analysis. New York: Wiley Interscience, 1973.
3. Clifford, H.T., and Stephenson, W. An Introduction to Numerical Classification, New York: Academic Press, 1975.
4. Hand, D.J. Discrimination and Classification. Chichester: John Wiley, 1981.
5. Duffy, F.H., Burchfiel, J.L., and Lombroso, C.T. Brain electrical activity mapping (BEAM): A method for extending the clinical utility of EEG and evoked potential data. Ann. Neurol. 1979; 5:309–321.
6. Duffy, F.H., Denckla, M.B., Bartels, P.H., and Sandini, G. Dyslexia: Regional differences in brain electrical activity by topographic mapping. Ann. Neurol. 1980; 7:412–420.
7. Bartels, P.H. Concepts in multivariate data analysis, In Environmental Pathology: An Evolving Field. R.B. Hill and J.A. Terzian, eds. New York: Alan R. Liss, 1982; 321-341.
8. Fukunaga, K. Introduction to Statistical Pattern Recognition. New York: Academic Press, 1972.
9. Anderberg, M.R. Cluster Analysis for Applications. New York: Academic Press, 1973.
10. Everitt, B. Cluster Analysis. London: Heinemann Educational Books, 1974.
11. Hartigan, J.A. Clustering Algorithms. New York: John Wiley, 1975.
12. Spaeth, H. Cluster-Analyse-Algorithmen zur Objektklassifizierung und Datenreduktion. R. Munich: Oldenbourg Verlag, 1975.
13. Beale, E.M.L. Euclidean cluster analysis. Bull. Int. Stat. Inst. 1969; 43:92.
14. Kruskal, W.H., and Wallis, W.A. Use of ranks on one-criterion varince analysis. J. Am. Stat. Assoc. 1952; 47:583–621 (addendum, 1953; 48:907–911).
15. Genchi, H., and Mori, K. Evaluation and feature extraction on automated pattern recognition system. Denski-Tsuchin Gakki, Part I, 1965.
16. Sherwood, E.M., Bartels, P.H., and Wied, G.L. Feature selection in cell image analysis: Use of the ROC curve. Acta Cytol. 1976; 20(3):254–260.
17. Bartels, P.H., and Olson, G.B. Computer analysis of lymphocyte images. In N. Catsimpoolas, Methods of Cell Separation. New York: Plenum Press, 1980; 1–99.
18. Kanal, L., and Chandrasekaran, B. On dimensionality and sample. In Statistical Pattern Classification, Proc. Nat. Electr. Conf., 1968; 2–7.
19. Kulkarni, A.V., and Kanal, L. An optimization approach to hierarchial classifier design. Proceedings of the Third International Joint Conference on Pattern Recognition. IEEE Trans. Comput. 1976; 76:459–466.
20. Foley, D.H. Consideration of sample and feature size. IEEE Trans. Inform. Theor. 1972; IT-18(5):618–626.
21. Lachenbruch, P.A. Discriminant Analysis. New York: Hafner Press, 1975.
22. Selin, I. Detection Theory. Princeton: Princeton University Press, 1965.
23. Klecka, W.R. Discriminant Analysis. In N.H. Nie, C.H. Hill, J.G. Jenkins, K. Steinbrenner, and D.H. Brent, eds., SPSS: Statistical Package for the Social Sciences, 2nd ed. New York: McGraw-Hill, 1975; 434–467.

24. Cooley, W.W., and Lohnes, P.R. Multivariate Data Analysis. New York: John Wiley, 1971.
25. Cover, T.M., and Hart, P.E. Nearest neighbor pattern classification. IEEE Trans. Inform. Theor. 1967; IT-13:21–27.
26. Goldstein, M. k^n-Nearest Neighbor Classification. IEEE Trans. Infor. Theor. 1972; IT-18:627–630.
27. Fisher, R.A. The use of multiple measurements in taxonomic problems. Ann. Eugenics 1936; 7:179–188.
28. von Mises, R. On the classification of observation data into distinct groups. Ann. Math. Stat. 1945; 16:68–73.
29. Rao, C.R. Advanced Statistical Methods in Biometric Research. New York: Hafner Press, 1952.
30. Mahalanobis, P.C. On the generalized distance in statistics. Proc. Nat. Inst. Sci. (India) 1936; 12:49.
31. Bartels, P.H., and Bellamy, J.C. Self-optimizing, self-learning system in pictorial pattern recognition. Appl. Opt. 1970; 9:2453–2458.
32. Henrichon, E.G., and Fu, K.S. A non-parametric partitioning procedure for pattern classification. IEEE Trans. Comput. 1969; C-18:614.
33. Voss, K. Hyperquader als kompakte Klassifikatoren. Electron. Inform. Kybernet. 1977; 13:633–642.
34. Voss, K. Ein rechentechnisches Verfahren zur Konstruktion hierarchisch strukturierter Klassifikatoren. Electron. Inform. Kybernet. 1980; 16:281–286.
35. Voss, K., Simon, H., and Wenzelides, K. Logical classifiers for image analysis in medicine. J. Anal. Quant. Cytol. 1981; 3:39–42.
36. Breiman, L., Friedman, F.H., Olshen, R.A., and Stone, C.F., eds. Classification and Regression Trees. California: Wadsworth, 1983.
37. Taylor, J., Bartels, P.H., Bibbo, M., Bahr, G.F., and Wied, G.L. Implementation of a hierarchical classification procedure. Acta Cytol. 1974; 18:515–521.
38. Wu, C., Landgrebe, D., and Swain, P. The decision tree approach to classification. In TR-EE West Lafayette, Ind.: Purdue University, 1975; 75–17.
39. You, K.C., and Fu, K.S. An approach to the design of a linear binary tree classifier. In Proceedings of Symposium of Machine Processing of Remotely Sensed Data. West Lafayette, Ind.: Purdue University, 1976; 3A-1–3A-10.
40. Taylor, J., Bartels, P.H., Bibbo, M., and Wied, G.L. Automated hierarchic decision structures for multiple category cell classification by TICAS. Acta Cytol. 1978; 22:261–267.
41. Swain, P.H., and Hauska, H. The decision tree classifier: Design and potential. IEEE Trans. Geosci. Electron. 1977; GE-15(3):142–147.
42. Anderson, A.C., and Fu, K.S. Design and development of a linear binary tree classifier for leukocytes. In TR-EE West Lafayette, Ind. Purdue University, 1979; 79–31.
43. Bartels, H.G., Bartels, P.H., Bibbo, M., and Wied, G.L. Stabilized hierarchic classifier in cytopathologic diagnosis. Anal. Quant. Cytol. 1984; 6:247–261.
44. Anderson, T.W., and Bahadur, R.R. Classification into two multivariate distributions with different covariance matrices. Ann. Math. Stat. 1962; 33:420–431.
45. Van Ness, J. On the effects of dimension in discriminant analysis for unequal covariance populations. Technometrics 1979; 21:119–127.

46. Gilbert, E.S. The effect of unequal variance-covariance matrices on Fishers's linear discriminant function. Biometrics 1969; 25:505–515.
47. Marks, S., and Dunn, O.J. Discriminant functions when covariance matrices are unequal. J. Am. Stat. Assoc. 1974; 69:555–559.
48. Krzanowski, W.J. The performance of Fisher's linear discriminant function under non-optimal conditions. Technometrics 1977; 19:191–200.
49. Johnson, M.E., Wang, C., and Ramberg, J.S. Robustness of Fisher's linear discriminant function to departures from normality. In LASL, Los Alamos, N.M.: LA-8068-MS, 1979; UC-32.
50. Randles, R.H., Broffitt, J.D., Ramberg, J.S., and Hogg, R.V. Discriminant analysis based on rank. J. Am. Stat. Assoc. 1978; 73:379–384.
51. Randles, R.H., Broffitt, J.D., Ramberg, J.S., and Hogg, R.V. Generalized linear and quadratic discriminant functions using robust estimates. J. Am. Stat. Assoc. 1978; 73:564–568.
52. Bradley, J.V. Distribution-free statistical tests. Englewood Cliffs, N.J.: Prentice Hall, 1968.

14

Single-Trial Event-Related Potentials: Statistical Classification and Topography

Donald G. Childers

The recognition of differences between averaged event-related potentials (ERPs) monitored during various experiments is a skill that can be learned despite the lack of clearly defined features in ERP waveforms, and variability of components within the waveforms. Not long ago components in averaged ERPs were recognized only by human examination. But now computerized algorithms exist that (1) use auditory evoked responses for conducting hearing tests, (2) help diagnose brain disorders, and (3) assist the study of human learning and image and language understanding.

While single-trial ERPs and the electroencephalogram (EEG) are more difficult to study, we can nonetheless, learn their characteristics. Computer algorithms exist that recognize some of their features as well; e.g., EEG sleep records can be scored automatically, and epilepsy can be detected.

Generally, however, the algorithms for either averaged ERPs or single-trial events are heuristic and thus imperfect. They differ from one laboratory to the next. Usually only two hypotheses are tested, e.g., normal and abnormal. Differential hypothesis testing is an approach of considerable importance but remains elusive because EEGs and ERPs vary from individual to individual, being affected by information processing and motor centers within the brain. We also lack considerable knowledge about the proper topological monitoring sites that should be used when trying to detect a brain disorder.

Most ERP researchers employ subjective pattern recognition techniques to reduce their data to a few summary interpretations. The process encompasses examining the data in the temporal, topological (spatial), and frequency domains. The investigator attempts to isolate the "signal" from the background activity. Multichannel comparisons are made so that hemispheric asymmetries or focal activity may be discerned. Frequently the researcher may find the data so complicated in the local analysis frame that only a general global interpretation of the overall pattern is used. Many of the algorithms employed are simple, such as peak picking, but others are more complex.

But before we examine the issue of feature extraction from measured data, let us consider some factors that may influence our choice of features to represent our reduced data set.

FACTORS AFFECTING FEATURE
SELECTION FOR ERP DATA

Numerous factors can influence our choice of features to represent ERP data. Unfortunately, most of these factors are incapable of being expressed mathematically in a feature extraction algorithm. However, we can account for many of these factors by carefully designing our experiments and interpreting our results.

1.   *Brain Models.* The changes in ERP patterns are presumed to reflect changes in functional connections between cortical neurons, i.e., the number and types of transactions taking place between different vertical and horizontal neuronal compartments. Our data reduction and interpretation techniques are dependent upon clinical signs, patient history, experimental design, and conceptual models of how the brain functions. These models should help us integrate past data and predict new results; they should serve as generators of hypotheses and form the framework for experimental design. But our models of the brain are too elementary. We need to study how neuronal ensembles function in both temporal and spatial coordinates. But with our present understanding of the anatomical organization of the brain and how it processes auditory, visual, and other sensory data simultaneously and selectively, we are severely taxed to interpret our data properly.

2.   *Multichannel.* Topological comparisons often seek confirmation (by a majority vote) that a particular event has occurred in the data record. Multiple recording sites may also be necessary in order to detect the locus of a particular cortical site.

3.   *Components.* One often hears that the understanding of components of evoked potentials is inversely related to their latency. As time progresses following the presentation of a stimulus, more and more data processing takes place within the nervous system, making data analysis and interpretation more and more difficult. Therefore, many researchers look at early components (events) in the responses. This is done despite the fact that the late components are perhaps the most informative as far as behavioral performance of the organism is concerned. We often consider the components of our temporal evoked response to be independently generated by disparate neuronal ensembles. But this may be a fallacious assumption. Numerous examples of time-connected oscillatory waveforms can be easily constructed. We must therefore be flexible in our interpretation of the temporal data.

4.   *Data translation.* Spectral analysis, for example, may often be of

assistance in illuminating data characteristics not readily apparent in the other domain. But peaks in the spectrum may not be independently generated.

5. *Dipole models.* In order to interpret results we need to compare histological and electrophysical data. We may conceive of dipole models as stationary or moving. These models may in turn be associated with different cortical layers and more than one dipole may be active at a time.

6. *Electrodes.* We must remember that a surface or scalp recording represents an average, is dependent upon electrode size, and is a composite of potentials close to and far from the recording site. There are multiple pathways within the nervous system by which the signal may reach the recording sites. The electrode montage and interconnections (monopolar or bipolar) also influences our interpretation.

7. *Biological variability.* The ERP to a particular stimulus for various subjects may

- Be compressed or expanded in time
- Vary in amplitude
- Have latency variations in components
- Have spectral component variations

Often variations in ERP waveshape are attributed to the background EEG (or noise), but may be caused by

- Changes in excitability of various neuronal regions
- Arousal
- Attention
- Habituation
- Orientation
- Motivation
- Memory
- Meaning or familiarity of the stimulus
- Variations in the ability of the individual to predict the stimulus which reflects expectancy and uncertainty.

8. *Artifacts.* Our signal interpretation is certainly influenced by the intrusion of muscle activity, arterial pulsations, eye movements, and electrode artifacts. One of the major challenges to signal processing is the automatic recognition of artifacts.

9. *Data verification and validation.* For source location the methods potentially most valuable are histological examination, surgery, and postmortem examination, but these procedures are often not available to the researcher. For memory and information processing studies, multiple measurements and repeated experiments offer some help. The experimental design may be varied. Agreement or departure from earlier results should be sought. The construction of models is an aid to structure one's thinking.

Few of these factors lend themselves to quantification, and thus, they have little influence on our development of algorithms for data reduction and processing. But they nonetheless influence the data we collect, so we must be aware that one or more of these factors may affect the features we ultimately select to represent our data.

PATTERN RECOGNITION

The process of pattern recognition attempts to establish rules for making correct classifications of signals or data. Typically, we measure data from known mutually exclusive data classes. Rules are then derived to classify the known classes using the data from our training (design or learning) measurements. Frequently, cluster analysis is included as part of pattern recognition.

Patterns may be defined in various ways. We might have just the physical data, e.g., an x-ray plate, a photograph, a sampled time series. In these cases pattern recognition may have different units, e.g., age, height, weight, sex. A typical pattern here might be a medical syndrome. The pattern recognition might use a decision tree that could also be used to identify the pattern. Another type of pattern is statistical and may include some nonnumeric information, e.g., answers to a true/false test or colors, that must be converted to numerical form.

For ERP studies, averaged ERP data records are usually used and are often compared, using such techniques as template matching. But averaging hinders the researcher who wants to vary the stimulus on a trial-by-trial basis. Template matching may prove ineffective if the signal-to-noise ratio is low

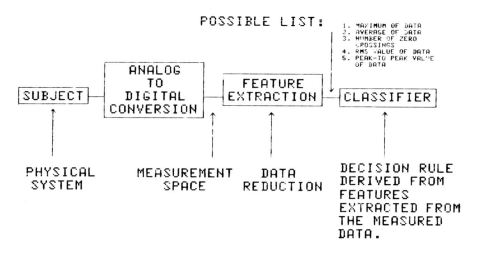

Figure 14.1. Feature extraction.

(i.e., ERP component variability is high). This occurs if too few ERPs are available to average. Consequently, researchers are presently looking for ERP single-trial tools that may be used to detect components in real time and change the stimulus during the experiment. However, to make decisions rapidly we must reduce the number of measurements to a few reliable features which adequately represent the data. This is the objective of feature extraction—that part of pattern recognition which attempts to reduce the size of the measured data in as few parameters as possible. (Figure 14.1).

Some authors have distinguished feature selection from feature extraction. Feature selection is any algorithm that chooses features without changing the coordinate system. The features are ordered by some criterion and then the best M features are chosen, such as in stepwise discriminant analysis. Feature extraction is any algorithm that chooses features from the measurements allowing changes in the coordinate systems. We make no distinction between feature selection and extraction.

Various methods exist for extracting features from data, including divergence, principal components, discriminant vectors, factor analysis, and others. We briefly discuss the relationships between these methods in Appendix 14A.

After we select the features, we design a data classifier. Classification often uses linear discriminant analysis to define a number that is a weighted combination of the original measurements. The weighting function is specific to a class of patterns and the value of the derived number allocates the pattern to a particular class when its value falls within the range associated with that class.

We often think of the sampled data as an n-dimensional vector that can be represented as a point in n-dimensional space. We then attempt to find methods by which we can circumscribe clusters of points as belonging to the same class, e.g., ERPs elicited by the same stimulus. The feature vectors can be plotted in the same manner, but their dimensions are usually smaller than the original data vectors. There are limitations to projecting our vectors into reduced dimensions, as shown in Figure 14.2. Very frequently a human observer

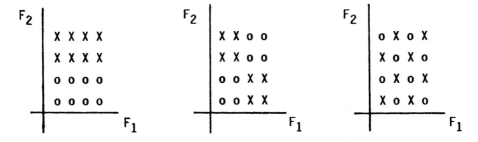

Figure 14.2. Three possible data clusters for two classes of data denoted by Xs and Os. The data may be separated in a higher dimensional space but when projected onto two dimensions, F_1 and F_2, in feature space the data may overlap.

can easily derive decision boundaries (or planes) for these situations, but it may be difficult to do so automatically.

Data reduction schemes use features that represent the data as well as possible. However, these features may not work well for classifying the data into their appropriate categories. Another problem often overlooked (or not known) is that the single best feature for a data set may not be a member of the set of two best features for classifying the data. This means that it is not easy to "grow" or extend a feature set with a recursive algorithm so that more refined or graded classifications may be developed.

FEATURE EXTRACTION

In designing a pattern classification system, complete knowledge of the underlying probability distribution is unknown; instead, only a small number of training samples is available. Thus the parameters of the class-conditional densities must be estimated from these training samples. In most practical situations the maximum likelihood estimates of the probability distribution parameters are used in place of the true values, but under these conditions the performance of the classifier is not necessarily improved as one increases the number of features [1–5]. In fact the pattern classifier performance may even deteriorate [2]. Thus, there exists an optimum number of features to be selected for a given pattern classifier system. This number is a function of both the number of training samples and the probabilistic structure of the data. The relationship between training sample size and the optimum number of features for a specific probabilistic structure has been studied [6–12]. However, the effect of the probabilistic structure of the data on the optimum number of features has remained unexplored. One of our objectives is to give a recursive algorithm for selecting a near optimal (suboptimal) feature set for the case of data with two classes described by two equiprobable multivariate normal densities with a common covariance matrix. In the next section the problem is formulated, the existing results are summarized, and we give our optimal exhaustive search feature selection algorithm. Then the suboptimal algorithm is discussed along with examples.

OPTIMUM NUMBER OF FEATURES

Consider the two-class classification problem. Let ω_1 denote the member set for class 1 and similarly ω_2 for class 2, with $x = (x_1, x_2, \ldots, x_m)^t$ being an m-dimensional column observation vector, and $p(\omega_1) = p(\omega_2) = 0.5$ being the a priori probabilities. Assume that the class-conditional probabilities $p(x|\omega_k)$ are normally distributed with mean μ_i and covariance matrix Σ for class ω_i ($i = 1,2$). It is well known [3,13] that if all the parameters of the class-conditional density functions are known, the minimum error classification rule for classifying an observation vector x is

$$\text{decide } x \in \omega_1 \text{ if } D_T = \left[x - \tfrac{1}{2} (\mu_1 - \mu_2) \right]' \Sigma^{-1} (\mu_1 - \mu_2) > 0$$

$$= x' \Sigma^{-1} (\mu_1 - \mu_2) - \tfrac{1}{2} (\mu_1 - \mu_2)'$$

$$\Sigma^{-1} (\mu_1 - \mu_2) > 0 \tag{14.1}$$

$x \in \omega_2$ otherwise

where x' denotes the transpose of vector x and Σ^{-1} the inverse of the covariance matrix Σ. Note, Fisher's discriminant function is $x' \Sigma^{-1} (\mu_1 - \mu_2)$ [3]. The other term in (1) is simply a constant, which determines the threshold for deciding if x belongs to ω_1.

If the parameters Σ, μ_1 and μ_2 are not known, and instead we have n_i training samples from class ω_i, $i = 1,2$, available, then the simplest and the most commonly used procedure is to replace the true values of the parameters in the decision rule given in (1) by their respective maximum likelihood estimates. The discriminant function, D_T, in (14.1) then becomes

$$D_S = \left[x - \tfrac{1}{2} (\hat{\mu}_1 + \hat{\mu}_2) \right]' S^{-1} (\hat{\mu}_1 - \hat{\mu}_2) \tag{14.2}$$

where μ_i and S are the sample mean of μ_i and the pooled unbiased estimate of the covariance matrix Σ respectively, i.e.,

$$\hat{\mu}_i = \frac{1}{n_i} \sum_{j=1}^{n_i} x_j^{(i)} \tag{14.3}$$

$$S = \frac{1}{n_1 + n_2 - 2} \sum_{i=1}^{2} \sum_{j=1}^{n_i} (x_j^{(i)} - \hat{\mu}_i)^2 \tag{14.4}$$

In the above expression $x_j^{(i)}$ refers to the jth training sample from class ω_i.

In order to determine the optimum number of features that maximizes the performance of the classifier, i.e., gives the lowest probability of error, we need to write the probability of error in terms of the number of features. The probability of error P_E when the discriminant function D is employed is

$$P_E = p(\omega_1)P_1 + p(\omega_2)P_2 \tag{14.5}$$

where $P_1 = Pr(D(x) < 0 \mid x \in \omega_1)$ \hfill (14.6)

$$P_2 = Pr(D(x) > 0 \mid x \in \omega_2)$$

$$D = D_T \text{ or } D_S$$

To determine P_i, $i = 1, 2$, one needs to know the conditional distribution of the discriminant function D when x is from ω_i. When all parameters are known the statistics of D_T are normally distributed with parameters.

$$E(D_T(x)|\omega_i) = \frac{(-1)^{i+1}}{2} (\mu_1 - \mu_2)^t \Sigma^{-1} (\mu_1 - \mu_2)$$

$$= \frac{(-1)^{i+1}}{2} \delta^2 \tag{14.7}$$

$$\text{Var}(D_T(x)) = E[D_T(x) - D_T(\mu_i)]^2$$

$$= (\mu_1 - \mu_2)^t \Sigma^{-1} (\mu_1 - \mu_2)$$

$$= \delta^2 \tag{14.8}$$

The quantity δ^2 is the Mahalanobis distance with known parameters. The probability of misclassification is

$$P_E = \Phi \left(-\frac{\delta}{2}\right) \tag{14.9}$$

where $\Phi(z)$ is the standard normal distribution function defined as

$$\Phi(z) = \frac{1}{2\pi} \int_{-\infty}^{z} \exp\left(-\frac{1}{2} u^2\right) du \tag{14.10}$$

When the parameters are unknown the statistic D_S is very complex. Many statisticians have studied this problem [14–28]. John [14–16] gave the exact distribution and the associated probability of misclassification of D_S when the covariance matrix is known. The unknown covariance matrix case has been studied by Sitgreaves [17]. Approximations have been given by various authors [20–28].

Jain and Waller [9] used the approximation of the probability of error given by Sitgreaves [27] for studying feature selection. They showed that an additional feature can be added to those already selected if its contribution to the Mahalanobis distance is greater than a certain proportion of the accumulated Mahalanobis distance. But no simple closed-form formula for the general case was given. To obtain a closed-form formula, another approximation of the probability of error must be employed. Lachenbruch [29] derived an approximation of the probability of error for D_S based on the expected means and variance of D_S which can be written as:

$$P_E = \Phi\left(-\frac{\Gamma}{2}\right) \tag{14.11}$$

$$\text{where } \Gamma = \left(\frac{(N - 2 - m)(N - 5 - m)}{(N - 3)(N - 3 - m)}\right)^{\frac{1}{2}} \frac{\delta^2}{\left(\delta^2 + \dfrac{4m}{N}\right)^{\frac{1}{2}}} \qquad (14.12)$$

N = total number of training samples
  = $n_1 + n_2$
m = number of features
δ^2 = Mahalanobis distance
$p(\omega_1) = p(\omega_2)$ = equal a priori probability = 0.5
$n_1 = n_2$ = equal number of training samples for each class

The case of unequal training samples for each class is studied in [30]. The estimate in (14.11) can be calculated by approximating the true Mahalanobis distance, δ^2 by the estimated Mahalanobis distance, Δ^2 where

$$\Delta^2 = (\hat{\mu}_1 - \hat{\mu}_2)^t \, S^{-1} \, (\hat{\mu}_1 - \hat{\mu}_2) \qquad (14.13)$$

Note from (14.11) that since $\Phi(\bullet)$ is a monotonically increasing function, then Γ monotonically increases with the probability of correct classification, i.e., the larger Γ the better the performance of the features used to classify the data. Therefore, Γ can be used as a performance index, and the problem of choosing the optimum feature set becomes the problem of finding a combination of features that gives the highest value of Γ among all the possible combinations. Note from (14.12) that for a fixed total number of training samples, N, Γ is a monotonically increasing function of δ^2 but a monotonically decreasing function of m. Thus for each value of m, Γ needs to be evaluated for only the best combination of features. In effect, the features are ordered from "best to worst" according to their contribution to the Mahalanobis distance. It is clear from this discussion that an exhaustive search is required for selecting features. Thus considerable calculation is required. Using these arguments we were able to derive the following optimal exhaustive search feature algorithm [30]:

1. Select the single best feature by calculating Γ_1 for the largest Δ^2.
2. Determine the best two-feature combinations by calculating Γ_2 for the largest Δ^2.
3. Continue until the desired number of features is obtained.
4. At each step we require that $\Gamma_n > \Gamma_{n-1}$.
5. Stop if $\Gamma_n < \Gamma_{n-1}$.

Unfortunately, there is no known optimal, nonexhaustive sequential feature selection procedure available [31]. In the next section we discuss an algorithm for obtaining a near optimal feature set solution of (14.12).

THE NEAR OPTIMAL ALGORITHM FOR FEATURE SELECTION

Note that the classification rule (14.1) can be written as

$$x \in \omega_1 \text{ if } D_T = x'W - c$$
$$= w_1x_1 + w_2x_2 + \ldots + w_mx_m - c > 0 \qquad (14.14)$$

$$x \in \omega_2 \text{ otherwise}$$

where $x' = (x_1, x_2, \ldots, x_m)$, the feature vector
$$W = (w_1, w_2, \ldots, w_m)$$
$$= \Sigma^{-1}(\mu_1 - \mu_2), \text{ the weighting vector}$$
$$c = \tfrac{1}{2}(\mu_1 - \mu_2)'\Sigma^{-1}(\mu_1 - \mu_2), \text{ a scalar threshold}$$

This rule can be interpreted as follows: If the weighted sum of features, x_i is greater than a threshold c we decide $x \in \omega_1$; otherwise $x \in \omega_2$. Thus, a "significant" feature x_i should be weighted more than an "insignificant" feature. Then, we can order the features by the values of the weighting factor w_i. A feature with the highest weighting factor should then be selected first.

By utilizing this feature-ordering technique instead of the exhaustive search in the last section, the near optimal feature set can be obtained. The flow chart of the procedure is shown in Figure 14.3. Note that Σ'^{-1} can be computed recursively.

Example 1

This example is from Jain and Waller [9]. The purpose of this example is to illustrate the method of suboptimal feature selection and to compare three feature selection methods, namely, the optimal method (exhaustive search), the suboptimal method just described, and a "natural" ordering [9]. For simplicity, let us assume that the difference between the means for each feature are the same (and they also have the same sign), i.e.,

$$\mu_2 - \mu_1 = (d, d, d, \ldots, d)'.$$

Thus, the Mahalanobis distance is simply the sum of all elements of Σ^{-1} times d^2. Also assume the covariance matrix has the following form:

$$\Sigma = \begin{vmatrix} 1 & r & r^2 & \cdot & \cdot & \cdot & r^{M-1} \\ r & 1 & r & \cdot & \cdot & \cdot & \cdot \\ r^2 & r & 1 & r & \cdot & \cdot & \cdot \\ \vdots & \cdot & \cdot & \cdot & 1 & \cdot \\ r^{M-1} & \cdot & \cdot & \cdot & \cdot & r & 1 \end{vmatrix} \qquad (14.15)$$

which means the correlation between features x_i and x_j is equal to $r^{|i-j|}$. For simplicity we will consider only the cases where $0 < r < 1$. Note that in this case, when each feature is used alone they are equally good. However, a different set of m features ($m > 1$) may not give the same value for the Mahalanobis

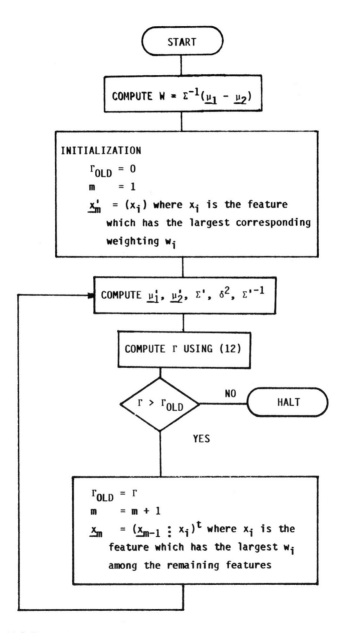

Figure 14.3. Recursive procedure for finding a set of near optimal features.

distance. For example, the Mahalanobis distance of any two features x_i and x_j is monotonically increasing with $|i - j|$, since the correlation between two features is lower if they are farther apart. Thus, the best combination of two features is the first and the last one, and the worst combination is any two consecutive features.

Jain and Waller [9] and El-Sheikh and Wacker [10] considered this problem. They found the optimal number of features, m_{opt}, to be the order m of the covariance matrix in (14.15) that minimizes the expected probability of error. In effect, they select the features in a natural order. The optimal number was found to be approximately (but always less than) $N/2 - 1$ [9]. In this case, the optimal number of features, m_{opt}, also depends on the total number of available features M, in addition to d^2, r, and N. The larger M the better the performance and the larger m_{opt} will be for a fixed r, d^2, and N. The optimal way of selecting features is to select features uniformly and maximally spaced. For example, for a set of one, any feature can be selected. The best set of two features is the combination of the first and the last feature. The best set of three features is the combination of the first, the middle, and the last feature. Note that it is a fortunate situation in this case that the covariance matrix is highly structured and the difference between the means for each feature is equal in both magnitude and sign. Thus the process of selecting the optimal feature set is rather simple. For this case, the computation of Γ in (14.12) is still a tedious task since a feature that is included in the set of m features may or may not be included in the set of $m + 1$ features. Thus the accumulated Mahalanobis distance δ^2 cannot be computed recursively.

Now let us apply the suboptimal method of the last section to this example. First we need to compute $\Sigma^{-1} (\mu_1 - \mu_2)$. It is shown in [9] that

$$\Sigma^{-1} = \begin{vmatrix} A & B & & & & \\ B & C & B & & & \\ & B & C & B & & \\ & & & & & \\ & & & B & C & B \\ & & & & B & A \end{vmatrix} \tag{14.16}$$

where $A = \dfrac{1}{1-r^2}$, $C = \dfrac{1+r^2}{1-r^2}$, and $B = \dfrac{-r}{1-r^2}$

Thus

$$w_i = \frac{1}{1+r} d \text{ for } i = 1 \text{ and } M$$

$$= \frac{1-r}{1+r} d \text{ otherwise} \tag{14.17}$$

The weighting factor w_i for $i = 1$ and M is larger than for any other i. This suggests that the first and the last feature should be selected first. The plots of Γ for various value of m for $M = 13$, $r = 0.5$, and $d = 1$ for all three methods are shown in Figure 14.4. We can see that the optimal method gives the best result and the natural ordering is the worst. The performance of our suboptimal method is somewhere between the optimal and natural methods. But the calculation for our method is much less involved than that for the optimal method.

Example 2

This example involves real data. Since in this situation it is impossible to find the optimal feature set we will compare the feature set obtained from our technique against the feature set composed of all available features. In this example we are trying to classify ERP patterns which correspond to a human subject making a binary decision, such as a true or false decision for a simple statement. The details of the experiment can be found in [32]. Each ERP pattern was 200 msec long and was digitized at the rate of 125 Hz. Thus there were 25 features for each pattern. The data were collected from eight subjects with 144 patterns for each subject; 72 patterns correspond to a true decision and 72 to a false decision. The error rate was determined by the hold-out method [33]. The data were partitioned equally into two mutually exclusive subsets, one subset for designing and another for testing the classifier. Two classifiers were designed using the design set. One classifier was obtained from the following procedure: (1) Obtain a feature set by our near optimal method. (2) If the number

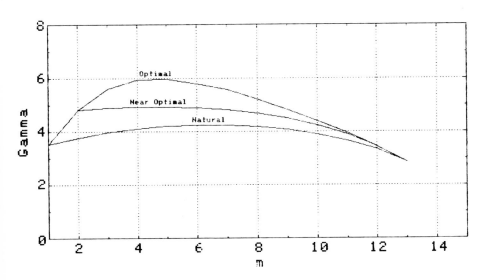

Figure 14.4. Comparison of feature orderings for example 1.

Table 14.1   Number of Errors Out of 72 Samples

	Optimal		All	
Subject	*Number of Features*	*Number of Errors*	*Number of Features*	*Number of Errors*
PJO	1		25	
D		10		3
T		17		22
VFH	7		25	
D		15		11
T		34		30
SMR	2		25	
D		28		7
T		30		43
DAT	3		25	
D		29		11
T		28		30
RHM	5		25	
D		18		11
T		29		26
JWB	1		25	
D		26		18
T		25		29
MPG	10		25	
D		15		15
T		36		38
JPM	10		25	
D		17		12
T		35		39
Average	4.87		25	
D		19.75		11.00
T		29.25		32.13

D, design; T, test.

of features in (1) is greater than two then reduce this number to two by the Foley-Sammon method [34]. This is done to aid the design of a linear classifier. Another classifier is obtained by directly reducing the number of features from 25 to 2 by the Foley-Sammon method [34]. Then a classifier is obtained in the same way as that used for the first classifier. Both classifiers are used to classify data for both the design and test sets. The number of errors for both classifiers for both the design and test sets are presented in Table 14.1. The first classifier is designated as "optimal" and the second as "all." It can be seen from Table 14.1 that the number of errors for the design set for the "all" method is always less and is usually much less than the error for the test set. This phenomenon is due to the sensitivity of the classifier when all the features are used in the design. This is caused by the dimensionality problem, i.e., the ratio of the number of samples in the data set to the number of features is too small. On the other hand, the number of errors in the design set for the "optimal" method is closer to the number of errors for the test set, and the number of errors in the test set for the "optimal" method is smaller than for the "all" method for the majority of the subjects (six of eight). A scatter plot of a sample set of the ERP data for both the design and test sets is shown in Figure 14.5. This example shows that in general our method for feature selection works reasonably well.

Example 3

There are numerous other theoretical examples that may be considered [9,30]. One such example is where each feature makes a contribution to the Mahalanobis distance that is a fixed multiple c of the contribution of the previous feature. In this case after m features are chosen, the accumulated Mahalanobis distance is

$$\delta_m^2 = d^2 + c^2 d^2 + c^4 d^2 + \ldots + c^{2(m-1)} d^2$$

$$= d^2 \frac{1 - c^{2m}}{1 - c^2}, \quad c > 0$$

where d^2 is the Mahalanobis distance of the first feature. An example of this occurs when the difference of the means is $(\mu_1 - \mu_2) = (d, cd, \ldots, c^{m-1} d)^t$ and the common covariance matrix is $\Sigma = I$.

When c is large, a large number of features is necessary to obtain the best classification. When c is small, the best classification is achieved with a small number of features, but the performance is inferior to that when c is larger. Thus, for large c the successive features contribute more significantly to correct classification. An example of this is shown in Figure 14.6.

In Figure 14.7 we see the effect of varying N, the number of training samples for this case. Increasing N improves the classification performance and increases the value of the optimal number of features required for classification. Table 14.2 shows the optimal number of features for various values of c, N, and d^2. When c is small, increasing N does not significantly increase the optimal number of features. When N is large changing d^2 does affect the optimal number of features. When c is large (on the order of unity or greater) the optimal number of features does not depend on d^2 but on the number of training samples N.

Note that for $c > 1$ the features are ordered from worst to best; for $c < 1$ the order is reversed. Figure 14.8 shows Γ versus m for both cases. We see a peaking phenomenon (optimal number of features) in both situations, with the peak for the worst to best occurring later. The performance of the best-to-worst ordering is always superior, except when all features are used; then both arrangements perform equally well.

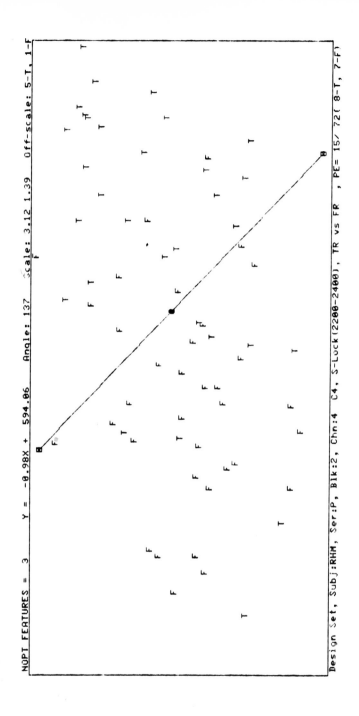

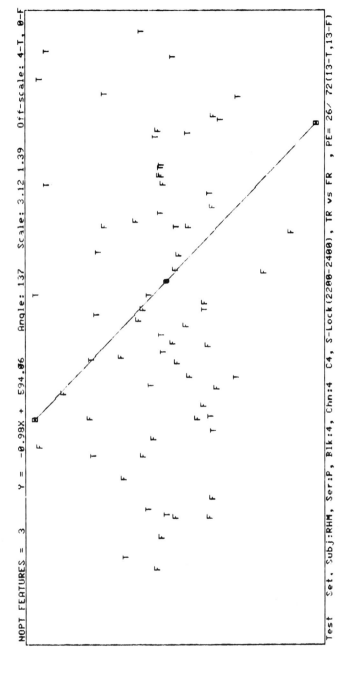

Figure 14.5. Scatter plot of ERP data for design and test data sets. Number of optimum features is three, but these were reduced to two.

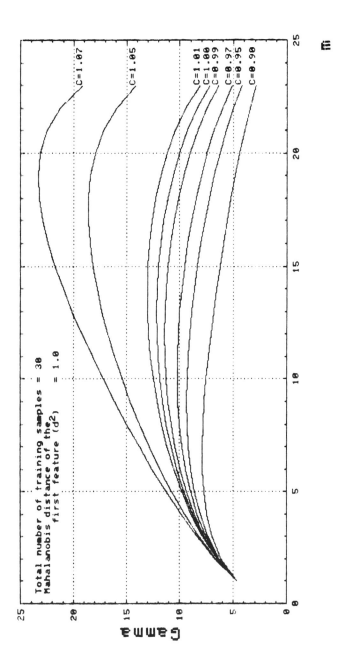

Figure 14.6. Effect of changing *C*, the fixed multiple of the contribution of the previous feature, to the Mahalanobis distance.

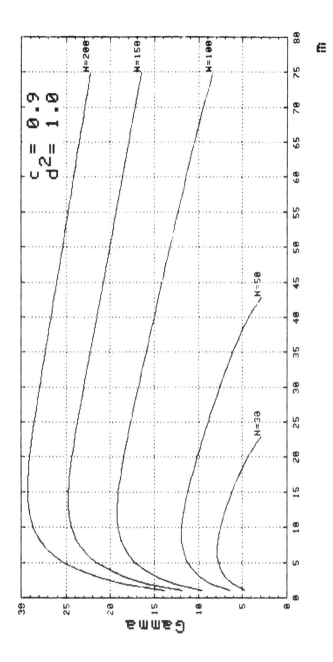

Figure 14.7. Effect of changing *n*, the total number of training samples.

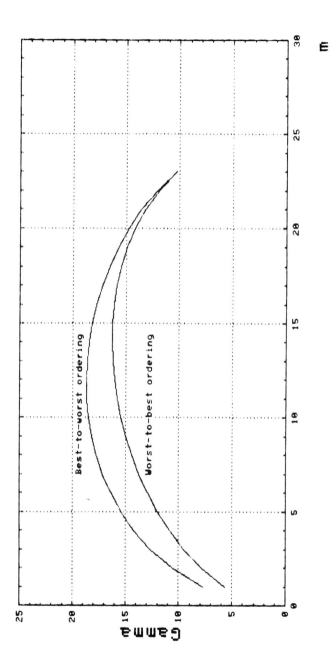

Figure 14.8. Comparison of feature orderings.

Table 14.2 The Optimal Number of Features for Example 3

d^2	N	0.001	0.01	0.1	0.3	0.5	0.8
0.1	20	8	7	5	2	1	1
	100	47	37	13	4	2	1
	200	93	66	18	6	3	1
	500	221	128	29	10	5	2
	1000	408	203	41	13	7	3
1.0	20	8	7	5	3	2	1
	100	47	39	19	9	5	2
	200	93	71	30	13	8	3
	500	223	142	50	22	13	5
	1000	412	227	74	31	18	8
10.0	20	8	8	6	4	3	2
	100	47	40	21	12	8	4
	200	94	72	33	18	12	6
	500	223	143	57	30	20	10
	1000	413	230	85	44	28	14

The column group spanning 0.001 through 0.8 is headed by *r*.

Example 4

Topographic factors in feature selection are dealt with extensively in Appendix 14C. Multichannel ERP data for feature selection and data classification using various design and test procedures are examined.

CONCLUSION

The dimensionality problem for equiprobable multivariate gaussian data with equal covariance matrices is studied. We have derived a recursive algorithm for selecting a near optimal feature set. An optimal exhaustive search feature selection algorithm is also presented and compared with our near optimal algorithm. Examples demonstrate that the algorithm works well. Our research addresses feature extraction that was optimal with respect to a Bayes classifier, i.e., the classifier with the minimum probability of error. Recall that the word "feature" in this chapter is synonymous with measurement or observation. It is not a weighted combination of measurements. Our examples are valid only when the difference between the means of the two classes is equal in both sign and magnitude in all directions and the correlation coefficients are positive. In general the best way to select features is through an exhaustive search, trying all combinations. However, the computation required is enormous even for a modest number of features. Consequently, we developed a recursive subopti-mal algorithm which works well.

In equation (14.1) we saw that the classification rule could be written in two ways. The second method compares a weighted sum of measurements to a threshold. A significant measurement would be one with a large weighting fac-tor. Consequently, one way to order the measurements is by their weighting factor $\Sigma^{-1} (\mu_1 - \mu_2)$. The measurement with the largest weighting factor should be selected first. For a fixed number of training samples, we suggest using an equal number of training samples for each class, i.e., $n_1 = n_2$.

In designing pattern classifiers, many factors are considered, e.g., the size of the training or design set and the number of measurements (observations, samples) in the data record (or vector). If the ratio of the available number of samples per class to the number of samples per data record is small, then data classification for both design and test sets may be unreliable [35]. This ratio should be on the order of three or larger [35]. This factor is important when only a small amount of data is available for designing the classifier. In this case there is an optimal number of features. Too few or too many features will de-crease the performance of the classifier. This is known as the peaking problem [2]. There are many causes for this, but one is that if you use too many features the added features may be unreliable or noisy and thus decrease the perfor-mance of the classifier. If you use too few features, then the classifier perfor-mance suffers because there is not sufficient data to properly classify the test samples.

While we did not show an example of this here, we point out that the fea-tures cannot always be ordered from best to worst. Further recall that the best features for a set of $(m - 1)$ features may not be included in the best feature of size m.

Appendix 14A gives an overview of the various methods for feature selec-tion; Appendix 14B outlines our algorithm for selecting features using parti-tioned data, which we have been applying to ERP data [36]. Appendix 14C presents extensive results related to the topography of ERPs. Basically we have found that by combining various channels in a "majority vote" configuration, we did no better than when we used the single best ERP channel. These results may be influenced by the experimental design, number of scalp electrodes and their configuration, and data processing. Our results suggest that each electrode channel contributes the same ERP information; therefore, the results using one channel were essentially as good as those obtained using multiple channels. One exception to this conclusion may be the use of ERP averaging across elec-trode channels. Presumably this would reduce the interference and improve the signal-to-noise ratio, giving a "better" topographically averaged ERP signal for feature selection. This possibility is presently being investigated.

The ability to detect single evoked responses (as distinguished from aver-aged evoked responses) will mean that real-time manipulation of the stimulus using signal processing will be possible. We should be able to design new experiments to better understand perception and cognition. The stimulus and response will reflect subtle shifts in meaning. We will witness the development of objective measures of learning, problem solving, and some aspects of behavior. And we should be able to trace the effects of drugs on brain function.

As we become more skilled at detecting the ERP and better able to tease out subtle "components" of the ERP associated with stimulus meaning and familiarity we should be able to enhance our human-machine communication capabilities. We might even be able to communicate with the computer via brain waves.

14A

Methods for Feature Selection

In this appendix we try to briefly show how various techniques for data reduction and feature extraction are related. Perhaps, we should start with *principal components*, introduced by Karl Pearson in 1901. The purpose of this statistical tool was to reduce the dimensionality of multivariate data. This technique is also known as the *Hotelling transformation*, the *Karhunen-Loeve expansion*, and *eigenvalue-eigenvector analysis*.

Principal components are linear combinations of random variables with special variances. The first principal component is the normalized linear combination of random variables (data samples) with maximum variance. The second principal component is the normalized linear combination that has the maximum variance of all such linear combinations which are uncorrelated with the first, and so on. This technique amounts to a rotation of coordinate axes to a new coordinate system which has the special statistical properties described earlier.

The principal components are the eigenvectors (characteristic vectors) of the data covariance matrix. The method of principal components was introduced to reduce the dimensions of the data set, but yet retain the spread (or variance) of the scatter of the data points as they were mapped from a higher dimensional domain to a lower dimensional domain.

The principal components may be ranked by various criteria and used as features of the data. For ERP time series the first principal component will be a time series waveform of the same number of samples and duration as the ERP; it might be something similar to the dc component of the ERP.

The Fukunaga-Koontz [37] method is a variation on the Karhunen-Loeve expansion. The best-fitting eigenvectors for class 1 are the poorest for class 2. This algorithm orders the eigenvectors according to their eigenvalues, which are normalized to the range 0 to 1. The eigenvector that is ranked first is the one whose eigenvalue differs the most from 0.5. This scheme rotates the feature space. The transform works well when the means of the two classes are equal and the covariances differ or when the means differ and the covariances are equal.

The Fisher ratio technique also transforms the data. This method works best when the means of the two classes differ and the covariances are equal. Data from two classes which have equal class means and equal covariances are not separable. The general case when the data for two classes is such that the class means and covariances are unequal is more difficult to solve.

Another way to approach feature selection is to maximize the distance between two classes in feature space. This is usually accomplished with a *divergence function*, which satisfies a number of properties. Let $D(\omega_i, \omega_j)$ be the divergence function for our data where ω_i denotes the ith class. Our feature vector is fixed in dimension to say, N. D is coordinate independent, additive for independent variables, and satisfies certain metric properties, such as

$$D(\omega_i, \omega_j) > 0,\ i \neq j$$
$$D(\omega_i, \omega_j) = 0,\ i = j$$
$$D(\omega_i, \omega_j) = D(\omega_j, \omega_i)$$
$$D(\omega_i, \omega_j)|_N \leq D(\omega_i, \omega_j)|_{N+1}$$

One such divergence function is the *discriminant vector* technique which selects features by sequentially maximizing a criterion based on Fisher's ratio.

Stepwise linear discrimination is a sequential search procedure that determines a subset of M features to represent the data. A feature selection criterion is adopted, perhaps Fisher's criterion. The feature vectors are selected sequentially. The single best feature vector with the highest selection criterion value is chosen first. This initial feature vector is then paired with all other features, one at a time, and the selection criterion is computed. The new feature vector which, in conjunction with the initial feature, produces the best criterion value is selected as the second feature, and so on. (Note that this method does not exhaustively compare all pairwise feature vectors, only those with the first feature. Thus, there may exist another pair which does not include the first feature with a higher criterion value.) As new features are selected, some features, previously selected, may lose their discriminatory ability because their information may now be contained in combination with other features. Such features are eliminated.

The set of M features may not be the best subset of M features. This is why it is called stepwise. But experiments have shown it works well. Similarly, experiments have shown that discarding some features does not greatly reduce the effectiveness of this technique.

This algorithm and others may, by chance, select features that work well with the design set but when applied to a test set may yield a poor classification. Therefore, algorithms should always be tested on a data set not used in the design.

According to Riccia and Shapiro [38] factor analysis puts more emphasis on discrimination than on representing the data accurately, as does principal components. The principal components approach tries to account for most of the feature variance, while factor analysis obtains a lower dimensional space that accounts for the correlation among the features.

One aspect of discriminant analysis (e.g., Fisher) is that we generally use a training set for the data. Factor analysis does not label the training and test data sets. All data samples are lumped together. Consequently, factor analysis is a good technique for cluster analysis since it uses all the data together in one set.

Riccia and Shapiro [38] have shown that Fisher discriminant analysis and factor *analysis* are related, with the Fisher optimal discriminant vectors being usually contained in the subspace found by factor analysis. This is important, since although these two approaches are conceptually quite different, they potentially have the same efficiency, with the additional advantage that factor analysis can be used in a wider range of pattern recognition problems.

14B

Summary of Our Feature
Extraction Procedure [36]

Each channel of our ERP data is partitioned into nine segments of 10 samples each. The duration between each sample is 8 msec (125 Hz sampling rate). Thus each partition is 80 msec long. The total data record is 720 msec in duration. The partition length was selected such that the correlation between adjacent partitions was small (less than 0.3 or so). We select one feature from each partition and rank-order these features. The two best features are then chosen for classifying the two classes of data, namely, the ERPs to true and false statements.

This feature selection is done as follows. Figure 14.B1 shows a sketch of our ERP and two partitions. For convenience we show only three samples in each partition. Figure 14.B2 shows a collection of ERPs for the true statements (class 1) and a collection of ERPs for the false statements (class 2).

In Figure 14.B3 we plot the data for one ERP for one partition in three-dimensional space, where each axis represents the amplitude of each sample. Thus, all three data samples end up being combined and represented as one point in this new three-dimensional space.

In Figure 14.B4 we show the result of plotting all the data for both classes of data. Here the responses for class 1 fall into one cluster with a centroid and the responses for class 2 comprise the other cluster with a corresponding centroid.

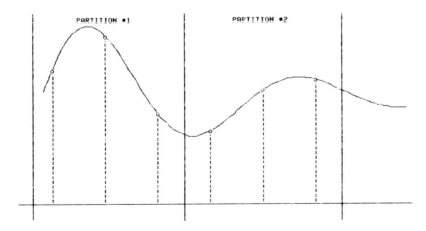

Figure 14.B1. Partition data.

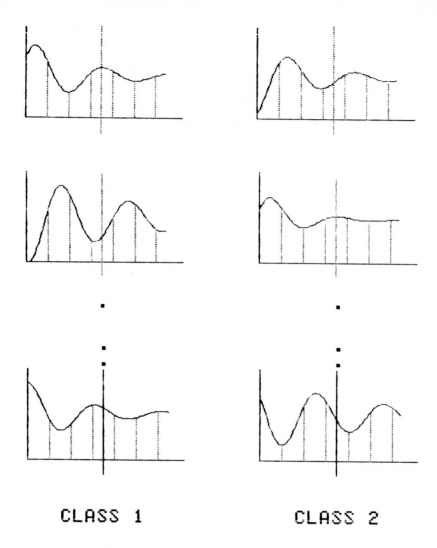

CLASS 1   CLASS 2

Figure 14.B2. Two classes of partitioned data.

Now these three features (or data samples or measurement values) can be reduced in several ways. First we could simply choose to use only two of the three data samples. This would mean that we would be in a two-dimensional space or a plane as shown in Figure 14.B5. Or we could even use just one data sample and have the data represented on a line as in Figure 14.B6.

Another way which makes use of all the data samples is to project the data clusters in a three-dimensional space onto a plane in such a way that the difference between the centroids (means) of the clusters divided by the sum of the variances of the clusters is maximized. This criterion is known as Fisher's criterion. Thus in Figure 14.B7 we might find that such a two-dimensional plane is as shown. We show the projected data

Figure 14.B3. Three-dimensional feature space.

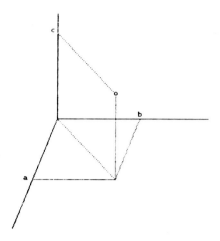

Figure 14.B4. Two classes of data plotted in three-dimensional feature space.

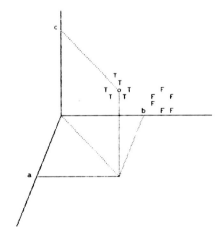

Figure 14.B5. Data for both classes projected into two-dimensional feature space.

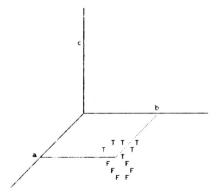

Figure 14.B6. Data for both classes projected into one-dimensional feature space.

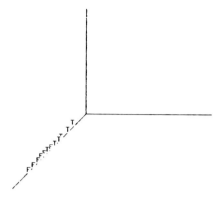

Figure 14.B7. Data for both classes in three dimensional feature space with decision plane separating the two data clusters.

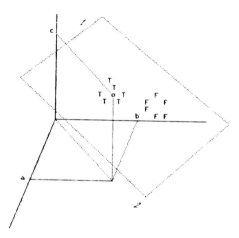

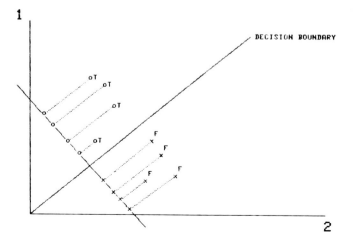

Figure 14.B8. Data for both classes in two-dimensional feature space with decision line separating the two data clusters.

onto this plane in Figure 14.B8. But we can repeat this step again by applying Fisher's criterion to reduce the number of features to just one by projecting the data onto the line shown. We now have one feature representing our original set of three samples taken from one partition. Each point in this feature space corresponds to data taken from an ERP. These data cluster in this feature space such that the ratio of the difference between the cluster means to the sum of the variances for each class is maximized. So we now have one feature to represent the data. We find the best such single feature. We may be fortunate enough to be able to successfully classify the data with a low probability of error using just this one feature. If not, we select the second-best feature from another partition of our data (because the data between two separate partitions are nearly uncorrelated) and use these two features to classify the data. An illustrative result is shown in Figure 14.5 of Example 2. Seldom do we use more than two features.

The features (as well as the original data samples) could be weighted (or linearly combined). We have investigated this to only a slight degree.

This feature selection scheme is basically a linear filtering of the data, e.g., classifying the data based on a linear weighting of the selected data features, and is not our recursive suboptimal method.

14C

Topological Factors

In one of our ERP studies we investigated the effects of multichannel recording on data classification. We were interested in the effect electrode placement and the number of electrodes had on data classification. As described for our other ERP studies, the subject's task was to read propositions and decide if the statement was true or false. We wanted to correctly classify the subject's responses using only ERP data. Did the use of multichannel data affect this classification?

The method we typically use is known statistically as the hold-out method for estimating the probability of error. This method designs the classifier using a design data set and then tests the classifier using a hold-out test data set. This method is known to give a pessimistic estimate of the probability of error.

An alternate classifier design method is the leave-one-out or jack-knife. Here one sample is left out, and the classifier is designed and then tested using the sample left out. This process is repeated for all members of the data set. An experimental upper bound on the classification probability of error is determined by this method.

Still another method we have examined is called resubstitution, which uses all the data to design the classifier. Then the complete data set is resubstituted as the test set and the classification probability of error is determined. This method essentially gives an experimental lower bound on the classification probability of error.

Tables 14.C1–14.C3 present the number of errors in classifying the data for the resubstitution, leave-one-out, and hold-out classifier design methods, where in each case we have reduced the number of features from the original 25 to only 1.

Table 14.C4 gives the number of errors obtained when a classifier is designed for each channel, but the decision for each subject is made using a "majority" vote obtained by pooling 3 and 5 channels, respectively. The column "best result" reflects the number of errors from the best channel for that subject. The channel 2 (Pz) column shows the results for our typically "best" electrode channel. Tables 14.C5–14.C7 are the near optimal feature selection versions of Tables 14.C1–14.C3 respectively. From these tables we have reached the following conclusions:

1. The probability of error lies between 25% and 33%. The resubstitution method gives a reliable estimate because the ratio of the number of samples to the number of features is $144/25 = 5.76$.
2. The ordering of the channels from best to worst is Pz, C3, C4, Fz, Cz, for resubstitution and leave-one-out methods, but is C4, C3, Pz, Fz, Cz for the hold-out method.

286

Table 14.C1 Number of Errors in Classifying 144 Response Trials of the Occupational "P" Experiment (2200–2400 msec) by the Resubstitution Method

Subject	Channel 1 (Fz)	Channel 2 (Pz)	Channel 3 (C3)	Channel 4 (C4)	Channel 6 (Cz)
PJO	29	22	25	23	27
VFH	47	29	32	37	40
SMR	50	51	37	49	51
DAT	45	36	44	40	44
MPG	40	41	45	51	47
JPM	44	38	45	55	43
RHM	35	32	36	27	39
JWB	38	41	37	39	45
Total number of errors for each channel	328	290	301	321	336
Average number of errors for each channel	41.0	36.25	37.63	40.13	42.0
Average errors in % for each channel	28.47	25.17	26.13	27.86	29.17

Table 14.C2 Number of Errors in Classifying 144 Response Trials of the Occupational "P" Experiment (2200–2400 msec) by the Leave-One-Out Method

Subject	Channel 1 (Fz)	Channel 2 (Pz)	Channel 3 (C3)	Channel 4 (C4)	Channel 6 (Cz)
PJO	35	29	29	30	32
VFH	51	36	37	40	46
SMR	54	53	42	52	54
DAT	47	41	47	46	48
MPG	44	47	48	54	53
JPM	50	43	47	60	47
RHM	43	38	44	34	46
JWB	46	48	46	43	46
Total number of errors for each channel	370	335	340	359	372
Average number of errors for each channel	46.25	41.88	42.50	44.88	46.5
Average errors in % for each channel	32.12	29.08	29.51	31.16	32.29

Table 14.C3 Number of Errors in Classifying 72 Response Trials of the Occupational "P" Experiment (2200–2400 msec) by the Hold-Out Method

Subject	(Fz)	(Pz)	(C3)	(C4)	(Cz)
PJO					
D	5	3	5	4	4
T	23	19	20	23	25
VFH					
D	10	7	8	9	12
T	35	32	24	30	36
SRM					
D	18	17	9	19	8
T	41	43	33	39	43
DAT					
D	14	8	16	14	16
T	36	29	27	25	31
MPG					
D	9	17	14	15	17
T	38	33	40	30	40
JPM					
D	18	10	15	20	15
T	36	29	39	36	40
RAM					
D	12	9	13	7	13
T	33	36	29	24	27
JWB					
D	24	24	18	15	21
T	26	33	27	28	31
Average number of errors					
D	13.75	11.88	12.25	12.88	13.25
T	33.5	31.75	29.88	29.38	34.13
Average errors in %					
D	19.10	16.49	17.01	17.88	18.40
T	46.53	44.10	41.49	40.80	47.40

D, design; T, test.

3. The results obtained using multiple channels is nearly the same as that using the best result for each subject. The results using the combination of three and five channels are essentially the same and are not substantially better than that for the single-best channel (Pz). It appears that all channels convey essentially the same information.

4. Our near optimal algorithm did not improve the probability of error (PE) for this experiment for the leave-one-out and resubstitution methods. It does slightly improve the PE for the hold-out method.

Table 14.C4   Number of Errors in Classifying 144 Response Trials of the Occupational "P" Experiment (2200–2400 msec) by the Leave-One-Out Method with Multiple Channels

Subject	All 5 Channels	3 Channels (Pz, C3, C4)	Channel 2 (Pz)	Best Result
PJO	28	21	29	29
VFH	40	36	36	36
SMR	47	47	53	42
DAT	40	41	41	41
MPG	44	44	47	44
JPM	42	45	43	43
RHM	33	35	38	34
JWB	46	41	48	43
Average number of errors	38.75	38.75	41.88	39.0
Average errors in %	26.90	26.90	29.08	27.08

Table 14.C5   Number of Errors in Classifying 144 Response Trials of the Occupational "P" Experiment (2200–2400 msec) by the Resubstitution Method with the Near Optimal Algorithm

Subject	Fz	Pz	C3	C4	Cz
PJO	38(1)	25(1)	29(2)	28(3)	33(3)
VFH	62(2)	42(5)	40(2)	43(3)	45(4)
SMR	60(1)	52(4)	60(2)	64(1)	63(1)
DAT	47(9)	45(12)	52(2)	64(2)	55(5)
MPG	40(6)	46(3)	49(3)	40(3)	57(6)
JPM	44(6)	60(3)	53(5)	64(1)	52(2)
RHM	46(6)	43(4)	46(6)	41(5)	48(5)
JWB	48(5)	50(4)	55(2)	51(4)	47(4)
Total number of errors for each channel	385	363	384	395	400
Average number of errors for each channel	48.13	45.38	48.0	49.38	50.0
Average errors in % for each channel	33.42	31.51	33.33	34.29	34.72

The number in parentheses for each subject and electrode location denote the number of features used.

Table 14.C6   Number of Errors in Classifying 144 Response Trials of the Occupational "P" Experiment (2200–2400 msec) by the Leave-One-Out Method with the Near Optimal Algorithm

Subject	Fz	Pz	C3	C4	Cz
PJO	38(1)	25(1)	30(2)	28(3)	33(3)
VFH	63(2)	44(5)	42(2)	44(3)	47(4)
SMR	62(1)	55(4)	61(2)	68(1)	68(1)
DAT	49(9)	48(12)	53(2)	66(2)	56(5)
MPG	42(6)	48(3)	50(3)	42(3)	60(6)
JPM	45(6)	62(3)	53(5)	69(1)	58(2)
RHM	49(6)	44(4)	46(6)	41(5)	50(5)
JWB	48(5)	53(4)	56(2)	52(3)	50(4)
Total number of errors for each channel	396	379	391	410	419
Average number of errors for each channel	49.5	47.38	48.88	51.25	52.38
Average errors in % for each channel	34.38	32.90	33.94	35.59	36.37

The number in parentheses for each subject and electrode location denote the number of features used.

REFERENCES

1. Allias, D.C. The problem of too many measurements in pattern recognition. IEEE Int. Conv. Rec. 1966; Part 7; 124–130.
2. Hughes, G.F. On the mean accuracy of statistical pattern recognizers. IEEE Trans. Inform. Theor. 1968; IT-14:55–63.
3. Duda, R.O., and Hart, P.E. Pattern Classification and Scene Analysis. New York: Wiley, 1973.
4. Trunk, G.V. A problem of dimensionality: A simple example. IEEE Trans. Pattern Anal. Machine Intell. 1979; PAMI-1: 306–308.
5. Chandrasekaran, B., and Jain, A.K. Quantization complexity and independent measurements. IEEE Trans. Comput. 1974; C-23:102–106.
6. Kanal, L., and Chandrasekaran, B. On dimensionality and sample size in statistical pattern classification. Pattern Recog. 1971; 3:225–234.
7. Van Ness, J.W., and Simpson, C. On the effects of dimension in discriminant analysis. Technometrics 1976; 18, (2):175–187.
8. Van Ness, J.W. On the effects of dimension in discriminant analysis for unequal covariance populations, Technometrics 1979; 21 (1):119–127.
9. Jain, A.K., and Waller, W.G. On the optimal number of features in the classification of multivariate Gaussian data. Pattern Recog. 1978; 10:365–374.

Table 14.C7 Number of Errors in Classifying 72 Response Trials of the Occupational "P" Experiment (2200–2400 msec) by the Hold-Out Method with the Near Optimal Algorithm

Subject	Fz	Pz	C3	C4	Cz
PJO					
D	18	10	8	15	9
T	21	19	20	18	17
VFH					
D	23	28	10	20	15
F	38	28	24	27	33
JMR					
D	30	27	30	28	31
T	34	33	27	31	32
DAT					
D	18	19	31	35	30
T	31	32	27	27	28
MPG					
D	14	15	20	20	17
T	38	35	41	26	38
JPM					
D	18	31	22	23	18
T	32	36	37	40	39
RAM					
D	34	10	15	16	18
T	29	34	32	30	30
JWB					
D	32	27	32	22	27
T	29	31	24	29	25
Average number of errors					
D	23.375	20.88	21.0	22.238	20.63
T	31.5	31.0	29.0	28.5	30.25
Average errors in %					
D	32.47	28.99	29.17	31.08	28.65
T	43.75	43.06	40.28	39.58	42.01

The typical number of features used for each subject and electrode channel was 3.

10. El-Sheikh, T.S., and Wacker, A.G. Effect of dimensionality and estimation on the performance of Gaussian classifiers. Pattern Recog. 1980; 12:115–126.
11. Raudys, S., and Pikelis, V. On dimensionality, sample size, classification error, and complexity of classification algorithm in pattern recognition. IEEE Trans. Pattern Anal. Machine Intell. 1980; PAMI-2; 242–252.
12. Roucos, S., and Childers, D.G. On dimensionality and learning set size in feature extraction. Proc. 1980 Int. Conf. Cybernet. Soc. 1980; 26–31.

13. Anderson, T.W. An Introduction to Multivariate Statistical Analysis, New York: Wiley, 1958.

14. John, S. The distribution of Wald's classification statistic when the dispersion matrix is known. Sankhya 1960; 21:371–376.

15. John, S. On some classification statistics. Sankhya 1960; 22:309–317.

16. John, S. Errors in discrimination. Ann. Math. Stat. 1961; 32:1125–1144.

17. Sitgreaves, R. Some results on the distribution of the W-classification statistic. In H. Solomon, ed., Studies in Item Analysis and Prediction. Stanford: Stanford University Press, 1961; 241–251.

18. Wald, A. On a statistical problem arising in the classification of an individual into one of two groups, Ann. Math. Stat. 1944; 15:145–162.

19. Anderson, T.W. Classification by multivariate analysis. Psychometrika 1951; 31–50.

20. Harter, H.L. On the distribution of Wald's classification statistics. Ann. Math. Stat. 1951; 22:58–67.

21. Sitgreaves, R. On the distribution of two random matrices used in classification procedures. Ann. Math. Stat. 1952; 23:263–270.

22. Teichroew, D. and Sitgreaves, R. Computation of an empirical sampling distribution for the W-classification statistic. In H. Solomon, ed., Studies in Item Analysis and Prediction. Stanford: Stanford University Press, 1961; 252–275.

23. Bowker, A.H. A representation of Hotelling's T^2 and Anderson's classification statistic W in terms of simple statistics. In H. Solomon, ed., Studies in Item Analysis and Prediction. Stanford: Stanford University Press. 1961; 285–292.

24. Bowker, A.H. and Sitgreaves, R. An asymptotic expansion for the distribution function of the W-classification statistic. In H. Solomon, ed., Studies in Item Analysis and Prediction. Stanford: Stanford University Press, 1961; 293–310.

25. Okamoto, M. An asymptotic expansion for the distribution of the linear discriminant function. Ann. Math. Stat. 1963; 34:1286–1301, (correction: 39, pp. 1358–1359).

26. Kabe, D.G. Some results on the distribution of two random matrices used in classification procedures. Ann Math. Stat. 1963; 34:181–185.

27. Sitgreaves, R. Some operating characteristics of linear discriminant functions. In T. Cacoullos, ed., Discriminant Analysis and Applications. New York: Academic Press, 1973; 365–374.

28. Anderson, T.W. Asymptotic evaluation of the probabilities of misclassification by linear discriminant function. In T. Cacoullos, ed., Discriminant Analysis and Applications. New York: Academic Press, 1973; 17–35.

29. Lachenbruch, P.A. On expected probabilities of misclassification in discriminant analysis, necessary sample size, and a relation with the multiple correlation coefficient. Biometric 1968; 24:823–834.

30. Achariyapaopan, T. Feature extraction and pattern recognition for realtime EEG processing. Doctoral dissertation, University of Florida, 1983.

31. Cover, T.M., and Van Campenhout, J.M. On the possible orderings in the measurement selection problem. IEEE Trans. Syst. Man. Cybernet. 1977; SMC-7: 657–661.

32. Fischler, I.S. Childers, D.G., Achariyapaopan, T., and Perry, N.W. Jr., Brain potentials during sentence verification: Automatic aspects of comprehension, unpublished paper.

33. Devijver, P.A., and Kittler, J. Pattern Recognition: A Statistical Approach. London: Prentice Hall, 1982.
34. Foley, D.H., and Sammon, J.W., Jr. An optimal set of discriminant vectors. IEEE Trans. Comput. 1975; C-24: 281–289.
35. Foley, D.H. Considerations of sample and feature size. IEEE Trans. Inform. Theor. 1972; IT-18:618–626.
36. Childers, D.G., Bloom, P.A., Arroyo, A.A., etal. Classification of cortical responses using features from single EEG records. IEEE Trans. Biomed. Eng. 1982; BME-29:423–438.
37. Fukunaga, K. and Koontz, W.L.G. Application of the Karhunen-Loeve expansion to feature selection and ordering. IEEE Trans. Comput. 1979; C-19:311–318.
38. Riccia, G.D., and Shapiro, A., Fisher discriminant analysis and factor analysis. IEEE Trans. pattern Anal. Machine Intell. 1983; PAMI-5:99–104.

15

Spatiotemporal Analysis of Cerebral Evoked Potentials

Giulio Sandini, Frank H. Duffy, and Paolo Romano

The measurement of brain electrical activity is based on the localized discrete sampling, both in space and time, of a biological variable. In multichannel evoked potentials (EPs) the underlying biological event is both space-and time-variant. To analyze the scalp-recorded activity generated by such events, spatiotemporal relationships must be explicit. This is readily apparent by inspecting the dynamic evolution of topographic maps generated by even simple sensory stimulations. Although topographic maps make biological events more comprehensible, they do not simplify the quantitative evaluation of the phenomenon; on the contrary, new and more complex features are made evident. Expressions such as slowing, lateralized, persistent, focal, and asymmetrical are often used to describe these complex phenomena. Such subjective terminology may be descriptive of the findings but is not easily amenable to a quantitative evaluation. How can we quantify these subjective judgments? How can we measure focality (a typical spatiotemporal event)? The answers to these quesions will enhance the diagnostic power of event-related potentials.

EVALUATION OF CORTICAL TOPOGRAPHY [1,2]

An analysis of the visual evoked response (VER) elicited by localized pattern reversal stimulation attempted to define the resolution achievable in the localization of brain activity with topographic methods of evaluation. Such resolution depends on a number of methodological and biological variables: (1) number, location, and spatial integration of recording electrodes; (2) position of the activated area with respect to the scalp; and (3) electrophysiological properties of the stimulated areas. Most of the biological variables depend heavily on the stimulation paradigm. To try to minimize some of these sources of error, a stimulation paradigm was designed in which (1) all twelve available electrodes were placed over the posterior quadrants; (2) the activated cortical area was limited to small portions of the primary visual cortex parallel to the scalp; and (3) the pattern of the stimulus was designed so as to normalize the activated area of the visual cortex irrespective of the location on the visual field.

Methods

The pattern used was generated on the TV monitor of an image-processing system (Figure 15.1*A*). The stimulus has a circular symmetry with a luminance profile defined by the difference of two gaussian functions. The ratio between the standard deviations of the two functions is 3. This corresponds in the spatial frequency domain to a range of about 1.6 octaves. As the integral of the stimulus profile is zero, the contrast reversal does not produce any change in the mean luminance. The mean luminance was set to 30 cd/m^2 and the contrast to 50%. The pattern reversal period was chosen randomly between 1.5 and 2.5 seconds.

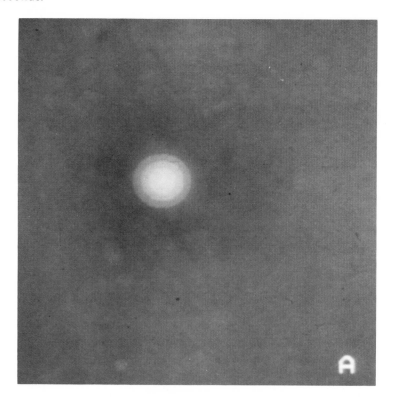

Figure 15.1A

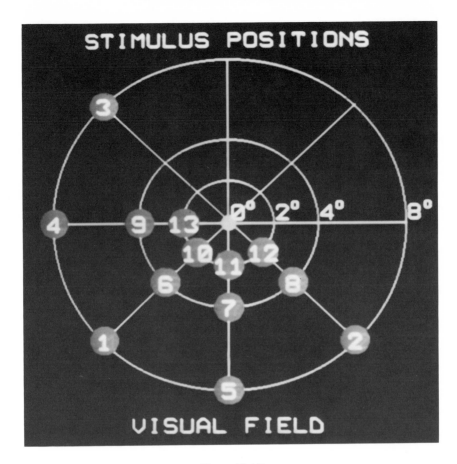

Figure 15.1B

Thirteen VERs were recorded from each subject by positioning the stimuli on 13 different locations of the visual field (see Figure 15.1*B*) at eccentricities ranging from 2 to 8 degrees. The size of the stimuli were varied as a function of foveal eccentricity such as to activate an approximately equal number of neurons irrespective of eccentricity. This was achieved by linearly varying the diameter of the stimulus as a function of eccentricity. Thus, at 2 degrees eccentricity the diameter was set to 1.5 degrees, while at 4 degrees it was changed to 3 degrees and at 8 degrees to 6 degrees in diameter. By considering the formula derived from experimental studies on the retinocortical projection in humans [3], the area of the primary visual cortex activated at each eccentricity was computed (see Table 15.1). Also the relative distance between nearby stimuli was computed in terms of millimeters on the surface of the visual cortex. Figure 15.1*C* presents the results of this computation. It is worth noting that by changing the size of the stimulus, the spatial frequency content also

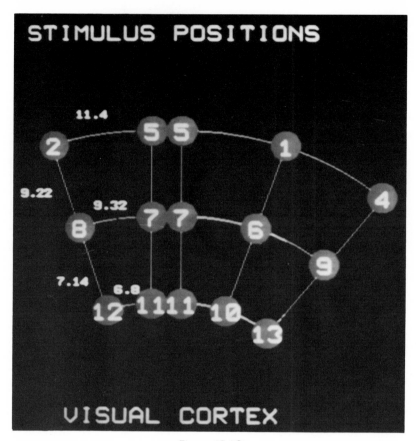

Figure 15.1C

changes: doubling the size causes the central frequency of the stimulus to decrease by 1 octave. This is an important parameter if we wish to normalize the stimulus with respect to the number of neurons actually activated, which depends not only on the projected stimulus area but also on the spatial frequency response of the cortical neurons.

Figure 15.1*D* shows the positions of the 12 recording electrodes. Some of the electrodes are in the standard 10–20 system positions, and others were

Table 15.1 Stimulus Radius at Different Eccentricities and Corresponding Cortical Size

Eccentricity (deg)	Retinal Radius (deg)	Cortical Radius (mm)
2	0.75	3
4	1.5	4
8	3.0	6

added to sample the occipital areas with higher spatial frequency. In this experiment a linked-ear reference was used. The experiment involved eight normal subjects ranging in age from 25 to 30. During the recording the subjects had to maintain fixation within a 0.5-degree circular area looking at the screen with both eyes. For each subject 100 trials for each stimulus were collected and averaged after visually inspecting all trials to remove artifacts for all subjects (the average number of trials for summation was not less than 80).

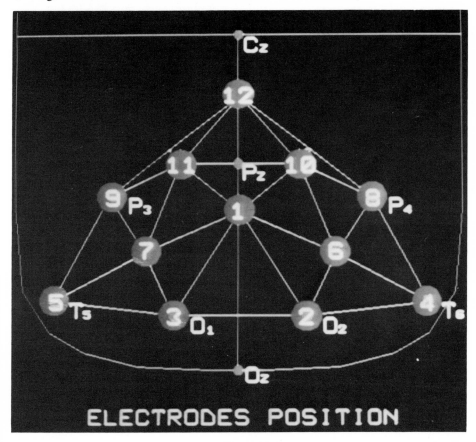

Figure 15.1D

Figure 15.1. *A.* Bidimensional shape of the stimulus used in the VER experiment. Average luminance was 30 c/m^2 and contrast 50%. The size of the target varied with eccentricity (see Table 15.1). *B.* Position of the stimulus on the visual field. *C.* Theoretical cortical projections of the stimuli (numbers are millimeters on the surface of visual cortex). *D.* Electrode configuration. The correspondence between the recording channel and some standard 10–20 locations are indicated. The vertex-to-inion distance was 64 pixels within the interpolation matrix used for bidimensional mapping. From Sandini et al [1], reprinted with permission from Martinus Nijhoff Publishers BV, The Netherlands.

Waveform Morphology and Topography

Figure 15.2 presents the VER of a subject to stimulus 5. Note that because of the central position of the stimulated area on the visual field, the morphology and the amplitude of the responses are quite symmetrical over the two hemispheres. On the other hand, if a left-field stimulus is used, the amplitude of the EP is higher over the contralateral hemisphere (see Figure 15.3). Stimuli do not produce a paradoxical lateralization [4] because of their localized nature and their positioning at eccentricities always lower than or equal to 8 degrees.

The mean response of the eight subjects to stimulus 5 is shown in Figure 15.4. During the study we noticed a considerable constancy of the EP waveform morphology among subjects. We attribute this constancy to the fact that,

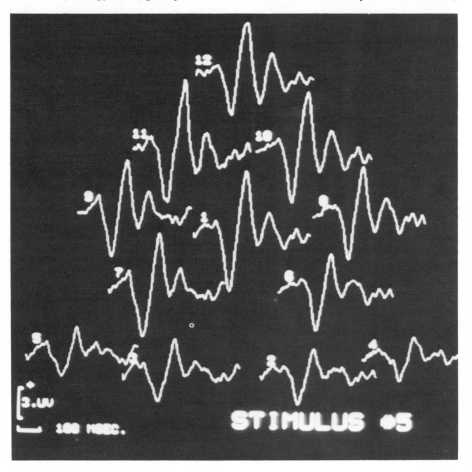

Figure 15.2. VEP of a single subject to a stimulus positioned on the vertical meridian (stimulus 5 in Figure 15.1*B*). The total duration of the averaged EP is 512 msec.

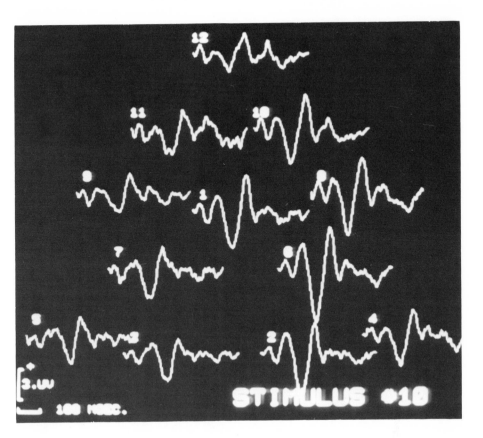

Figure 15.3. Response of the same subject to a laterally positioned stimulus (stimulus 10).

as the stimuli are very localized, the anatomical differences between the subjects do not cause distortion of the EP waveform as in full-field or half-field stimulation. In order not to bias the experimental results, the data from the eight subjects were averaged and stored in archive files in a form suitable for statistical processing [1]. The following analysis was performed on these averaged data.

The mean response of the eight subjects to a laterally positioned stimulus (10) is shown in Figure 15.5. Comparing Figures 15.4 and 15.5 two points are worth mentioning. The first is related to the "correct" lateralization of the response; the second, to the fact that, the maximum amplitude of the response, even if detected at different electrodes, is approximately equal for the two stimuli. This second finding is related to the normalized cortical activation achieved by varying the size of the stimulus as a function of eccentricity. The greatest difference was found for the EP elicited by the stimuli positioned over the vertical meridian (stimuli 5, 7, and 11) where the maximum amplitude was

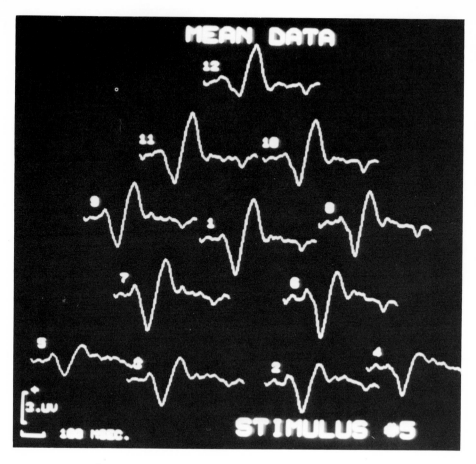

Figure 15.4. Mean VEP of the eight subjects to stimulus 5.

higher than that elicited by the other stimuli because the vertical meridian has a double projection of the visual field onto the visual cortex.

The primary morphological signature of the EP elicited by our stimuli was the presence of two main peaks, the first at about 160 msec with a negative polarity (N160), followed by a positive polarity peak at about 224 msec (P224). Analysis was limited to these two components. Apart from the findings described thus far, the analysis of the VER from monodimensional tracings does not allow for an accurate localization of cortical activity because monodimensional tracings account only qualitatively for the relative distance between the recording electrodes. Topographic techniques require quantitative evaluation of the spatial positions of the recording electrodes in order to produce a two-dimensional map of the superficial electrical activity. The approximation necessary to translate the three-dimensional spatial coordinates of the recording electrodes into coordinates within a flat surface (the interpolation matrix),

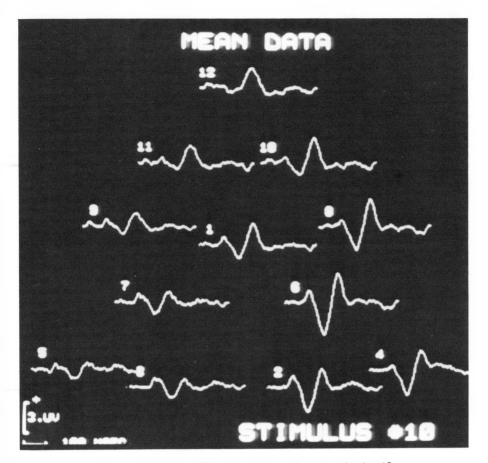

Figure 15.5. Mean VEP of the eight subjects to stimulus 10.

along with the choice of the spatial sampling frequency (proportional to the density of recording electrodes), actually limits the resolution achievable in the localization of focal brain activity. Given these limitations, the quantitative evaluation of spatiotemporal characteristics of the EP is certainly improved by explicitly considering interelectrode distances.

Figure 15.6 shows the spatiotemporal distribution of two VER to stimuli 6 and 7. Each single map represents the distribution of the electrical activity with a 4-msec time span (only the range 60 to 284 msec is shown). The basic spatiotemporal evolution of the two VERs does not differ significantly: activity of negative polarity originating from the central region spreads toward the occipital areas and is substituted by a positive polarity wave. The basic difference is represented by the movement of the positive and negative wave over the scalp, which is symmetrical for central stimuli. For lateralized stimuli this movement tends to be skewed toward the contralateral hemisphere. On the

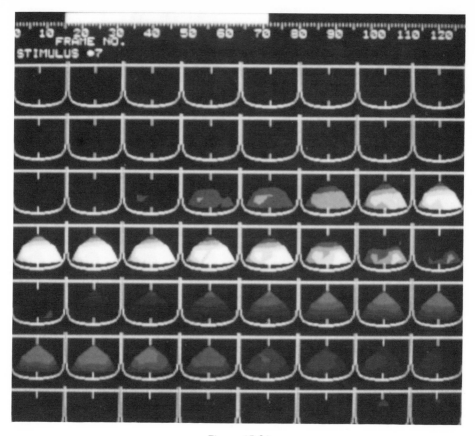

Figure 15.6A

other hand, the set of stimuli used in this study should, theoretically, produce different electrical fields according to not only the laterality of the stimulus position but also its meridian and eccentricity values. In order to test the possibility of performing such fine discrimination, a spatiotemporal measure must be capable of quantitatively evaluating the position of the superficial electrical field in time and space.

Spatiotemporal Analysis and Feature Extraction

The analysis of scalp-recorded EPs is based on the assumption that different intracranial electrical events generate different superficial electrical fields. While it is possible to describe particular situations in which this hypothesis is certainly false, in most practical situations the hypothesis can be assumed to be true. This does not mean that the relationship between intracranial and super-

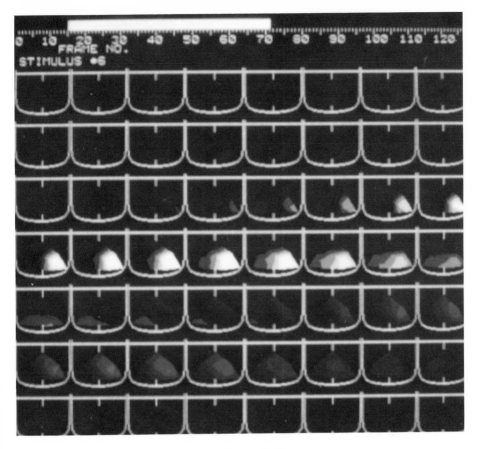

Figure 15.6B

Figure 15.6. Spatiotemporal evolution of the VEP topography for stimuli 6 (*A*) and 7 (*B*). Each map represents the distribution within 4 msec in a range 60 msec to 284 msec from the stimulus onset.

ficial variations is simple, nor that this relationship is space-invariant. It certainly depends on how deeply a given electrical event is generated. As to our experimental protocol the theoretical cortical changes are known and the deepness of the stimulus-activated areas is approximately constant. For this reason the data are well suited to study the relationship between internal and superficial changes of electrical activity. Conversely, it should be pointed out that the feature extraction algorithms described in the following paragraphs are designed to measure the superficial projection of the electrical event and not to determine the internal-to-superficial transfer function. For this reason terms such as movement and focal refer only to the features of the superficial projection of the intracranial electrical event. In the following analysis stimulus 3 (Figure 15.1B) was not included due to technical problems.

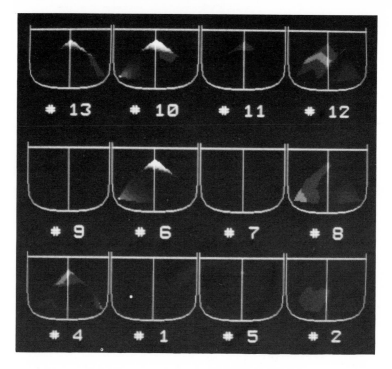

Figure 15.7. Latency maps. Each map represents the distribution of the latencies from stimulus reversal to the N160 component. The distribution is shown as the difference between the average latency of a particular EP and the latency at each electrode. (In the original color display blue areas corresponded to latencies shorter than the average; red areas represented latencies longer than the average). For example, for stimulus #6 the left posterior of the map is red while the central anterior is blue, meaning that over the posterior region a latency longer than the mean was measured while over the central anterior part the latency of the N160 component was shorter than the mean. Similar results were found for the P224 component.

Latency Maps

One way to measure the spatiotemporal properties of the EP is to measure the latency, or the time-to-peak, of a given component of the EP and to display these results topographically. By using this procedure, a measure of the timing of the spread of the electrical potential over the scalp can be derived. A "peak-finding" algorithm was implemented in order to identify the instant in time where a local maximum (or minimum) of each EP waveform is detected. The same procedure is applied for all electrodes. The matching between the maxima of different electrodes is performed by selecting the absolute maximum and searching for the closest (in time) maximum of all other electrodes. The matching procedure is then repeated on the remaining maxima until all the measures are matched or the current absolute maximum falls below a given threshold (selected as percentage of the absolute maximum of the EP). This hierarchical procedure assures that wrong matchings, if any, are most likely to occur only on low-amplitude peaks. For our data, for example, the two main components of the EP were always matched correctly. Figure 15.7 shows the latency maps for the N160 components. In order to determine the relative difference in latency between the electrodes, zero latency shift is assigned to the mean value computed over all electrodes. It can be readily noted that the peak of the activity is reached first over the regions contralateral to the stimulation site. This measure and display modality highlights both time and space characteristics of the EP. However, this measure does not provide information about the "focality" of the electrical event. In fact, the same latency map can be obtained, in principle, either by focal activity "spreading" over the scalp or by a localized maximum "shifting" over the scalp. To distinguish between these two requires a simultaneous measure of time, space, and amplitude.

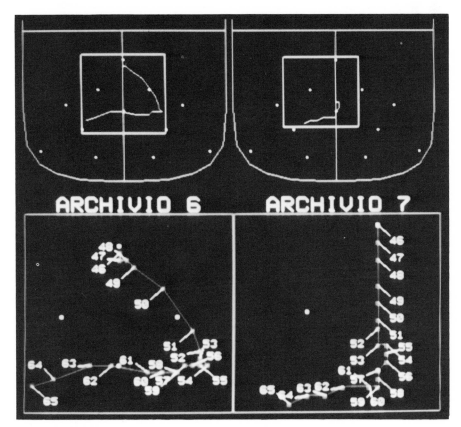

Figure 15.8. Trajectories of the CoG of the P224 component. *Left.* The trajectory for stimulus 6. *Right.* The trajectory of stimulus 7. The time span was 184–260 msec. Archivio = archival data averaged for 8 patients.

Center of Gravity and Trajectories Analysis

This set of features is aimed at measuring the position in time and space of the distribution of the electrical field. To this purpose, the position in space of the center of gravity (CoG) of the potential distribution is computed for each instant of time by computing for each frame the center of gravity of the area (or areas) whose amplitude exceeds a given threshold. For each frame the CoG of positive and negative polarity areas are computed separately. The threshold is preset as a percentage of the maximum amplitude for each frame and is computed adaptively by the program. If the CoG of successive frames derives from partially superimposed areas, the two CoG are said to be linked in time. The movement of linked CoG defines the trajectory of the superficial distribution of the electrical potential. Figure 15.8 shows the trajectories measured on two stimuli at P224 (in the range 184–260 msec). Each dot marks the position of the CoG for the corresponding frame (the frame number is also indicated). It can be seen that the trajectories describe synthetically the movement of the peaks of the electrical potentials presented in Figure 15.6. In addition to this graphic output, quantitative measures can also be derived. Among them the most useful in characterizing the spatiotemporal evolution of brain wave activities are:

1. Direction of movement
2. Velocity of movement
3. Area and spatial extent of the region above threshold
4. Measures of the spatial extent of the trajectory (i.e., maximum and minimum X and Y coordinates, area, etc.)
5. Focality score (FS) (the ratio between amplitude of the EP and velocity of the movement)

The FS proved very useful in clinical applications in locating abnormal focal activity in patients with supratentorial brain tumors [2].

The trajectory analysis described so far provides information about positive and negative polarities independently. In order to measure the combined evolution in time and space of both positive and negative polarities, a different feature extraction algorithm was implemented.

Zero-Crossing Analysis

During the spatiotemporal evolution of the superficial electrical activity elicited by sensory stimulation, the simultaneous presence of both positive and negative polarity activity is often found. In order to measure the relative position of positive and negative areas, the border between those areas, or the zero-crossing lines (ZCL), is identified in successive frames of the EP. The output obtained from different stimuli (10, 11, 12, and 13) is shown in Figure 15.9.

Descriptors for this feature other than the graphic output include:

1. Spatial orientation (computed as the angle of the best-fitted line throughout the ZCL)
2. Bending energy (measuring the error between the actual ZCL and its best fit)
3. Gradient at the point of zero-crossing (measuring the steepness of the potential distribution at the point of zero-crossing).

Results and Discussion

These feature extraction algorithms were designed in order to quantify the perceptual impressions of a human observer inspecting the dynamic evolution of a surface-recorded EP and they were not specifically aimed at describing the underlying intracranial event. On the other hand, the careful design of the stimulation protocol simplifies the internal-to-surface transfer function in such a way that the superficial electrical field should be a good approximation of the intracranial event. Certainly, the stimulation protocol allows for the testing of the experimental results from a point of view of the sensitivity to small changes in

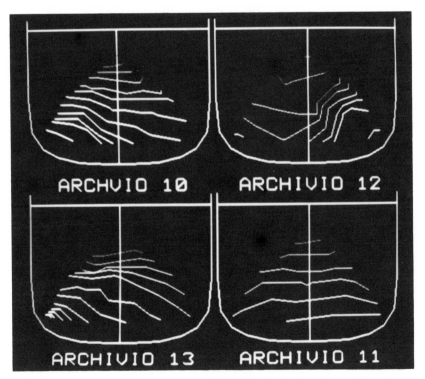

Figure 15.9. Positions of zero crossing lines for stimuli 10, 11, 12, and 13 in the interval 104–152 msec. Archivio = archival data averaged for 8 patients.

the cortical electrical activity [1]. Figure 15.1*C* presents the theoretical cortical projection of the array of stimulus positions derived from human experimental data positions. The ultimate goal is the development of a superficial measure consistent with these theoretical results. This implies not only a spatial measure, but also the selection of the particular latency at which to perform this spatial measure. The time-to-peak of the principal components of the EP is related to the electrode where the measurement is performed and varies with the stimulus position on the visual field. For this reason, instead of choosing a particular latency, the spatial measure of the superficial distribution was performed at the latency corresponding to the absolute maximum of each EP. These latencies are listed in Table 15.2 for both N160 and P224. The spatial measure performed was the computation of the CoG for all 12 stimuli. Table 15.2 lists these positions relative to the 64-x-64 matrix used for bidimensional interpolation. The results for N160 and P224 are presented in Figure 15.10. The results for P224 are qualitatively similar to what we predicted from the topography of human primary visual cortex. On the other hand, the results obtained for the N160 component are not well separated. The only clear information is the hemispheric lateralization.

There are a number of points worth discussing about this result. First, using our localized stimuli, the peaks showing higher repeatibility across subjects were at long latencies (about 160 and 224 msec). The P100 component showed a greater variability across subjects, as is demonstrated by its absence from the averaged EP. Moreover, the morphology of the EP is quite similar for all EPs. Generally speaking, we observed that the use of small, localized stimuli produces responses with a smaller variability than large target sizes, eventually producing a "paradoxical" lateralization [4–7] caused by the spread of the response from the hemisphere contralateral to the stimulated hemifield over the ipsilateral electrodes.

Figure 15.10 presents the positions of the CoG at N160 and P224. It is clear that while the mapping at P224 is consistent with the theoretical predictions, the distribution of the CoG at N160 does not show a good approximation. Taking the latencies of the peaks into consideration, it is quite possible that this mismatch at 160 msec is because at that instant in time distant neural processors are active simultaneously, summing their activity at the scalp. At longer latencies, however, the activity may be limited to cortical areas acting as localized current sources. In other words, while the electrical activation is reaching the primary cortex, electrical activity may still be present at the tectum and along the optic radiation (and possibly at the retina and along the optic nerve). For this reason, the only "uncontaminated" cortical activity is at longer latencies. The reason why we are able to correctly perform the retinocortical mapping in spite of the multiplicity of cortical projections of the visual field is still unclear. A tentative explanation may be based on the difference in processing performed by the different cortical areas [8] and the relative simplicity of the adopted stimulus, causing the main response to be produced at the primary visual cortex.

Table 15.2   Latencies Corresponding to Maximum Amplitude for All Electrodes for Both N160 and P224 Components. (Also indicated is the channel number where the maximum amplitude was detected and the value of the maximum amplitude. The coordinates of the CoG are relative to the 64-×-64 matrix used for the interpolation of the electrical data.)

Stimulus Number	Channel	Latency (msec)	Amplitude (μV)	Position X	Y
N160					
1	6	168	− 3.59	45.6	26.5
2	7	160	− 3.14	18.1	27.4
4	6	168	− 3.00	46.4	27.0
5	6	164	− 3.42	34.8	27.8
6	6	172	− 3.25	46.5	24.4
7	6	172	− 3.47	34.7	26.3
8	7	160	− 2.64	17.0	28.2
9	6	172	− 3.04	46.5	26.0
10	6	172	− 2.87	46.9	25.0
11	6	160	− 3.17	32.2	27.8
12	7	160	− 3.06	15.1	26.1
13	6	168	− 2.30	46.3	24.6
P224					
1	10	216	2.56	36.8	36.2
2	11	228	3.23	26.5	36.7
4	10	224	2.36	36.5	36.3
5	11	228	4.14	29.8	36.2
6	6	232	2.68	40.6	31.7
7	11	232	3.44	31.1	34.2
8	7	228	2.70	23.9	35.9
9	8	220	2.75	39.4	36.1
10	6	228	2.78	42.3	31.7
11	1	236	2.68	30.6	31.7
12	7	220	2.67	23.3	34.2
13	8	224	2.70	40.6	35.4

SPATIOTEMPORAL FEATURES IN CLINICAL STUDY

Very often the responses evoked by different sensory modalities carry different information about a particular pathological condition. In clinical application it is almost impossible to predict which sensory modality will be most useful for diagnostic purposes. This is due to the nature of the pathological condition, to its location within the scalp, and to intersubject variability. The aim of this research was to study the clinical usefulness of multimodality sensory stimulation associated with topographic data analysis. In order to perform such a task, the pathological condition must be known in advance. To test the localizing

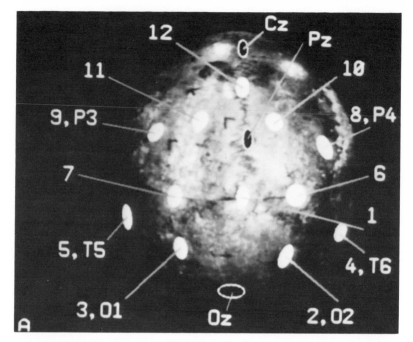

Figure 15.10A

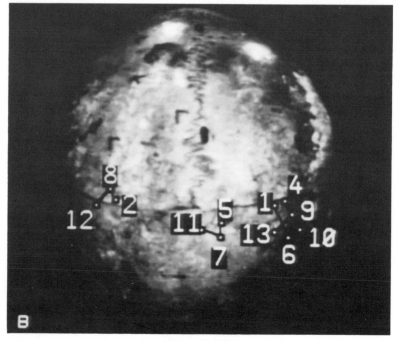

Figure 15.10B

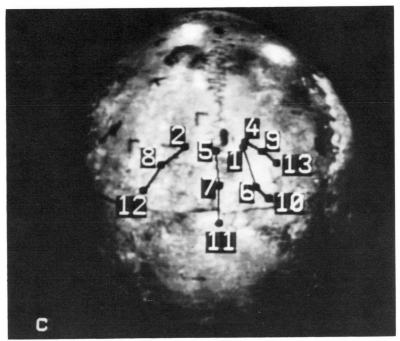

Figure 15.10C

Figure 15.10. Measured cortical projections for N160 component and P224 component. *A.* Mapping of the electrode positions over a human skull. *B.* Mapping over the skull of the N160 component. *C.* Mapping over the skull of the P224 component. Each dot in *B* and *C* represents the position over the scalp of the CoG of the distribution of the electrical potential at the time of maximum amplitude. A good approximation to the theoretical cortical projection (Figure 15.1*C*) is found for the P224 component (see text). See also table 15.2 for numerical values.

power of the stimulation-analysis paradigm, information about the position within the brain of the abnormality must also be available. A natural choice is thus to study the EP of brain tumor patients with positive findings on computed tomography (CT) scans. The choice of the stimulation modality is also important. One factor affecting this choice in a clinical environment is the attempt to simplify, as much as possible, the task required of the patient. Four different stimulation protocols, with three sensory modalities, were selected for study:

1. VER to flash stimuli
2. VER to checkerboard pattern reversal
3. Auditory evoked response (AER) to a pip of 1000 Hz, 20 msec duration
4. Somatosensory evoked response (SER) to bilateral stimulation of the medial nerve at the wrist

It is clear that the task of measuring the discrimination power of four different EPs involves the simultaneous processing of topographic numerical and visual data. Moreover, the spatiotemporal features considered diagnostically useful are usually expressed as verbal impressions rather than mathematical procedures. For example, a clinical evaluation of an evoked potential might read: "Initial negative vertex wave within normal limits but exhibiting tendency toward greater activation over right frontal area." The computational definition of a suitable algorithm capable of measuring such subjective judgments is by no means simple. An attempt was made to specify in computational terms some feature extraction algorithm capable of quantifying these subjective judgments. As an alternative to an exhaustive search checking each possible feature for its discrimination power, it was decided to derive from these experience-based features a set of numerical descriptors. Feature reduction and automated classification techniques were then employed to determine the best descriptors from this set. It is worth noting that this procedure, far from being a blind search is based on experience-derived observations and the statistical evaluation of their discriminating power.

Some of the features presented were formed by a statistical comparison between a given subject and a population of normal controls. Using such reference groups is mandatory in a clinical environment if one is interested not only in a quantitative measurement of specific features, but also in a statistical measure for classification purposes. To this extent, even if the diagnostic process is a far more complex procedure involving the correlation between the result of multiple observations and different clinical tests, if we restrict ourselves to a single specific examination, the task of deciding whether the data are within normal limits is a well-defined statistical procedure [9]. We were interested in more than a yes/no classification. For example, we were interested in classifying an EP as either globally or locally abnormal, as characterized by ipo- or iperactivity, and finally, as asymmetrical only or focally abnormal as well. These characteristics all require different measures of the topographic distribution.

Cross-Correlation Analysis

A first set of feature extraction procedures was aimed at providing a map of the spatial distribution of the EP irrespective of time. This was achieved by means of a cross-correlation analysis (CCA) technique based on the computation of the correlation coefficient between each of the 20 EP waveforms of a given subject and the waveforms of a reference group. These 20 numerical values (the correlation coefficients at time zero, or CCt0) can be used to produce a map. Plate 5 represents the distribution of the correlation coefficient for a subject with a tumor in the left frontal region. The region of poor similarity is clearly evident. This image represents a measure of difference irrespective of time: it is impossible to tell if the poor correlation is due to latency or amplitude differences. In order to measure latency shifts, a lagged correlation technique was used and two further features were obtained: the first mapping the maximum value of the correlation obtained within 100 msec lag time (MaxC) and the second showing the time delay to highest correlation (TMaxC). The mapping of MaxC for the same subject shown in Plate 5 is presented in Plate 6. In "pure" delay (i.e., not involving a morphological difference) on one or more channels, this map would have been uniformly distributed. The mapping of TMaxC is presented in Plate 7. This last feature aimed more at quantifying the latency shift, as well as its position on the scalp. In addition to the clinical meaning of each feature, it is important to consider the combined results of different cross-correlation features. For example, a pure latency shift would be indicated by a simultaneous high value of CCA features MaxC and TMaxC, while a low value of MaxC associated with a high value of TmaxC would indicate both a morphological and a latency abnormality of the EP. Obviously other combinations are possible (and were in fact found for some subjects).

Numerical descriptors can also be defined for CCA-generated features. From the more than 1500 EP features, the most important selected by automated classification techniques include the mean value computed over the electrodes of the CCtO and the minimum and maximum values of the TMaxC. These proved the most powerful in discriminating among normal persons and tumor patients. A combination of these two alone was sufficient to classify correctly 90% of patients. Of these features one was derived from AER, the other from flash VER.

Time-Only Related Features

An additional algorithm was designed for time-related features (EP score or EPS), which measured the average deviation from normal for each instant of time, irrespective of space. The result of this computation is presented, for a normal subject, in Figure 15.11A. The abscissa is time; the ordinate, the average value of the Z-statistic [10]. It is worth noting that in this normal subject, while no consistent deviation from normal is found, brief periods of statistically significant deviation from normal can be seen. Far from being rare, this testifies to the fundamental importance of multimodality stimulation and analysis of EP data. It is quite common in clinical practice for a single EP of a normal subject to show abnormal statistical behavior (e.g., above 2.5 standard deviations). No one of the EP modalities studied was sufficient by itself to correctly classify normal and tumor patients level significantly different from simple chance.

The information extracted by the EPS feature allows the determination of different classes of latency abnormality. Two of these are presented in Figures 15.11*B* and *C*. The former demonstrates a medium and long latency abnormality of a VER, the latter a long latency abnormality. Other classes include diffuse as well as highly localized latency abnormalities.

Spatial Trajectory Analysis

In examining the application of spatial trajectory analysis (STA) to clinical situations, we have found the main difference between patients and normal control subjects is that the spatial evolution of the trajectory is much more complex in the clinical population. Quite often more than one region of both positive and negative polarity is present. Some of these regions eventually merge or split during their evolution. From a computational point of view, we were forced to modify the original algorithm to allow for the determination of multiple CoG in a single frame.

Some examples of normal EP trajectories are presented in Figure 15.12. The basic pattern of all modalities is symmetrical with occasional slowing over the central and occipital areas: flash VER is mainly central-occipital; pattern-reversal VER, occipital; AER, central; and SER, centroparietal. For abnormal EP, the basic pattern is a long-lasting asymmetry, often over the position of a tumor. Some examples of abnormal trajectories are presented in Figure 15.13. In addition to the evident asymmetries, the focality measure (i.e., amplitude divided by velocity) proved particularly useful in determining latency and location of abnormal focal activity. For example, in Figure 15.13*D*, the maximum of the focality measure exactly pinpoints the location of the tumor. This exact localization is not always found. In fact, in other situations the focal ac-

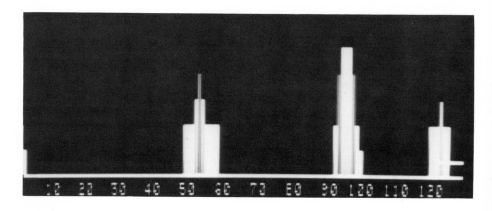

Figure 15.11A

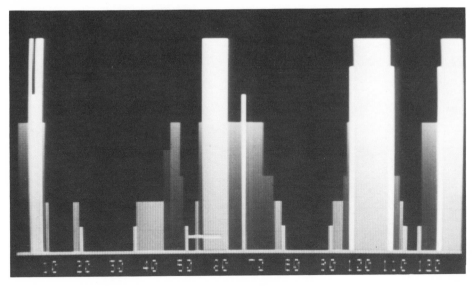

Figure 15.11B

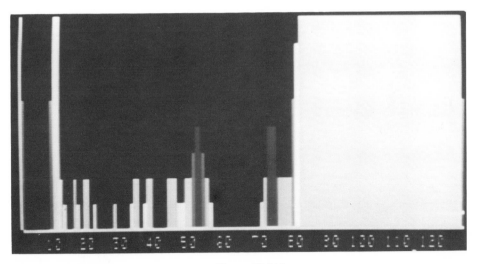

Figure 15.11C

Figure 15.11. Histograms of the EP score. This parameter represents the mean Z score computed over all the electrodes at each instant in time. This feature is space independent. *A.* Normal AER (see text). The maximum deviation was, for this subject, 2.5 SD (the highest bar of the histogram). *B.* Abnormal EP showing medium and long-latency abnormality (VER). *C.* Abnormal EP restricted to long latencies (AER). For both *B* and *C* the deviation from normal was higher than 3.5 SD (the highest bars in the histograms).

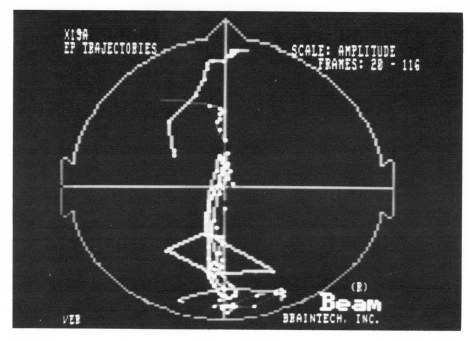

Figure 15.12A

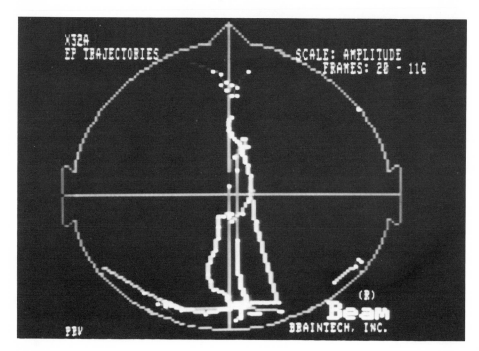

Figure 15.12B

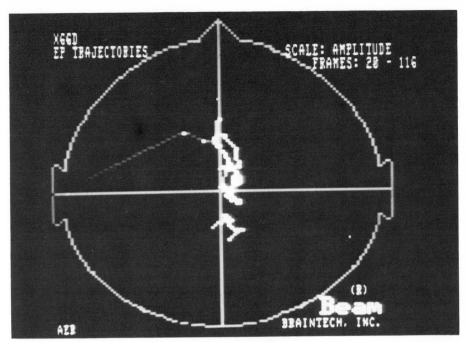

Figure 15.12C

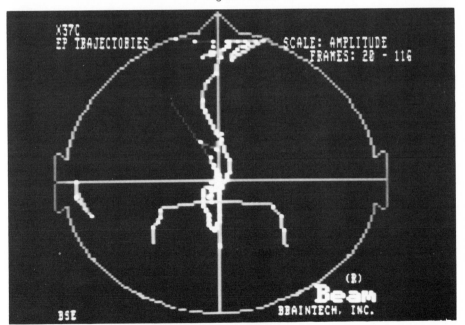

Figure 15.12D

Figure 15.12. Normal trajectories for the EP used in the present study. *A.* Flash VER. *B.* Pattern-reversal VER. *C.* AER. *D.* SER.

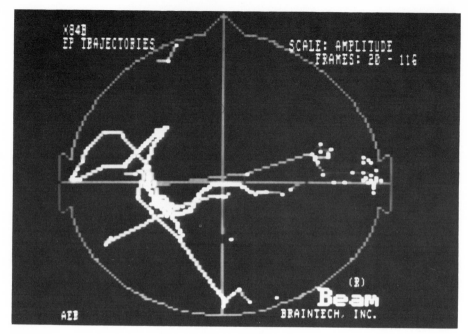

Figure 15.13A

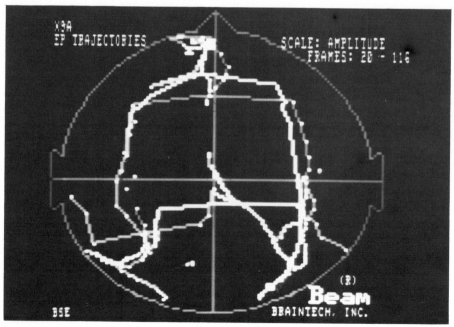

Figure 15.13B

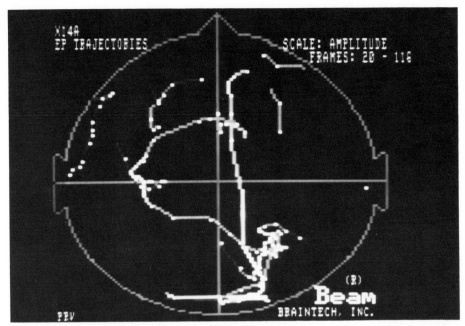

Figure 15.13C

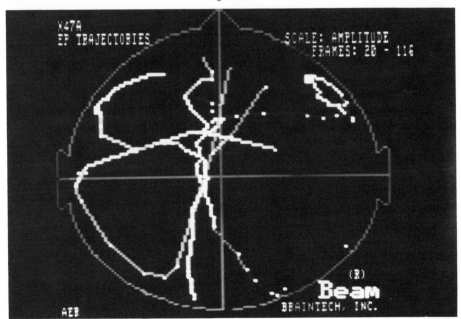

Figure 15.13D

Figure 15.13. Abnormal trajectories: *A*. AER for a patient with a left posterior quadrant tumor. *B*. BSE for a patient with a right posterior quadrant tumor. *C*. Pattern-reversal VER for a patient with a right posterior quadrant tumor. *D*. AER for a patient with a right anterior quadrant tumor.

tivity does not have any spatial correlation with the location of the tumor. This lack of correlation, far from being a disadvantage of EP analysis, is actually a useful measure of the functional involvement of an anatomical lesion, an indication of abnormality in regions other than in the locus of the tumor.

By using features derived from the STA we have been able to classify correctly 20 of our 21 tumor cases according to the location of the tumor (i.e., right or left, anterior, central, or posterior).

Discussion

A population of patients with CT-scan-diagnosed supratentorial brain tumors were studied to provide an evaluation of spatiotemporal features in a clinical application. Four different sensory modalities were used to test the classification power of multimodality-derived features. As anticipated, no EP modality proved sufficient by itself. The reduction of the number of features performed by feature selection and automated classification techniques allowed for the determination of the best combination of features from at least two EP modalities. With these techniques a total of more than 3000 features were reduced to the two best. It would have been possible, in principle, to forego the automated classification techniques and to attempt to hypothesize the best features according to some experience-derived rule. Our approach was chosen mainly for practical reasons. First, there are too many variables which need to be taken into account and, second, in a multimodality situation, it has been our experience that the combined use of more than one feature is probably the best classification method. This task cannot be reasonably performed without feature reduction and automated classification techniques. Moreover, the basic characteristics of our features are derived from experience in the analysis of clinical EP topography, thus ensuring physiologically and diagnostically meaningful features.

This chapter stresses the importance of a quantitative evaluation of EP characteristics from the standpoint of spatiotemporal analysis. Feature extraction algorithms are aimed at quantifying the subjective impressions gained by visually inspecting EP data in topographic form. The relevance of these numerical descriptors in a clinical environment is examined. We are furthermore convinced that even without application of visual inspection of these techniques, the EP data in topographic format allows for easier detection of brain electrical abnormality then does the inspection of polygraphic tracings. The basic aim here is to demonstrate that visual inspection procedures can be translated into computational procedures that eventually increase the timely resolution of the entire diagnostic process. Obviously the subject is far from being fully examined and even within the framework of the present study a considerable amount of work is still necessary.

The field of computer science is now at the stage where it is becoming feasible to outline and model the 'intelligent" behavior involved in the diagnostic process. Terms such as artificial intelligence, expert systems, and knowledge engineering are becoming more and more prevalent in the medical literature. Why are these techniques often linked to diagnostic applications? It is, we feel, because expert systems are capable of 'reasoning" with uncertain information. More than simply providing automated diagnosis, these procedures are designed to model the decision process by which the expert consultant performs a diagnosis. Modern medicine has become a technically complex process; more and more medical knowledge is developed each year either by the use of new methods of examination (for example, the explosion of imaging techniques) or by the development of new drugs or therapeutic procedures. Yet the cognitive capabilities of the clinician are pretty much fixed. How can he acquire, incorporate, and use this expanding body of knowledge? From an educational point of view the response has been to create specialties and subspecialties. The figure of the 'expert" serving as shared consultant is becoming more and more common in modern medical centers. This fact creates a broad heterogeneity in the quality of the medical service. The goal of artificial intelligence in medicine is to translate into computer programs the knowledge of expert consultants in order to provide advice to less expert physicians. In spite of the relative newness of this field compared to most clinical research areas, clinically useful examples have already been developed [11].

The interpretation of brain electrical data is undoubtedly a task requiring a great deal of expertise. On the other hand, this expert reasoning is based on quantitative data as well as perceptual impressions acquired during visual inspection of the EEG or EP data. These perceptual impressions need to be translated into objective measures in order to eventually build an expert system in the field of neurological examination (we would call this the "eyes" of the expert system).

This research area, along with the definition of the reasoning processes, is most probably going to be an important topic, not only in the field of brain topography but also in the broader areas of medical diagnosis based on imaging techniques. The feature extraction algorithms described here lead toward that goal.

ACKNOWLEDGMENTS

Part of this research was funded by the Special Project on Biomedical Engineering of the Italian National Council of Research and the National Institute of Communicative Disorders and Stroke grant NS 1467 (Dr. Duffy, principal investigator).

REFERENCES

1. Sandini, G., Romano, P., Scotto, A., and Traverso, G. Topography of brain electrical activity: A bioengineering approach. Med. Prog. Technol. 1983; 10:5–19.
2. Duffy, F.H., Sandini, G., Hochberg, F.H., and Burchfiel, J.L. Tumor detection from topographic maps of long latency evoked potentials: Spatial trajectory analysis and cross correlation analyses, unpublished paper.
3. Rovamo, J., and Virsu, V. An estimation and application of the human cortical magnification factor. Exp. Brain Res. 1979; 37:495–510.
4. Barrett, G., Blumhardt, L., Halliday, A.M., Halliday, E., and Kriss, A. A paradox in the lateralization of the visual evoked response. Nature 1976; 261:253.
5. Lesèvre, N. Potentiels evoques par des patterns chez l'homme: Influence de variables caracterisant le stimulus et sa position dans le camp visuel. In A. Fessard and G. Lelords, eds., Activities Evoques et Leurs Conditionnement. Paris: INSERM, 1973.
6. Cobb, W.A., and Morton, H.B. Evoked potentials from the human scalp to visual half field stimulation. J. Physiol. 1970; 208:39–40.
7. Lehmann, D., and Skrandies, W. Multichannel mapping of spatial distributions of scalp potentials evoked by checkerboard reversal to different retinal areas. In D. Lehmann and E. Callaway, eds., Human Evoked Potentials. New York: Plenum Press, 1979.
8. Zeki, S.M. Functional Specialization in the Visual Cortex of the Rhesus Monkey. Nature 1978; 274:3:423–428.
9. Duffy, F.H., Bartels, P.H., and Burchfiel, J.L. Significance probability mapping: An aid in the topographic analysis of brain electrical activity. Electroenceph. Clin. Neurophysiol. 1981; 51:455–462.
10. Dowie, N.M., and Heath, R.W. Basic Statistical Methods. New York: Harper and Row, 1974.
11. Szolovits, P., ed. Artificial Intelligence in Medicine. Boulder: Westview Press, 1982.

16

Geometric and Scaling Issues in Topographic Electroencephalography

Monte S. Buchsbaum, Erin Hazlett, Nancy Sicotte, Ron Ball, and Steven Johnson

The electrical activity generated on the surface of the brain may be recorded with electrodes placed on the scalp. This activity is not uniform over the entire scalp but differs from brain region to region. These regional differences have long been visually observed and deviations from a normal pattern taken as indicative of dysfunction. Electroencephalographic (EEG) tracings have been typically displayed as a single vertical series of lines, making spatial relationships of adjacent areas especially difficult to perceive. Interpolation and mapping make visual interpretation easier. A second problem historically has been the difficulty of detecting small quantitive differences in EEG activity at specific narrow bands of frequency. Spectral analysis techniques provide this assessment with precision. Together the two methods have provided a valuable new tool for the clinical investigation of the functional activity of the brain. These techniques, pioneered by Lehmann, Shipley, Rémond, and others, have been automated and brought to clinical fruition by Duffy, ourselves, and other groups in the past few years.

SCALP PROJECTION

In order to develop a representation of the surface of the scalp and brain that would be suitable for mapping of electrical activity, as well as information derived from blood flow or positron emission tomography, it was first necessary to represent the three-dimensional curved surfaces of the scalp and cortex on a two-dimensional surface. To provide a lateral view of the scalp and cortex, a series of coronal sections cut at 1-cm intervals were used (Figure 16.1). These cuts were taken from a whole-head atlas.

The work of Lehmann [1] and Ragot and Rémond [2] suggested the need for more than a standard international 10–20 system array. Their contour

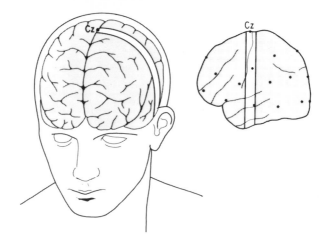

Figure 16.1. Generation of a brain lateral projection. The approximately equal area projection is derived from a series of coronal whole-head slices [12]. The lengths of the strip segment traced along the scalp were measured for each slice for the left hemisphere. The base point of each section was formed by the line connecting the nasion with the external auditory meatus and the meatus with the occipital protuberance. The succession of lengths measured at 1 cm intervals formed a surface when laid out flat as shown (*right*). The electrodes were then located on the map according to the international 10-20 system for electrode placement with four additional electrode locations in posterior cortex as shown in Figure 16.2. These positions were then projected downward at right angles to a line tangent to the scalp surface.

maps of visual evoked potentials (EPs) showed higher spatial frequencies in posterior cortex, manifested by a much closer spacing of contour lines. We therefore placed four additional electrodes in posterior cortex (Figure 16.2).

In order to compute a continuous surface density map for EEG or EP amplitude data, a four-nearest-neighbor interpolation algorithm was chosen since the 10–20 system is basically a square grid. For every picture element within the outline, the four nearest electrodes are identified by standard analytic geometry (Figure 16.3). Next, values for each picture element are calculated to provide a continuous surface map (Figure 16.4).

The technique is demonstrated for a group of 16 normal controls who had EEGs recorded and analyzed [3]. Increments of 1 cycle per second (cps) were chosen to reveal the boundaries of the classical delta, theta, alpha, and beta frequency bands. So that the relative regional distribution could be seen, each map was normalized. To do this, we calculated the mean amplitude and standard deviation across all 16 electrodes for each map. Then each electrode value was transformed by subtracting the hemisphere mean and dividing by the standard deviation. This produces a map of mean value = 0 and standard deviation = 1. Without this transformation, the high amplitude maps (e.g., alpha,

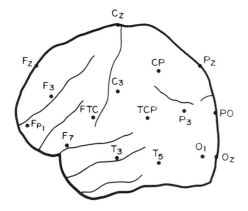

Figure 16.2. The left lateral brain outline is displayed showing electrode locations according to the international 10–20 system. Four additional electrode locations were added to provide greater resolution of the posterior cortex. These interpolated electrodes were placed in the centers of squares formed by connecting P3 – Pz – Oz – O1 (PO), C3 – Cz – Pz – P3 (CP), T3 – C3 – P3 – T5 (TCP) and F7 – F3 – C3 – T3 (FTC).

20–50 µV) would be black all over and low amplitude maps (e.g., beta, 7–12 µV) would be all white. Figure 16.5 shows the 20 steps from 1 to 20 cps and provides some visual confirmation of classical EEG frequency bands. Thus, frontal delta activity spans 1 to 3 cps, a central theta appears at 4–8 cps, occipital alpha at 9–14 cps, and diffuse beta at 15 cps and above. The topographic distribution tends to lump 8 cps with theta rather than alpha, as is often done. An occipital distribution appears up to 15 cps, but typical alpha blocking may not. Both functional and topographic criteria may be needed to define and understand frequency differences.

TOP-DOWN VIEW FOR CLINICAL APPLICATIONS

To provide the clinician with a view of the head from the top down, we used sagittal brain slices in the same way as the coronal ones in Figures 16.1 and

Figure 16.3. Interpolation from four electrodes to calculate the value for a position between electrode points. In this example, a location at distances (in arbitrary units) of 1, 2, 3, and 4 units are measured. Weights are then calculated with values inversely proportional to the distances as developed in Buchsbaum et al. [3]. The weights are scaled to be proportions of 1.00.

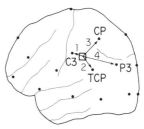

LEAD	DISTANCE	WEIGHT
C3	1	.48
TCP	2	.24
CP	3	.16
P3	4	.12

FILLING A SURFACE

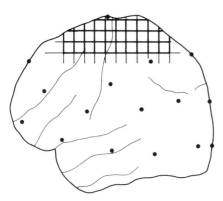

Figure 16.4. The surface of the brain lateral outline is filled by a succession of interpolated values. The value for each interpolated picture element or pixel is computed as the sum of the weighted contributions from the four nearest electrodes and the map is generated. The numeric values for each pixel are then assigned a color or gray level for visual presentation on a computer screen. A typical brain map comprises 2000–4000 pixels.

16.2. The strip from which the projection is derived is shown in Figure 16.6 and the arrangement of electrodes in Figure 16.7. This view is advantageous for examining cortical asymmetry in regions near the midline. However, the temporal lobe is less clearly seen than on the lateral view.

SCALING AND MAPPING DEVIANCE

Topographic maps can present EEG amplitude much as the colors on a geological survey map present altitude above sea level. Currently, it is standard to use a color or gray value scale representing absolute amplitude in microvolts (Figure 16.8, left). An advantage of quantitative electroencephalography is that by providing numeric quantification, comparable data on control populations with means and standard deviations can be gathered. Duffy and co-workers [4] have skillfully used this approach to provide maps that compare a single clinical case to a reference population. We have adopted this convention as well. An example is shown in Figure 16.8 (middle), where data on an individual are rescaled so that the values displayed and mapped for each electrode represent the deviance from the control population in SD units. Thus, for example, if the control population's mean alpha at Oz is 40 μV and its SD 20 μV, then an individual patient with a value of 60 μV is mapped as follows: patient minus control divided by control SD; i.e., $(60 - 40)/20$, or 1.00. This is usually sufficient to find major abnormalities, but may be insensitive: (1) to shifts in regional focus, (2) in low amplitude individuals, and (3) for low amplitude regions. These insensitivities stem from individual differences in mean amplitude and the skewed distribution of EEG amplitudes with a tail of large values. These create large SDs, making it nearly impossible for low EEG values to reach the -2 SD limit. For example, at Oz, our population mean is 35.1 μV and SD is 17.5; a zero amplitude (essentially unobtainable) is necessary to be abnormal. Further,

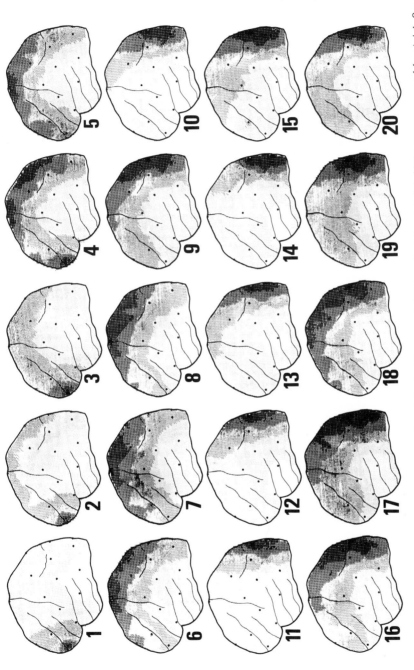

Figure 16.5. Mean topographic distribution of EEG activity in 16 normal controls from 1–20 cps. Maps are all normalized to the same scale to allow visual comparison; black = +2 SD, white = −2 SD (see text for details). Note appearance of frontal 1–3 cps delta, central 4–8 cps theta, occipital 9–15 cps alpha and central and occipital 16 cps and above beta.

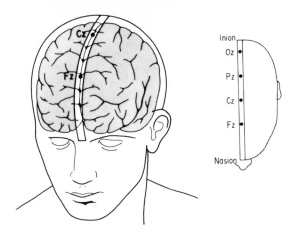

Figure 16.6. Formation of top-down of cortical surface from strips of the head created by sagittal sections. Because of the greater steepness of slope as the slices move outward from the midline, this projection tends to reduce the area of the inferior temporal lobe.

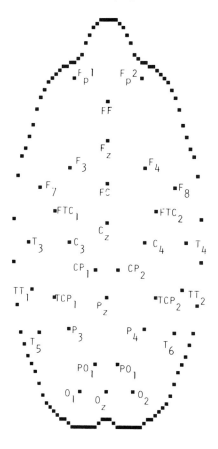

Figure 16.7. Placement of 32 electrodes on top-down map. Additional coverage of temporal poles and midline frontal areas is given as compared to Figure 16.2. Electrode placement uses the international 10–20 system locations plus five interpolated locations (FTC, CP, TT, TCP, and PO) on each hemisphere and two interpolated midline positions (FF, FC).

in individuals with generally low-amplitude EEG, even a substantial topo-graphic shift may result in a small SD shift. These problems are illustrated in Figures 16.8 and 16.9. A transformation of the individual maps as in Figure 16.5 before comparison with normal populations assists us; in the normalized map we emphasize the shape of the distribution rather than only its amplitude.

POLYNOMIAL SMOOTHING AND DATA REDUCTION

Polynomial surface fitting provides the possibility of reducing the number of values necessary to represent a map and to provide parameters that describe the surface in simple terms. Since both EEG and evoked potentials may have front-to-back gradients, a model as simple as a first-degree polynomial plane could fit some data. An equation of the form $z = a_0 + a_1 x + a_2 y$ could represent

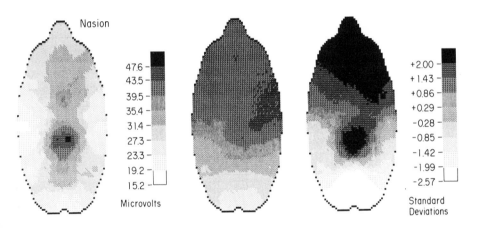

Figure 16.8. Top-down 32-channel alpha topographic maps are shown for a 32-year-old man with a history of psychiatric symptoms. Patient was resting with eyes closed for 3 minutes of recording. (*Left*) Map is full scale, and gray scale gives alpha magnitude in microvolts. Note alpha is of normal amplitude for the occipital region but peaks in parietal and posterior frontal cortex at the midline. (*Middle*) The patient's map was compared to a mean map of 10 normal controls, lead by lead. The entire frontal half of the map has high alpha activity (approximately 1.5 SD above normal range). However, nothing reaches ± 2.0 SD range. (*Right*) The patient's map is normalized as follows: the mean and SD of the 32 leads were calculated; next, from the value of each lead we subtracted the mean and divided by the SD. Thus, his map had a mean 0.0, SD = 1.0. His normalized map is then compared to the normalized control group map (mean of 10 normalized maps) and clearly shows abnormal alpha activity with values exceeding 2 SD in frontal and anterior parietal regions. This map appears more consistent with the visual impression from the raw data of an individual with an unusually central and frontal alpha distribution.

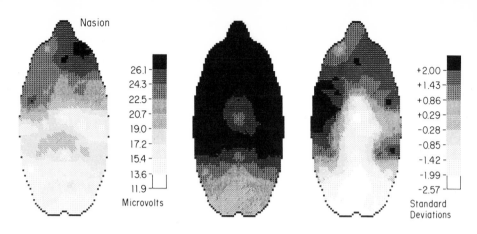

Figure 16.9. Top-down 32-channel delta topographic maps are shown for a 26-year-old man who had suffered an injury in the left temporal lobe area. Patient was resting with eyes closed for 3 minutes of recording. (*Left*) Full scale; gray scale gives delta amplitude in microvolts. (*Middle*) Patient's normal deviate map as compared to mean map for 10 normal controls. Patient shows high delta activity in the 2.0 SD above normal range in frontal and temporal areas. (*Right*) Data are expressed as within subject normalized scores. Delta activity is clearly abnormal, with values exceeding 2.0 standard deviations in left temporal region (*right*). This version appears to match clinical history in a superior manner. Comparison of these two scaling techniques is an area of ongoing research.

a visual EP or an alpha maximal at the occiput and minimal at the front, with the coefficient x (for anteroposterior position) describing the rate of decrease. This x coefficient, a_1, could be clinically useful in describing alpha abnormalities. In Figure 16.8 this shape description parameter would be abnormally low. However, as shown in Figure 16.10, surface fitting may require higher degrees of polynomials.

CORRELATIONS BETWEEN EEG AND BRAIN METABOLISM

In general, with alerting and mental activity, the slower rhythms of brain (alpha and the still slower theta and delta activity) are replaced by faster beta activity (3–20) cycles. Since local functional activity of the brain is closely tied to the use of glucose, the major energy source of the brain [5], one might expect relationships between EEG activity and local cerebral glucose use.

This relationship has been studied indirectly, taking advantage of the close coupling of blood flow to glucose use [5]. Correlations between EEG frequency and cerebral oxygen uptake, as well as blood flow assessed by the xenon clearance technique have been reported [6,7]. Electrical impedance rheoencephalography has revealed high alpha and increased blood flow [8]. In these studies, individuals are at rest, with their eyes closed and without a specific mental task. In this state, considerable individual differences are seen, with some individuals showing almost continuous alpha and others little or none: the correlations observed depend on this variation. The three studies indexed did not actually assess the region-by-region relationships between blood flow and EEG, as only a single EEG lead was recorded.

We have directly measured local cerebral glucose use by positron emission tomography (PET) with simultaneous topographic recording of EEG. The subjects were four men and two women (mean age 26) volunteers. All were right-handed and selected as controls for PET studies reported elsewhere [9]. Subjects were seated, slightly reclining, in an acoustically treated darkened room. Intravenous lines for injection of the radioisotope and withdrawal of blood sample were placed well in advance of the procedure and subjects were allowed to relax. Room lights were extinguished at 5- to 10-minute intervals before injection of 2-deoxyglucose (2DG) labeled with ^{18}F. Subjects were asked to close their eyes and keep them closed throughout the 30–40-minute post-injection period. Blood sampling, time keeping, and other activities were done by the light of a small low-intensity lamp and flashlight, and subjects were monitored for eye closure. Blood samples for ^{18}F-2DG and glucose were withdrawn from the left arm which was warmed to arteriolize the venous blood. Thirty-five minutes after injection, subjects were transferred to the scanner and seven to eight scans parallel to the canthomeatal (CM) line from +90 to +15mm in 12–15-mm increments were done as quietly as possible with lights off in the scanner area. The slices were reconstructed [9], and raw counts of each PET image were transformed into glucose use in micromoles of glucose/100 g brain tissue per minute [10].

Polynomial Regression Mapping

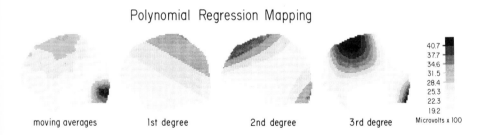

| moving averages | 1st degree | 2nd degree | 3rd degree | Microvolts x 100 |

40.7
37.7
34.6
31.5
28.4
25.3
22.3
19.2

Figure 16.10. Left lateral view of N120 visual evoked potential component using 16 electrodes and the standard interpolation (moving averages) technique is shown at far left. Next, a linear (first-degree) polynomial least squares fit of the form $z = a_0 + a_1x + a_2y$ is shown. Quadratic polynomial (second-degree) fit is of the form $a_0 + a_1x + a_2y + a_3xy + a_4x^2 + a_5y^2$ These six coefficients reduce the 16 lateral electrodes to six data points, a useful simplification in data analysis. Last, on the right, a cubic polynomial (third-degree) fit yields 10 coefficients but an improved fit to the image derived from the moving averages technique (*far left*).

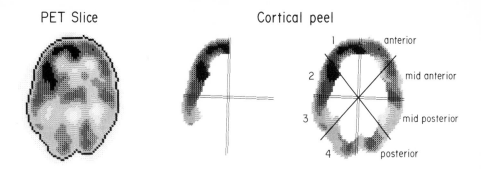

Figure 16.11. Technique for measurement of surface glucose metabolic rate. PET image is outlined by boundary-finding algorithm (*left*) and vertical and horizontal meridians are fit by the least squares method. Next, a radial scan defines a 2.3-cm-thick peel of cortical area (*middle*). The cortical peel is then divided into four sectors in each hemisphere, termed L1 to L4 for the left and R1 to R4 for the right. Typical localization of the highest glucose use cortical area within each zone is seen (*right*). PET scan is presented as a 9-level dot-density gray scale.

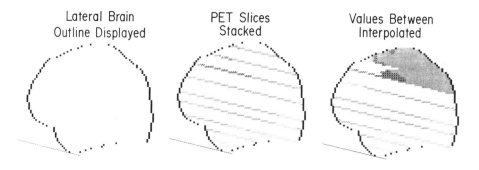

Figure 16.12. Technique for creating lateral cortex surface maps from PET slice images (Figure 16.11). Hemisphere cortical peels are placed on the brain lateral outline (see Figures 16.1 and 16.6) and values are interpolated between them. The resulting cortical map is then available for group statistical analysis.

EEG epochs following the ^{18}F-2DG injection were selected to occur during the period of most rapid FDG uptake (generally 2 to 8 minutes postinjection). The recordings were screened for eye movement and muscle artifacts, and 10 epochs were selected for analysis.

The transverse PET glucose images were reconstructed into a lateral cortical equal-area projection developed for EEG topographic mapping [11]. First, each PET slice had a 2.5-cm (8-pixel, or picture element) cortical strip peeled off the left hemisphere as shown in Figure 16.11. Values were then averaged across an 8-pixel depth. The proportional height of the slice from the CM line was calculated and the strip positioned and scaled anteroposteriorly on the lateral brain outline. Values between strips were interpolated forming a solid lateral view (Figure 16.12). From the known EEG coordinate positions on this view, a glucose value was thus obtained for the cortex approximately underlying each of the 16 EEG leads.

As individual differences in mean-slice glucose were greater than within-slice differences, we also normalized each subject's glucose values. This was done by calculating the subject's mean and SD across the 16 positions and then expressing each value as (absolute value − mean)/SD. Correlations were calculated between EEG power for the four frequency bands and the normalized glucose values (Figure 16.13) for $r = 0.75$, $p < 0.05$, two-tailed. A negative association between beta amplitude and glucose use was observed, reaching statistical significance in the temporal lead ($r = 0.871$). A negative correlation between alpha and normalized glucose was observed at the occiput (Oz, $r =$

NORMAL SUBJECTS
(n=6)

ALPHA   DELTA

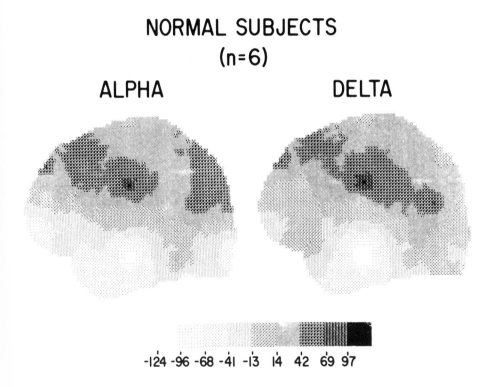

-124 -96 -68 -41 -13 14 42 69 97

Figure 16.13. Correlation coefficients between EEG activity and metabolic rate of glucose displayed as topographic map. Scale is Z-transform of product movement correlation coefficient x 100. Note significant negative correlation at occipital pole, indicating that the higher an individual's alpha, the lower his metabolic rate for glucose. This is consistent with the concept of alpha as an idling cortical rhythm.

-0.76) and temporal cortex ($r = -0.83$). Positive correlations were seen in central cortex (C_3)($r = 0.805$).

Analysis of the relationship of the functioning of the brain to spontaneous EEG rhythms has previously been approached through examination of EEG change during behavioral states without simultaneous measurement of glucose use. EEGs reveal that individuals who clearly show the occipital alpha pattern at rest associated with no visual stimulation exhibit regional lows in glucose use. Our correlation was extremely similar to that reported by Jacquy [8] ($r = 0.75$ in his report as in ours) despite his recording the REG from posterior but not occipital leads. An association between increased slow EEG (mainly delta) and low blood flow was noted by Ingvar et al. [6] and Tolonen and Sulg [7], although the latter findings were limited to patient's damaged hemispheres. Our finding that both positive and negative correlations appear in different cortical areas suggests that the physiological interpretation of these rhythms may differ by area. The harmlessness, repeatability, and low cost of EEG topography give it some advantages over the high cost of PET or isotopic regional blood flow techniques. Extended studies will be necessary to define further regional relationships; simultaneous PET and EEG studies may be able to better characterize metabolic information available in scalp electrical activity. Nevertheless, the studies here support the use of EEG topographic mapping as a way of inferring functional brain activity in brain regions directly below the electrode—a common supposition behind much of the work presented in this book.

REFERENCES

1. Lehmann, D. Multichannel topography of human alpha EEG fields. Electroenceph. Clin. Neurophysiol. 1971; 31:439–449.
2. Ragot, R.A., and Rémond, A. EEG field mapping. Electroenceph. Clin. Neurophysiol. 1978; 45:417–421.
3. Buchsbaum, M.S., Rigal, F., Coppola, R., et al. A new system for gray-level surface distribution maps. Electroenceph. Clin. Neurophysiol. 1982; 53:237–242.
4. Duffy, F.H., Bartels, P.H., Burchfiel, J.L. Significance Probability Mapping: An aid in the topographic analysis of brain electrical activity. Electroenceph. Clin. Neurophysiol. 1981; 51:455–462.
5. Sokoloff, L. Relationships among local functional activity, energy metabolism and blood flow in the central nervous system. Fed. Proc. 1981; 40:2311–2316.
6. Ingvar, D., Sjolund, B., and Ardo, A. Correlation between dominant EEG frequency, cerebral oxygen uptake and blood flow. Electroenceph. Clin. Neurophysiol. 1976; 41:268–272.
7. Tolonen, U., and Sulg, I.A. Comparison of quantitative EEG parameters from four different analysis techniques in evaluation of relationships between EEG and CBF in brain infarction. Electroenceph. Clin. Neurophysiol. 1981; 51:177–185.
8. Jacquy, J., Charles, P., Piraux, A., and Noel, G. Relationship between the electroencephalogram and the rheoencephalogram in the normal young adult. Neuropsychobiology 1980; 6:341–348.

9. Buchsbaum, M.S., Ingvar, D.H., Kessler, R., et al. Cerebral glucography with positron emission tomography. Arch. Gen. Psychiat. 1982; 39:251–259.

10. Sokoloff, L., Reivich, M., Kennedy, C., et al. The ^{14}C deoxglucose method for the measurement of local cerebral glucose utilization: Theory, procedure and normal values in the conscious and anesthetized albino rat. J. Neurochem. 1977; 28:897–916.

11. Buchsbaum, M.S., Cappelletti, J., Ball, R., et al. PET image measurement in schizophrenia and affective disorders. Ann. Neurol. 1984; 15:157–165.

12. Thompson, J.R., and Hasso, A.N. Anatomy of the head and neck. St. Louis: C.V. Mosby, 1980.

17

Issues in Topographic Analysis of EEG Activity

Richard Coppola

The surge of interest in the topographic mapping of electroencephalography (EEG) data is reflected by the several commercial systems that are now available and the many clinical and basic research studies under way. Some of these studies have as their direct interest the topographic (or spatial) analysis of the EEG; others are merely using topographic presentations of the data as an adjunct to the study. We know that there is considerable spatial variation in EEG patterns, thus topographic analysis and presentation has considerable potential for enhancing the value of EEG to both the clinician and the basic scientist. However, the ability to produce color maps of EEG patterns does not in itself overcome the many thorny problems of EEG analysis. The purpose of this chapter is to comment on some of the issues facing both the researcher involved in refining topographic methods and the clinician interested in application [1].

It is first necessary to distinguish among the possible uses of topographic EEG information. One use is for communication. Maps may be used as a succinct way to rapidly demonstrate focal activity, changes in activity over time, or different spatial patterns between clinical groups or between different conditions [2]. For this use the maps do not tell us any more than what we can already read off the paper EEG recording, but they do allow for a more graphic representation of that information. A second use is for localization of activity. Here the map provides information about the location of some activity or abnormality [3,4]. The map is the instrument for locating some region of interest and not just the graphic representation of already understood results. The distinction here is formed by the need for anatomical accuracy: for localization we require an anatomical map projection; for graphic illustration we need only a schematic representation. Both uses are of clinical concern. A third possibility is to make use of image or map projections to show spatial-temporal patterns in a way presently unavailable from only the paper record or the usual quantification methods. Here, we are interested in basic brain mechanisms relating both to normal and abnormal function. Temporal analysis is an important means of following the interaction between brain regions in a dynamic manner [5].

The issues around mapping include not only the details of how the spatial projections or graphic representations are derived but also how brain electrical data is to be analyzed. Further, there are a host of problems related to EEG data collection and analysis in general that are still present if not magnified by use of the map representations.

DIRECT TOPOGRAPHIC ISSUES

The accuracy of the map presentation is very important to localization of activity. For schematic presentation the concerns are more aesthetic, but we must also be sure that the methods employed do not introduce any artifacts or confuse interpretation or readability. For some systems the maps form the front end of the data path, that is, analysis proceeds upon the map. For other systems the map forms the final output; after quantification and analysis, the map is generated to illustrate the results. The map only exists as a computer representation of some model of the distribution of electrical activity at the scalp. This model must be kept in mind when analysis is carried out with map values.

For localization, the accuracy of the map is crucial; however, even for illustrative purposes map accuracy is desirable if it is not too expensive. The issue of map accuracy can be divided into three concerns: the choice of the projection geometry for map presentation and associated display characteristics; the interpolation method used to fill in the map; and the montage used to derive the electrical information. This last item includes the choice of reference electrode(s) and the transformation to be worked upon the recorded EEG, if any, prior to map generation.

The one salient issue about map choice is that of projection geometry. The three-dimensional head must be represented by a two-dimensional surface in order to generate the map view. This is a cartography problem and the choice of projection will affect the amount of distortion in the two-dimensional view. The only choice which does not introduce gradient distortions is an equal area projection, that is, the projection of an area from the three-dimensional surface that is represented by an equal area on the two-dimensional surface. This makes the metric for distance equal in all parts of the map and allows comparison of gradients (potential change per centimeter) at any place on the map. Once the projection geometry and viewpoint has been selected, it must be represented within the limits of the computer display to be used. Fortunately computer technology has reached the point where these limits do not provide any significant constraints [6]. Most display systems represent images as an X and Y grid of image points, or pixels. We have used a 60-by-80 pixel grid to represent the lateral view of the head, as shown in Figure 17.1. The issue here is to have a pixel resolution comparable to the spatial resolution of our data. Either a gray scale or color scale must then be used to represent the data value at each pixel. Choices of scale can drastically change the impact of the image. Smooth transition in both intensity and hue is necessary for color coding.

Given our choice of map geometry and display format it is next necessary to arrive at a number representing the appropriate EEG measure for each pixel. Regardless of whether we are displaying the instantaneous amplitude of the EEG or a derived value such as those using spectrum analysis, we have real data at only the original recording leads. Most mapping schemes use some form of interpolation from nearby electrodes, usually 3 or 4, to compute the value for pixels other than those at the electrode sites. Usually linear interpolation, based on a weighting by the inverse of the distance to the neighboring electrodes, has been the preferred method. Walter and Etevenon [7] have argued for using inverse distance squared or cubed as weighting factors. Others have looked at the number of electrodes to use for the interpolation [8]. The best plan would be to choose the method empirically. We are currently working on determining a regional model based on 32-lead recordings performed on one hemisphere, as shown in Figure 17.1. Due to various heterogeneities, the number and choice of electrodes, as well as the appropriate weighting, varies considerably in different regions of the scalp. It appears that the pattern of elec-

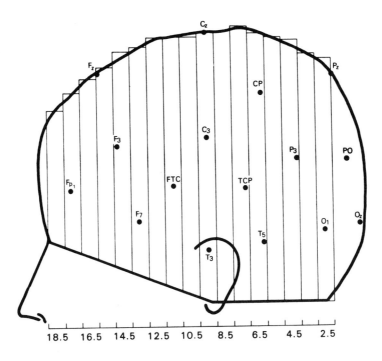

Figure 17.1. Lateral view of the left hemisphere showing equal area projection and electrode placements for 16 lead recording.

trodes in this regional model will follow lobe boundaries. Also, any model developed empirically for one brain state may introduce errors when applied in another condition.

This discussion of interpolation (and most currently applied topographic mapping) is based on referential EEG recordings where the multiple electrode sites are all recorded and referenced to the same electrode. That is, in order for the mapping to make sense, the data at each electrode must be determined relative to the same reference point. Linked ears, a noncephalic reference, or common average electrode have been the usual choices [9–11]. Each has its disadvantages and considerable effort has gone into finding a reference-free method in order to overcome these. The source derivation method of Hjorth [12,13] is one such attempt, but when approximated by the distance-weighted sum of all the recording electrodes, it is basically equivalent to the common average reference method. The source derivation was meant to be an approximation to the Laplacian of the potential field, thus representing the current source density distribution [14]. This requires having electrodes in a special arrangement in order to achieve the necessary directional sensitivity. This directional sensitivity is lost in the distance-weighted source derivation method because electrode orientation is not taken into account. Another way to compute the Laplacian would be based upon an improved interpolation model being developed using each pixel as if it were an electrode. Even if a reference-free derivation is arrived at, it will not immediately solve all our problems. We will still have to learn to interpret our results in this new framework and to develop further models about how this surface distribution relates to underlying activity.

ANALYSIS ISSUES

Topographic maps may be a useful means of illustrating our data but by themselves do not constitute an analysis of that data. One aspect of analysis may, of course, be localization, for example, of a spike focus, and the map produced by the proper topographic methods may demonstrate the result so dramatically that little further analysis is necessary.

Analysis issues may be considered in three parts: those methods applied before the data is mapped such as spectrum analysis; spatial analysis such as used to produce the map itself; and group analysis, including the various statistical methods needed to demonstrate differences among clinical populations.

Most topographic EEG studies have utilized spectrum analysis (SA) as the initial data-processing step. The choice of the proper parameters for SA has been under discussion for many years [15, 16]. When the SA results can be examined across time and for all frequencies, the exact choice of parameters is not so crucial; however, producing maps from SA telescopes a lot of data into one or more maps. A map represents the activity in a specific frequency band for some specific period of time. Thus, the choice of band and time length is critical to the map appearance and interpretation.

The bands are usually chosen at the classical divisions of EEG into delta, theta, alpha, and beta. The exact frequencies comprising the bands are somewhat arbitrary and many investigators have subdivided both alpha and beta into low- and high-frequency ranges. This frequency structure has been examined in several studies by factor analytic techniques in an attempt to arrive at more rigorously defined bands [17,18]. However, most of these studies have used only one, or just a few, EEG leads. It may be useful to use topographic data to better determine the frequency structure. In preliminary data we found that low and high alpha bands had considerably different topographic distributions. In 20 subjects at rest with eyes closed, low alpha (7 to 10 cps) showed a parietal maximum, where alpha in the band 10 to 13 cps showed an occipital maximum. The SA was averaged over 1 minute with linked ears as reference. Plate 8 shows this result for the left hemisphere lateral view. The suggestion is that the EEG spectrum can be segmented on frequency as well as topographic structure and that both will be necessary to define normative SA.

Spectrum analysis requires first choosing some epoch length of EEG for which the activity at different frequencies is computed, usually by fast Fourier transform methods. The length of the epoch is inversely related to the width and spacing of the frequency bins so that temporal resolution can only be obtained at the expense of frequency resolution. Unless very narrow frequency components are of interest, only a resolution sufficient to define the edges of the frequency bands to be analyzed is necessary. We have chosen a basic epoch of 2.56 seconds for a frequency resolution of about 0.4 Hz. (1/2.56). Bands are then computed by summing across these basic or raw frequency bins. For analysis of longer pieces of EEG, the SA results are averaged for several 2.56-second epochs. The size of the longer piece of EEG to be used will depend on how long a subject's EEG remains stationary, which in turn depends on the subject's behavioral state. This will be related to how well we can define or control this state, perhaps by activation procedures.

After the initial processing steps for individual data, further statistical analysis is usually required. Such analysis may be designed to compare a specific subject's data with normative values or to compare between-group data. Significance probability mapping, as developed by Duffy and Bartels [19], is a way of accomplishing both these comparisons by performing the statistical analysis directly on the EEG maps on a pixel-by-pixel basis. The combination of statistical and classification techniques can be a very powerful way to quantify topographic differences. However, when statistics are being computed on a pixel basis, it means that interpolated points form most of the data base. Topographic results can be misleading due to reduction of variance at interpolated points, yielding a spuriously higher statistic. On the other hand, the clustering of significance is more easily recognized, thus helping to follow areas of interest through the analysis.

Multilead EEG data can be analyzed in a more conventional statistical approach using standard software packages. Multivariate analysis of variance (MANOVA) is an approach that can be used to demonstrate statistical differences and to verify topographic distributions. The model used is that of the usual factorial design, for example, treatment by group and condition with repeated measures if appropriate. The multivariates are the leads. A separate MANOVA using this model is then performed for each frequency band of interest. The frequencies could also be analyzed as multivariate, but usually the number of subjects is too low. If the multivariate interaction is significant, then the univariate statistics for each lead can be examined to determine the topographic structure. Other multivariate methods may be employed to describe the regional pattern of spectral information [20].

ACTIVATION PROCEDURES

Eyes closed, resting—the usual condition for baseline EEG recording—is essentially an uncontrolled state. One subject may relax in such a situation, another may remain anxious or keep his or her mind active with some problem. Many investigators use, in addition to baseline, some activation procedure in order to have a more uniform recording condition among subjects [21,22]. This is becoming increasingly important as topographic mapping takes its place with positron emission tomography and regional cerebral blood flow as an imaging technique for the study of brain function [23].

One place to start is by the use of an activation procedure provided by nature, an example of which is epilepsy. Recordings from epileptic patients provide an excellent data base from which to refine our topographic techniques [24]. Plate 9A shows the map for the raw amplitude of the EEG at the peak of an interictal spike from a patient with complex partial epilepsy. This is a graphic illustration of an event that the clinical electroencephalographer would have had no trouble in reading from the paper record. However, a series of maps made at 5-msec intervals during the spike reveals that it builds up and recedes in place with no movement of the maximum, something that would have been almost impossible to ascertain from the paper record. Plate 9B also shows the map of the activity in the beta band (13–20 Hz) for a 2.56-second epoch centered on this spike. Again, this is exactly what we would expect from the EEG paper record. However, in Plate 9C we see something that was not at all apparent on the paper. The beta band for an epoch that was free of spikes is mapped. We see an excess of fast activity at this same focal point. The combination of quantitative EEG and graphic mapping shows a chronic EEG abnormality that might have been missed by the usual clinical EEG. This type of analysis could be a powerful way of following the effects of medications on this patient.

The effect of drugs on brain activity constitutes another form of activation. Pharmaco-EEG has for some time appreciated the fact that there are important regional differences [25,26]. It remains to be seen whether advanced topographic methods can quantify these differences in a useful way.

The choice of cognitive activation procedures presents a particular challenge to both the researcher and the clinician. It does not appear that there would be any way to standardize on a particular paradigm. Different clinical groups would need to have tasks tailored to the particular deficits or abnormalities to be expected. The effect of task difficulty on EEG is often greater than the effect of the cognitive manipulation making it difficult to parcel out results due to nonspecific factors such as an arousal from more central cortical factors. This area constitutes a challenge for cognitive psychophysiology to develop paradigms that will work in concert with developing neurophysiological methods.

Topographic analysis of EEG holds great promise for research into brain function as well as for the clinician looking for a more sensitive instrument to monitor central nervous system function. The hope is that underlying functional components may be revealed by brain imaging technique. However, even if such components cannot be localized specifically we should remember the central dogma of EEG as given by Donchin [27]; namely, different topographic patterns of EEG activity reflect different functional states of the brain. This will still give us a strong empirical tool to work with in brain research. As neuroscientists we necessarily hope that the partition of cognitive space will be correlated with that of neurophysiological space.

REFERENCES

1. Coppola, R. Topographic methods of functional cerebral analysis. In A.R. Potvin and J.H. Potvin, eds. Frontiers of Engineering in Health Care. New York: IEEE Press, 1982.
2. Coppola, R., Buchsbaum, M.S., and Cappelletti, J. Presentation of multilead EEG by topographic maps of electrical activity. In Proceedings of the 9th Annual Bioengineering Conference. New York: Pergamon Press, 1981.
3. Duffy, F.H., Burchfiel, J.L., and Lombroso, C.T. Brain electrical activity mapping (BEAM): A method for extending the clinical utility of EEG and evoked potential data. Ann. Neurol. 1979; 5:309–321.
4. Duffy, F.H., Denckla, M.B., Bartels, P.H., and Sandini, G. Dyslexia: Regional differences in brain electrical activity by topographic mapping. Ann. Neurol. 1980; 7:412–420.
5. Petsche, H. Topography of the EEG: Survey and prospects. Clin. Neurol. Neurosurg. 1976; 79:15–28.
6. Coppola, R., Buchsbaum, M., and Rigal, F. Computer generation of surface distribution maps of measure of brain activity, Comput. Biol. Med. 1982; 12:191–199.
7. Walter, D.O., Etevenon, P., Pidoux, B., Tortrat, D., and Guillou, S. Computerized topo-EEG spectral maps: Difficulties and perspectives. Neuropsychobiology 1984; 11:264–272.
8. Buchsbaum, M.S., Rigal, F., Coppola, R., et al. A new system for grey-level surface distribution maps of electrical activity. Electroencephalogr. Clin. Neurophysiol. 1982; 53:237–242.

9. Lehmann, D., and Skrandies, W. Reference-free identification of components of checkerboard-evoked multichannel potential fields. Electroenceph. Clin. Neurophysiol. 1980; 48:609–621.

10. Ragot, R.A., and Rémond, A. EEG field mapping. Electroenceph. Clin. Neurophysiol. 1978; 45:417–421.

11. Wolpaw, J.R., and Wood, C.C. Scalp distribution of human auditory evoked potentials. I. Evaluation of reference electrode sites. Electroenceph. Clin. Neurophysiol. 1982; 54:15–24.

12. Hjorth, B. Source derivation simplifies topographic EEG interpretation. Am. J. EEG Technol. 1980; 20:121–132.

13. Wallin, G., and Stalberg, E. Source derivation in Clinical EEG. Electroenceph. Clin. Neurophysiol. 1980; 50:282–292.

14. MacKay, D.M. On-line source-density computation with a minimum of electrodes. Electroenceph. Clin. Neurophysiol. 1983; 56:696–698.

15. Coppola, R. Isolating low frequency activity in EEG spectrum analysis. Electroenceph. Clin. Neurophysiol. 1979; 46:224.

16. Gasser, T., Bacher, P., and Mocks, J. Transformations towards the normal distribution of broad band spectral parameters of the EEG. Electroenceph. Clin. Neurophysiol. 1982; 53:119–124.

17. Herrmann, W.M. Electroencephalography in Drug Research. Stuttgart: Gustav Fischer, 1982.

18. Andresen, B., Stemmler, G., Thom, E., and Irrgang, E. Methodological conditions of congruent factors: A comparison of EEG frequency structure between hemispheres. Multivar. Behav. Res. 1984; 19:3–32.

19. Duffy, F.H., Bartels, P.H., and Burchfiel, J.L. Significance probability mapping: An aid in the topographic analysis of brain electrical activity. Electroenceph. Clin. Neurophysiol. 1981; 51:455–462.

20. Tucker, D.M., and Roth, D.L. Factoring the coherence matrix: Patterning of the frequency-specific covariance in multichannel EEG. Psychophysiology 1984; 21:228–236.

21. Dolce, G., and Waldeier, H. Spectral and multivariate analysis of EEG changes during mental activity in man. Electroenceph. Clin. Neurophysiol. 1974; 36:577–584.

22. Gevins, A.S. Analysis of the electromagnetic signals of the human brain. IEEE Trans. Biomed. Eng. 1984; BME-31:833–850.

23. Coppola, R. EEG imaging of brain activity: Methods and potentials. In Proceedings International Symposium on Medical Images and Icons. New York: IEEE Press, 1984.

24. Coppola, R., Salb, J., and Chassy, J. Topographic analysis of epileptiform discharges. Epilepsy Int. Symp. 1983: 474.

25. Kunkel, H., Luba, A., and Niethardt, P., Topographic aspects of spectral EEG analysis of drug effects. In P. Kellaway and I. Petersen, eds., Quantitative Analytic Studies in Epilepsy. New York: Raven Press, 1976.

26. Sannita, W.G., OHonello, D., Perria, B., et al. Topographic approaches in human quantitative pharmaco-EEG. Neuropsychobiology 1983; 9:66–72.

27. Donchin, E. Use of scalp distribution as a dependent variable. In D. Otto, ed., Multidisciplinary Perspectives in Event-related Brain Potential Research. Washington, DC: Government Printing Office, EPA-60019-77-043, 1978.

18

Clinical Application of Computed EEG Topography

Richard N. Harner

Computed EEG topography (CET) is a term which may be applied to any of several computer-based methods for the computation and two-dimensional display of electrical activity of the brain, whether spontaneous or evoked by stimulation, and in which varying intensities of a specified parameter are indicated by a corresponding isopotential contour line, or a change in density or color of the display image. Most often data are recorded from 16 to 64 points on the head and an interpolating algorithm is used to create 256 to 4000 or more points in order to produce an acceptable map.

To the clinical electroencephalographer (accustomed to constructing field maps of EEG and evoked potential data in his own head and drawing sketches to aid in understanding complicated field structures or to communicate with colleagues), interpolated maps of brain activity, particularly when displayed in color, can produce a surge of excitement concerning possible clinical applications. Manufacturers are currently racing to implement proprietary methods of CET. However, to date, the majority of applications of CET have emphasized specialized areas of research, particularly in relation to cognitive or psychiatric disorders. There have been fewer articles where CET has been applied to stroke, epilepsy, and tumor. The following discussion covers methodology, artifacts and pitfalls, and potential clinical applications of CET and then evaluates the prospects for future clinical application.

METHODS

Input data may be divided into two categories, time domain and frequency domain. The time domain is that in which we ordinarily record raw EEG or evoked potential data. Time flows along the X-axis and amplitude varies along the Y-axis. Reduction of EEG into individual waves, each having a measurable wavelength and amplitude, may be performed without leaving the time domain. Averaging of evoked potentials by resetting time to zero at the beginning of each stimulation and summing EEG data over a specified time segment is all done within the time domain. The cardinal characteristic of such data is that information concerning waveshape and latency between events is retained in an easily recognizable form.

In the frequency domain, a different tack is taken. An analog signal, such as an EEG or evoked potential, is represented by a number of sinusoidal waves, each having a specified frequency, amplitude, and phase. Since the original theoretical elaboration by Fourier, it is widely accepted that any waveform, however complex, can be transformed from the time domain into the frequency domain without loss of information given a sufficient number of frequency components. In practice, the number of frequencies available is limited, often to less than 100, resulting in a certain level of information loss when complex waveforms are present.

Amplitude in the frequency domain is represented on the Y-axis and frequency is represented on the X-axis. By discarding phase information, one produces a power spectrum in which the amplitude measure used is power. It is important to remember that once data has been reduced to a power spectrum one can no longer reconstruct the original waveform in the time domain. Thus any retrospective interest in the waveform of the original signal would have to be resolved in some other fashion.

Transformation of data from the time domain into the frequency domain was time-consuming and laborious until a fast computer algorithm was developed by Cooley and Tukey [1] in 1965. Since that time the fast Fourier transform (FFT) has been widely implemented in microcomputer software and is now even available in a hardware chip. Thus, time domain and frequency domain analyses are currently almost equally easy to obtain, making the choice of which domain in which to study a signal class one of theoretical suitability rather than practical availability.

Some time domain waveforms are easily represented in the frequency domain. For example, a single sine wave or a mixture of several sine waves will each show up as a peak at the corresponding frequency in the power spectrum. But what about a step function, the sudden rise from one level of signal to another such as occurs at the onset of a square wave? This will require an infinite number of frequencies, each with its phase aligned so that peaks occur at the onset of the step function. In practice we have nonsinusoidal spikes and a limited number of frequencies, say 30, with which to represent them. Spikes or muscle activity will be represented as a broad-band increase in power across a broad range in the power spectrum.

What if we have a power spectrum from 1 to 30 Hz and attempt to represent time domain data at frequencies above 30 Hz? This results in a phenomenon known as aliasing in which progresive increases in frequency outside the range of a particular power spectrum will be represented by peaks of decreasing frequencies within the power spectrum. This results in a high order of misinformation. Clearly, assiduous filtering of analog data to keep it within the chosen range of a power spectrum must be done to avoid this unfortunate consequence of implementation of the FFT in a digital computer.

Modern signal processing often takes advantage of both time domain and frequency domain processing. For example, averaging of evoked potentials in the time domain produces useful information concerning waveform and latency. However, the FFT may also be used to construct a digital filter to further improve the signal-to-noise ratio of an evoked potential by selecting only those frequency components of the input signal which are found to be prominent in the evoked potential when compared with the background noise.

One point deserves emphasis. Frequency values in a power spectrum are real in the mathematical sense but may not be visible as such in the raw tracing. Remember the square wave represented by an infinite number of sine waves. None of those sine waves can be seen in the original signal. Similarly low-frequency activity in the power spectrum may be related to subtle shifts of baseline or irregularity of waveform that have little to do with what clinical electroencephalographers call delta activity in the EEG. The ambiguity of increased power at low frequencies sometimes needs to be resolved by resort to the original analog EEG signal.

Ordinarily data is recorded from the scalp from a relatively small number of points. The need for at least 64 equally spaced locations on the head to provide adequate spatial resolution of EEG signals has been suggested. The international 10/20 system provides 19 commonly used scalp locations with provision for intermediate electrodes which could double that number. Commercially available CET methods use input channels ranging in number from 16 to 32. The practical choice of number of channels will probably range around 20 or 21, providing sufficient spatial resolution for major segments of EEG activity, i.e., slow wave foci and alpha activity.

In order to make informative maps with smooth transitions from one level of intensity to the next, a minimum of 1000 points is desirable, thus leading to the need to fill in the spaces between recording electrodes. This is performed by an interpretive algorithm which may be either linear or nonlinear. Linear algorithms plot an interpolated point between adjacent data points as a direct function of distance. A few researchers prefer nonlinear methods, chosen because they believe the field to be curved and therefore a curved line should fit better. Interpolated points are plotted as a quadratic or higher order polynomial function, fitted to nearby data points. These nonlinear algorithms are more time consuming but can produce a map with fewer irregularities of contour than that produced by the linear interpolation. Such a method was developed by Dubinsky and Barlow [2]. In most cases the linear interpolation is satisfactory.

Early methods of CET represented intensity using contour lines [3]. Recent emphasis has been on representation by density (gray scale) or color. The former produces a more trustworthy display. Each density chosen represents a corresponding value on a linear scale. Color displays are much more dramatic but can be misleading since sudden shifts of color may occur even with only a small increment in intensity. For this reason medical imaging of the brain has remained with the gray scale in computed tomography (CT) and magnetic resonance imaging (MRI). However, color scales appear to be developing as the *de facto* standard in CET, requiring the interpreter to be constantly alert for overemphasis of minor differences among different brain areas.

Considerable discussion can often be elicited among CET specialists concerning the best type of map projection, some insisting that equal-area projections are essential to "realistic" mapping. However, since the electrical potentials being mapped do not have exact anatomical correlates, no exact anatomical representation should be expected. Some displays show the lateral views of the left and right hemispheres separately. While this has certain advantages for localization within lobar regions of the brain, there is a significant loss in ability to judge asymmetries of brain activity. Since symmetry or variations from symmetry are so important in evaluating brain function it may be that this loss is crucial in some instances. For these reasons the simplest displays, in the form of an ovoid showing the head as seen from above, are probably sufficient.

There are several important issues concerned with the analysis of CET data. How does one decide that a regional variation is significant? What standard does one use? The standard most widely used, suggested by John [4] and by Duffy and colleagues [5], is the comparison of regional values for a test subject with those obtained from a number of age-matched controls. This approach can be misleading if one concludes that deviation from a set of normals, however great the difference, constitutes an abnormality in the sense of disordered brain function. The use of multiple measures increases the likelihood that a significant difference may be found at a given site in a given individual. Performing such analysis not only at the points of data collection but also at the interpolated points multiplies the problem of multiple measures. Perhaps it is best to view such attempts at determination of statistical significance as a method of normalization, highlighting areas of unsuspected variability for attention and further analysis rather than as abnormalities.

There are other methods of normalization that can be used. For example, one may study the effect of a test state by expressing activity in each region as percent change from a resting state. This technique can be quite useful in localizing the suppression of alpha activity that occurs in the motor region following contralateral motor activity (Figure 18.1). Even more simply, one may express the amplitude at each point in the map as a function of the variability among all points in that same map, thus localizing areas which are particularly prominent compared to all others. Or one may use each hemisphere as the control of its opposite, looking for measures of symmetry as was originally done by Butler and Glass [6] in the localization of alpha suppression related to language function.

The crucial issue is not which method of normalization is best, but that a method of normalization must be chosen that provides the most utility in a particular clinical or research setting. In the case of dramatic asymmetries, for example, simple visual comparison of the two hemispheres may be sufficient to determine which is abnormal.

Selection of the appropriate parameters for mapping is also problematic. There has been gravitation toward the use of power within specified frequency bands as a measure of spontaneous activity and wave amplitude as a measure for evoked potentials. However, it may be that coherence, for example, is a better measure in both cases or that phase lag is an important time domain parameter if one wants to study wave propagation. In the latter case, as seen in Figure 18.2, maps of interpeak latencies across all combinations of channels show marked disruption in interhemispheric "connections" following section of the corpus collosum. This information could not be obtained utilizing the two commonly mapped parameters noted above.

In summary, it will probably be as important to store original analog data in normal as well as test subjects for some time in order to allow for the reanalysis of data in light of new information concerning methods of normalization and parameter selection.

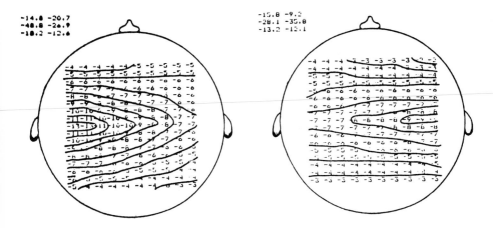

Figure 18.1. Contour maps of percent reduction of alpha power (reactivity) compared with resting state, eyes closed, mean of 5 subjects. *Left map.* Effect of repetitive right fist clenching (RFist), *Right map.* Left fist clenching (LFist). Montage: LF-LC, LC-LO, LO-LT and RF-RC, RC-RO, RO-RT. Raw percent are shown at upper left of each map. Scaled map values are divided by 4. Maximum reactivity occurs in the contralateral C-O derivation: RFist = −48.8%, LFist = −35.8% (From R.N. Harner, and D. Samson-Dollfus, unpublished).

BEFORE OPERATION,EC.REST(SEQ.)

AFTER OPERATION,REST,EC(SEQ.)

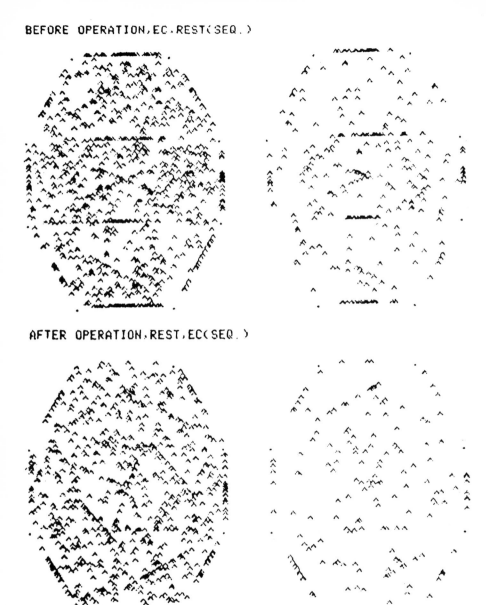

Figure 18.2. CET of inphase interaction in a young epileptic before and after complete section of the corpus callosum (CCX). Each caret represents the occurence of a peak-to-peak correspondence (+/− 20 msec) and is plotted along the line connecting the corresponding channels. After CCX, intrahemispheric interaction is abolished but intrahemispheric interactions persist. From R.N. Harner, N.M. Sussman, and H. Meleis, unpublished.

ARTIFACTS

The same types of artifact that plague the clinical electroencephalographer (eye movement, muscle, drowsiness, electrode artifact, active reference, etc.) also plague the interpreter of a map generated by CET. However, the separation of the map from the original analog data and the apparent spatial coherence of certain elements of color or density may be quite misleading to the uninitiated. This will require frequent cross-reference between the analog recording and the simultaneously generated map in order to learn the discrimination of artifact from alterations of brain function.

One of the most troubling types of artifact is that of eye movement. It simply cannot be removed by filtering. Perhaps the best approach is to hold the eyes so that no movement artifact is visualized in electrodes placed near the eye, thus giving the strong presumption that eye movement artifact will not be present in electrodes more distant from the eye. Failing that, delta activity sharply localized to the frontal polar regions on maps should be presumed to be of ocular origin unless proven otherwise.

In some cases artifact can be reduced by chosing an appropriate montage so that the orientation of a derivation or the selection of a reference is such as to reduce the likelihood of noncerebral potentials appearing in the map. Use of the Laplacian transformation of EEG data [7], now easily performed in a small computer, may be helpful in this regard. Areas of local interest may be seen in a field that resemble monopolar recording in some ways but have no artifact contributed from reference electrodes since each area is referred only to its immediately surrounding regions.

The problem of drowsiness is everpresent so that symmetrical differences in slow activity occurring suddenly out of a background of faster activity must be presumed to be related to drowsiness. The best way to obtain an alert subject is to use an alert technologist to ensure that samples are collected from the most stable, highest alpha portion of the recording. Multiple samples of FFT and evoked potential data should be obtained in order to measure their variability within the same recording session to compare with data collected at other times in the same subject as well as with control groups collected at distant times or even in distant cities.

It is quite clear that, far from eliminating artifact, brain maps only increase the need for vigilance against surreptitious entrance of noise into the topographic arena where we search for signals of special interest.

CLINICAL STUDIES

In the beginning, Berger had as a primary goal the use of electroencephalography in understanding mental function. Thereafter the EEG was applied to a broad spectrum of brain disorders: tumor, stroke, epilepsy, metabolic encephalopathy, etc., but attempts to understand disorders of mental function through electroencephalography met with failure.

As pneumoencephalography, cerebral angiography, and, finally, computed tomography of the brain became available, clinicians have found increasingly less need for EEG in the diagnosis of focal brain lesions. At present, the main value of clinical EEG is for the diagnosis of epilepsy and the detection of those focal or diffuse metabolic disturbances that have not (yet) produced structural alteration of the brain.

With the advent of CET, hopes for a window into the mental processing of the brain rise once again, because we believe that EEG mapping techniques may be more sensitive than routine EEG to local alterations in brain function. But, do we know that CET is more sensitive? And if so, what parameters should be used to maximize this sensitivity? Given that we know so little about how CET should be applied to study of brain function and that we know even less about the localization of mental processes in the brain, should the application of CET to the study of brain function not begin with localization of lesions of the brain which can be known by recourse to the routine EEG, CT scan, or other imaging technique in order to best understand how CET can be optimized for localization of brain function?[8,9]

In our initial approach to this problem we have studied 70 patients with tumor, stroke or epilepsy, either primary or generalized. CET maps have been computed (Biologic Systems, Inc.) for power spectra from two to four separate 4-sec. samples of waking EEG recorded from 20 electrodes (each of the 19 standard 10–20 scalp locations plus 0z) and two trials of flash-evoked responses obtained using 100 samples each and an epoch length of 512 msec. The power spectral samples are brief but are chosen by the technologist to be representative, i.e., taken during samples of EEG recorded simultaneously that have a minimum of muscle, movement, and eye blink artifact and that appear to be most "representative" of the much longer clinical waking EEG recorded at the same time. Automatic artifact rejection occurs when samples exceed the maximum of the analog-to-digital converters. Much less technician input goes into the collection of evoked potential data, which also uses automatic artifact rejection.

It is too early to do more than list the preliminary observations that may serve as the basis for subsequent hypotheses:

1. In the cases of stroke and tumor, localized slow activity and depression of rhythmic alpha and beta activity correlate well with the localization and lateralization of similar changes in the routine EEG.
2. In one case of a right frontal tumor, EEG lateralization was not clear but repeated power spectral maps showed localization to the right frontal region in the area where a 6×6 cm glioma was seen on CT scan and subsequently confirmed by surgery.
3. Epileptic foci seen in the clinical EEG show, in nearly every case, a broad-

band increase in alpha, beta, theta, and delta activity at the site of spike and slow activity (Plate 10). Correspondence with clinical EEG localization is excellent so far. In the case of bilateral 3/sec spike-wave activity, shifting lateralization from left to right frontal regions is seen. The significance of this finding is unknown and not yet clarified by recourse to the raw EEG.

4. Flash evoked potential maps show alteration in 70–150 msec components with posterior or temporal lesions. Sometimes this disturbance is present in epilepsy even when the spike focus is located more anteriorly in the temporal region.

5. Epileptogenic foci and tumors located in the frontal regions show asymmetry of late components of the flash evoked potential in the 200–400 msec latency range (Plate 11).

6. There is good general correlation between localization on evoked potential and power spectral maps.

7. In one man with a 30-year history of epilepsy, power spectral and evoked potential data combined to suggest a left front lesion, but the simultaneous routine EEG showed no focal disturbance anywhere, including the left frontal region.

Each of these observations is the result of visual interpretation of power spectral and evoked potential maps using persistent asymmetry across several trials as a predominant criterion of abnormality. There appeared to be a good correlation between visual interpretation of the maps and the raw clinical EEG. The apparent value of the flash evoked potential maps in far anterior lesions of the brain was surprising. With these observations it should be possible to proceed with a blind study of maps recorded from patients with known lesions and known localizations. Then the value of rough criteria of asymmetry can be further assessed.

Whether recourse to statistical computation will improve our ability to detect localized lesions of the brain or even localized disorders of function is still open to question. There are now commercially available systems which analyze FFT and evoked potential data in a test subject with reference to data obtained from a group of age-matched normals. It would be helpful to see such methods (and others) widely applied to patients with known brain lesions in order to determine the accuracy and reliability of a more automated diagnostic process. Further, the results of such studies would provide important information concerning the selection of parameters for evaluation of more subtle disturbance of brain function about whose nature and localization we know so much less.

Some general aspects of computed EEG topography and its application to clinical disorders of the brain have been reviewed. It is clear that CET is a major advance in EEG and holds great promise for the evaluation of brain lesions and disordered brain function. Even at this time, when we know so little about clinical application of CET, communication with referring physicians should be improved by the topographic method. Pilot clinical studies suggest a good correlation between CET and clinical EEG. The diagnostic value of broad-band increases in power in the epileptic focus in these initial studies will have to be evaluated. At the present time the raw EEG signal is essential for artifact detection, sample selection, and best interpretation of CET data. Much research is needed before CET can be applied directly to clinical diagnosis, but the prospects in this area are good.

REFERENCES

1. Cooley, J.W., and Tukey, J.W. An algorithm for the machine calculation of complex Fourier series. Math. Comput. 1965; 19:297–301.
2. Dubinsky, J., and Barlow, J.S. A simple dot density topogram for EEG. Electroenceph. Clin. Neurophysiol. 1980; 48:473–477.
3. Rémond, A., and Lesèvre, N. Variations in average visual evoked potentials as a function of the alpha phase ("auto-stimulation"). Electroenceph. Clin. Neurophysiol. suppl. 1967; 26:42–52.
4. John, E.R. Neurometrics. Hillsdale, NJ: Erlbaum Associates, 1977.
5. Duffy, F.H., Bartels, P.H., and Burchfiel, J.L. Significance probability mapping: An aid in the topographic analysis of brain electrical activity. Electroenceph. Clin. Neurophysiol. 1981; 51:455–462.
6. Butler, S.R., and Glass, A. Asymmetries in the electroencephalogram associated with cerebral dominance. Electroenceph. Clin. Neurophysiol. 1974; 36:481–491.
7. Hjorth, B. An adaptive EEG derivation technique. Electroenceph. Clin. Neurophysiol. 1980; 54:654–661.
8. Harner, R.N., and Ostergren, K.O. Computed EEG topography. In Cobb, W.A., and Van Duijn, H., Eds., Contemporary Clinical Neurophysiology. Amsterdam: Elsevier, 1978: 151–161.
9. Harner, R.N. Computed EEG Topography—theory, implementation, and application. In Wilkinson, A.W., ed., Investigations in Brain Function. New York: Plenum Press, 1981:79–102.

19

Topographic EEG Correlates of Cerebral Blood Flow and Oxygen Consumption in Patients with Neuropsychological Disorders

Ken Nagata, Koichi Tagawa, Fumio Shishido, and Kazuo Uemura

Since Gibbs and Gibbs [1] described alpha electrical activity depressed on the side of cerebral ischemia, electroencephalography (EEG) has been applied to investigate cerebral ischemia as a parameter reflecting cerebral electrical function, contrasting with the neuroradiological approaches used in demonstrating anatomical lesions [2,3]. The relationship between cerebral electrical activity and cerebral circulation has been of great interest in understanding the pathophysiological mechanisms of cerebral ischemia. Two-dimensional measurements of regional cerebral blood flow (rCBF) using radioactive inert gas enabled in vivo investigation of cerebral circulation. The results of these rCBF measurements were compared with the findings of conventional EEG readings [4,5]. There were, however, technical limitations to these methods in investigating severe cerebral lesions [6,7]. With the advent of positron emission tomography (PET), which uses positron-emitting radionuclides, quantitative transverse section images of cerebral blood flow (CBF) and metabolism have been demonstrated in patients with various neurological disorders [8–11]. The PET scan has great promise for understanding the dynamic aspects of the underlying processes in brain pathology. On the other hand, topographic representation of EEG data has made it possible to extract objective and quantitative features from the multichannel EEG waveforms, even though the source of the data is the same as in the conventional EEG reading [12–14]. Our previous reports [14–17] used computerized mapping of EEG (CME) and showed that topographic analysis of EEG data could provide additional useful information when correlated with computed tomography (CT) and rCBF data in patients with ischemic cerebrovascular disease or brain tumors. Although our current experience is based on a limited number of patients with ischemic cerebrovascular disease, it includes a comparative study between PET and topographic EEG data. In this chapter, we take a preliminary look at the correlation between CBF and oxygen consumption on PET images and cerebral electrical activity on CME images in patients with a neuropsychological syndrome.

MATERIALS AND METHODS

This study was based on 21 patients with cerebral infarction whose diagnoses were confirmed on CT and cerebral angiography. PET studies were carried out between 12 days and 33 months after onset: the examination was within 15 days of onset in 6 patients, between 16 days and 1 month in 6 patients, and later than 1 month in 9 patients. All PET studies were carried out with informed patient consent. CME studies were performed within 24 hours of PET studies. Neuropsychological assessments were performed within 7 days of PET and CME studies.

Computerized Mapping of the EEG

Two kinds of topographic EEG analyses were carried out in this series of studies with the CME system. First, square root of the average power spectra was defined as an equivalent potential over the desired EEG frequency domain. The scalp distribution of the equipotential contours was displayed with color gradation. Second, we used scalp topography of the power ratio index (PRI), defined as the ratio of slow-wave to fast-wave components. The results were displayed in 11 color-coded levels on a color TV screen.

From the 16 scalp electrodes placed according to the international 10–20 system, the electrical activity was recorded by referential derivation with the reference electrodes on both ear lobes. A 16-channel EEG polygraph was connected to the computer system (CME-100 Japan System and 7T17 NEC Sanei), which consisted of computer, color TV display, keyboard, and printer. Both conventional reading of the EEG by visual inspection and computer-assisted topographic analysis were available. In this study, we used an EEG epoch of 60 or 120 seconds, which proved to have good replicability [14]. Fast Fourier transformation was used to obtain the power spectrum. For the frequency domain equipotential maps, the EEG frequency was divided into six categories: delta, theta, alpha-1 (slow alpha), alpha-2 (fast-alpha), beta-1 (slow beta), and beta-2 (fast beta). The PRI was calculated by dividing the slow component including delta and theta by the fast component from alpha-1 to beta-2. The results of both frequency domain equipotential maps and PRI maps were displayed in the same fashion. The 10–20 system was distributed onto a 25-point grid (5 points × 5 points). Values calculated from the EEG data at the 16 scalp electrodes were used for 16 points out of 25 points, and the values at the remaining 9 points were calculated from the average values of the adjacent points. The values between the 25 points of the grid were interpolated according to the modified algorithm of Ueno and Matsuoka [18]. The results were displayed in 11 color-coded levels on a color TV screen: the red color designated the highest value (either frequency or ration of frequency) and the dark blue color designated the lowest value.

For topographic comparison with CBF and oxygen consumption percentage frequency fraction was calculated from the equivalent potentials defined as square roots of the average power spectra. Percentage delta fraction is the percentage of delta equivalent potential to the total equivalent potentials over all frequency domains. Percentage theta fraction was calculated in the same manner, and percentage alpha fraction was defined as percentage of alpha-1 and alpha-2 equivalent potentials to the total equivalent potentials.

Plate 12 shows normal CME images obtained from a healthy volunteer. In the frequency domain equipotential maps, alpha-1 and alpha-2 activities were symmetrically distributed and predominant in the occipatal regions, with a mild increase of theta activity in these regions. There was no significant increase of delta activity. The distribution of PRI values was symmetrical and the values were slightly higher in both frontal regions compared with the occipital regions. This PRI image was considered to be a typical normal pattern.

Positron Emission Tomography

Quantitative transverse section images of CBF and oxygen use were measured using HEADTOME III [19,20], which is a dedicated positron emission computed tomography using small and deep bismuth germanate crystals arrayed on a large ring diameter to achieve high resolution and accuracy. The HEADTOME III has a capacity of five simultaneous slices. The PET imaging was performed during continuous inhalation of three kinds of oxygen-15-labeled compounds: oxygen-15-labeled carbon dioxide for determination of CBF, oxygen-15-labeled molecular oxygen for determination of cerebral metabolic rate of oxygen ($CMRO_2$), and oxygen-15-labeled carbon monoxide for determination of cerebral blood volume (CBV) [21,22]. The positron-emitting radionuclides were produced by the in-house cyclotron (BC-168). Ten transverse section images parallel to the orbitomeatal line were obtained for one examination. The thickness for the transverse section was 14.0 mm and the space resolution was 7.0 mm in these oxygen-15 studies. We measured four parameters of cerebral circulation with this system: CBF, CBV, $CMRO_2$, and oxygen extraction fraction (OEF), which is defined as a ratio of $CMRO_2$ value relative to CBF value at the corresponding picture element (pixel) on PET image. The anatomical landmarking of PET images was confirmed on x-ray CT sections which were taken at the same testing.

For the topographic comparison with percentage frequency fraction of the EEG power data, eight regional cortical values of CBF and $CMRO_2$ were calculated from 6-×-6 pixels on PET images corresponding to the location of the EEG electrodes: medial front (Fp1, Fp2), posterior frontal (F3, F4), and anterior temporal (F7, F8), posterior temporal (T5, T6), Rolandic (C3, C4), parietal (P3, P4), and occipital (O1, O2) regions. The mean of these regional values was regarded as a hemispheric mean value.

CASE REPORTS AND RESULTS

Case 1

This 56-year-old right-handed man was admitted to the hospital with right hemiplegia and speech disturbance. Neuropsychological evaluation demonstrated a severe impairment in both verbal expression and verbal comprehension. He was unable to understand either written or spoken sentences and he could only start one- or two-word emotional phrases. He was unable to repeat even short phrases. The patient was evaluated as having a global aphasia. Cerebral angiography revealed occlusion of the left internal carotid artery and poor collateral blood supply to the left internal carotid arterial system. CT scan demonstrated an extensive low-density area from the left frontal lobe to the left temporal lobe. There had been no significant recovery in his aphasic syndrome, and he continued to present a global aphasia in the chronic stage. PET studies were performed 109 days after onset. Plate 13 shows PET images of CBF, $CMRO_2$, and OEF. As compared with the right hemisphere, a marked reduction of both CBF and $CMRO_2$ was seen in the left hemisphere and the left basal ganglionic region. The most severe reduction was in the left frontal lobe. The OEF was reduced in the lower part of the left frontal lobe, suggesting a relative luxury perfusion syndrome, reflecting that the reduction of $CMRO_2$ was relatively greater than that of CBF in this part of the brain. Plate 14 shows this patient's CME images: frequency domain equipotential maps and PRI map. There was a marked increase of delta activity in both frontal regions and in the left centroparietal region. Theta activity was diffusely distributed in both hemispheres. Alpha-1 activity was depressed in the left hemisphere and highest in the right occipital region. The PRI values increased diffusely in both hemispheres although the right occipitotemporal region was spared.

Comments

This patient displayed all features of severe nonfluent aphasia and would be expected to have an extensive destructive lesion in the left frontal and temporal lobes. The PET images of left hemispheric depression of CBF and $CMRO_2$ could explain the clinicopathological relationship of this patient. The left hemispheric increase of delta activity accompanied by suppression of alpha-1 activity was considered to correlate with the left hemispheric depression of blood flow and oxygen utilization. Although there was no significant reduction of CBF or $CMRO_2$ in the right frontal lobe on PET images, the CME demonstrated a bifrontal delta focus.

Case 2

This 51-year-old right-handed man had a previous history of mild hypertension and experienced a sudden onset of weakness in the right extremities and speech disturbance. On admission, the patient displayed a right hemiparesis, right hemihypesthesia, right homonymous hemianopsia, and nonfluent aphasia. Neuropsychological evaluation demonstrated a severe impairment in his verbal expression. His spontaneous speech was agrammatical and telegraphic. In contrast, his verbal comprehension was relatively preserved, and he was able to carry out one part in response to verbal commands. He could read a couple of characters and he could follow short written directions. He was unable to write words. He was evaluated as having a complete occlusion of the left internal carotid artery. PET study was carried out 39 days after onset. Both CBF and $CMRO_2$ were markedly reduced in the left frontal lobe (Plate 15). There was a mild reduction of CBF and $CMRO_2$ also in the left basal ganglionic region including the left thalamus. The OEF was mildly reduced at the left frontal lobe. On CME images, there was bifrontal high-amplitude delta activity, and theta activity was increased diffusely (Plate 16). Alpha-1 activity, which was regarded as background activity, was suppressed focally in the left frontotemporal region. The focus of PRI was seen in both frontal regions while the left hemisphere showed higher PRI values as compared with the right side.

Comments

The clinical syndrome of this patient suggested a destruction of Broca's area. There was concurrence between the clinical pictures and the results of PET studies. In contrast to the localized lesions on PET images, the CME demonstrated diffusely extended abnormalities in the left hemisphere. Furthermore, a bifrontal delta focus was shown on CME image, although the right frontal lobe was spared on PET images. The PRI map reflected these extensive abnormalities. In this patient with motor aphasia, the EEG abnormalities on CME images were more widely spread as compared with CT and PET findings.

Case 3

This 71-year-old right-handed woman suddenly developed speech disturbance. On admission, she exhibited no motor weakness and was able to walk independently. Neuropsychological assessment indicated a severe impairment in verbal comprehension and inability to understand complex commands and conversation. Her spontaneous speech was fluent, but it contained numerous paraphasias that provided no information. Repetition was poor, even for single words. Reading and writing were also impaired. Her aphasic syndrome was classified as a sensory aphasia. The trajectory of her aphasic syndrome was not favorable and she continued to experience symptoms. The cerebral angiography revealed an occlusion in a branch of the left middle cerebral artery. There was a wedge-shaped localized low-density area in the left temporal lobe. PET studies were carried out 1002 days after onset, a point at which she continued to exhibit sensory aphasia. At this time, there was coupling between CBF and $CMRO_2$: OEF images were homogeneous in both hemispheres (Plate 17). PET studies demonstrated a localized reduction of both CBF and $CMRO_2$ in the left temporal lobe. The left basal ganglionic blood flow and metabolism were relatively preserved. There was a high-amplitude focus of delta activity in the midline regions, and theta activity was increased diffusely in both hemispheres (Plate 18). Alpha-1 activity was diffusely suppressed, and the focus of alpha-1 activity was found in the right parietal region. The PRI was increased diffusely in both hemispheres, with the highest values in the left centroparietal and midline regions.

Comments

This patient displayed sensory aphasia, the causative lesion of which was considered to be in the left upper temporal region. Both CBF and $CMRO_2$ maps indicated a localized lesion in the left temporal lobe. The CME studies, however, demonstrated diffusely spread abnormalities, and the PRI image failed to localize the EEG abnormalities. In this patient with sensory aphasia, localization of EEG abnormalities did not correlate with the focal ischemic lesion on PET images.

Case 4

This 67-year-old right-handed man was admitted to the hospital complaining of visual disturbance and reading difficulty. The patient displayed a right homonymous hemianopsia, with no sensory or motor disturbance. Neuropsychological evaluation revealed a striking deficit in reading ability in spite of preserved writing ability. He was unable to read aloud or understand his written productions a few minutes later. An attempt to facilitate reading by having him trace component characters of the words improved his performance. Conversational speech and other cognitive functions seemed relatively intact. The patient was considered to have pure alexia (alexia without agraphia). Cerebral angiography showed an occlusion of the left posterior cerebral artery. CT scan demonstrated a low-density area in the lower medial part of the left occipital lobe. PET studies were carried out 638 days after onset, when he still displayed pure alexia. The reduction of both CBF and $CMRO_2$ were confined to the lower portion of the left occipital lobe (Plate 19). The homogeneous OEF images suggested a coupling between CBF and $CMRO_2$. Plate 20 shows this patient's CME images: there was no abnormal increase of slow-wave electrical activities. Alpha-1 activity, which was regarded as background activity, was markedly lateralized to the right side, with the highest amplitude in the right parietal region. There was no lateralization of alpha-2, beta-1, and beta-2 activies. The PRI was diffusely increased in the left hemisphere: the highest PRI was demonstrated in the left frontal region whereas the lowest PRI was seen in the right occiptal region.

Comments

This patient had pure alexia and was expected to have the causative lesion in the left occipital lobe. The results of PET studies was consistent with the clinicopathological relationship in the literature [23,24]. The marked suppression of background activity in the left occipital region on CME could explain the left occipital involvement, although the highest PRI was not seen in that area.

STATISTICAL CORRELATION BETWEEN EEG POWER DATA AND CBF: GROUP DATA

Our analysis of group data on 21 subjects suggests an interrelationship between cerebral blood flow and certain frequencies of electrical activity in the brain. Figure 19.1 shows a relationship between regional CBF values and regional $CMRO_2$ values at the corresponding 16 cortical areas. There was a strong linear correlation between CBF and $CMRO_2$ measured from 12 days to more than 3 years after onset ($r = 0.86$). Such correlation suggested a coupling of two kinds of parameters at this time period, although some patients showed relative luxury or misery perfusion syndrome.

The relationship between regional CBF values and percentage alpha fraction at the 16 cortical areas corresponding to the EEG electrode placement is shown in Figure 19.2. There was a linear correlation between regional CBF values and percentage alpha fraction ($r = 0.76$). In contrast, Figure 19.3 shows a negative correlation between regional CBF values and percentage delta fraction ($r = -0.76$). An inverse relationship was seen between percentage alpha frac-

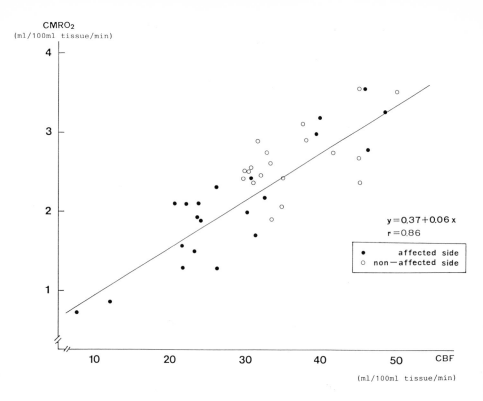

Figure 19.1. Relationship between regional CBF and regional CMRO$_2$ values. A linear correlation (r = 0.86) suggests a coupling of blood flow and oxygen utilization in cerebral ischemia. Closed circle represents data on the affected side and open circle represents data on the nonaffected side.

tion and percentage delta fraction. There was no particular correlation between percentage theta fraction and regional CBF values (Figure 19.4). These statistical and topographic comparisons may suggest that an increase of delta activity and decrease of alpha activity closely correlated with reduction of CBF in subchronic and chronic stages of cerebral infarction.

DISCUSSION

In this study of a limited number of aphasic patients, localization of hypoperfusion and hypometabolism on PET images correlated well with the lesions suspected through the clinical pictures of aphasias. The results of PET studies confirmed the classic clinicopathological correlation. These results were also in accordance with previous rCBF studies using two-dimensional measurements [25,26]. With an 18-F-2-fluoro-2-deoxy-D-glucose PET study, Metter and associates [8] showed an extensive cortical, basal ganglionic, and thalamic hypometabolism in aphasic patients with no CT abnormalities. Specifically, the left thamamic region was consistently involved in various types of aphasia. They speculated that the thalamic metabolic changes were secondary to the alteration of the language cortices. Out of our aphasic patients, cases 1 and 2, who had hemiparesis in addition to the aphasic syndrome and were examined between 39 and 109 days after onset, showed obvious reduction of $CMRO_2$ in the left thalamic region, whereas Cases 3 and 4, who did not exhibit either motor weakness or sensory disturbance and who were examined more than one year after onset, did not have marked reduction of $CMRO_2$ at the left thalamic region. We are not willing to extract any strong conclusions from these results. We feel that the location of the main involvement and the timing of examination would be associated with the remote metabolic influence on structurally intact tissues.

Degree of slowing of EEG activity has been considered to reflect the magnitude of the metabolic depression and the reduction of blood flow in cerebral

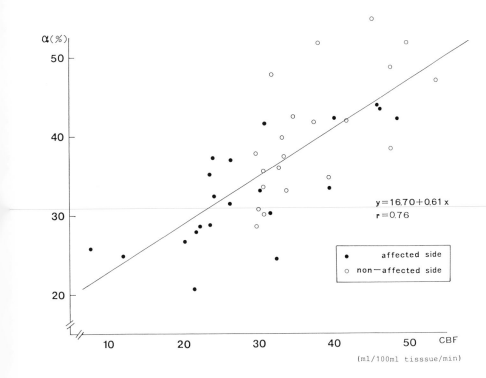

Figure 19.2. Relationship between percentage alpha fraction (%alpha) and regional CBF values. A positive linear correlation existed between the two parameters ($r = 0.76$). Closed circle represents data on the affected side and open circle represents data on the nonaffected side.

ischemia except for the period of luxury perfusion syndrome [4]. Polymorphic delta activity is known to have a localizing effect in cerebral ischemia and the slowest electrical activity often coincides with the most ischemic lesion [27]. Our previous report [14] with CME and two-dimensional rCBF measurements documented a potentially positive correlation between the focus of slow-wave activity and location of cerebral ischemia in patients with aphasia due to cerebral infarction. When the lateralization of background activity was not accompanied by high-amplitude slow-wave activity, CME did not indicate intrahemispheric localization of the lesion.

Electrical abnormalities demonstrated on CME were, however, more extensive than PET evidence of blood flow and oxygen use in all four patients. In cases 1 and 2, there was a bifrontal high-amplitude delta activity on PET, reflecting polymorphic delta activity on CME, whereas the depression of CBF and $CMRO_2$ was unilateral on PET images. Polymorphic delta activity is known to indicate a destructive lesion in the cerebral white matter [28,29]. Deafferentation or isolation of the cerebral cortex from afferent influences is

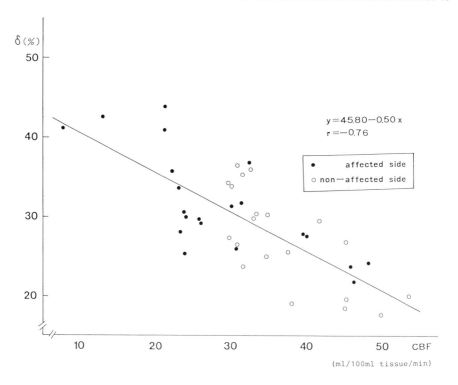

Figure 19.3. Relationship between percentage delta fraction (%delta) and regional CBF values. A negative linear correlation was seen between the two parameters ($r = -0.76$). Closed circle represents data on the affected side and open circle represents data on the nonaffected side.

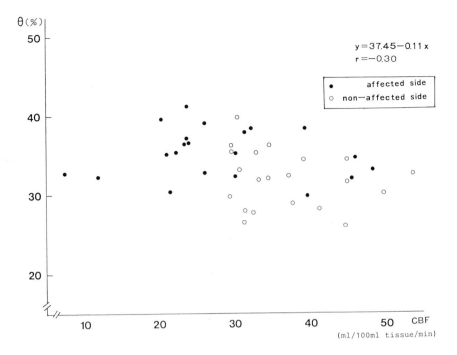

Figure 19.4. Relationship between percentage theta fraction (%theta) and regional CBF values. No particular correlation was seen between two parameters ($r = -0.30$). Closed circle represents data on the affected side and open circle represents data on the nonaffected side.

considered to correlate with the occurrence of polymorphic delta activity. The extensive cortical and subcortical ischemic lesion might have suppressive influences on electrical activity in the noninfarcted brain on the side opposite the lesion, although there was no such metabolic suppression as contralateral diaschisis at that area. At this time, we do not have enough data to explain this discrepancy betwen two kinds of parameters. In case 3, who exhibited sensory aphasis, the CME showed diffuse abnormalities, whereas localized metabolic lesion was shown on PET images. D'Alton and associates [30] showed that EEG abnormalities were more often detected with PET studies then with CBF and $CMRO_2$ measurements, and they concluded that EEG was a more sensitive measure of cerebral dysfunction than PET. We cannot fully agree with this conclusion, because our statistical comparison demonstrated a tight correlation between the EEG power data and regional CBF values on PET. Nevertheless, the topographic dissociation between electrical alteration and metabolic changes needs to be explained by an extensive comparative study with PET and topographic EEG.

Unilateral depression of alpha activity was seen in all patients. The polymorphic delta activity accompanied by a contralateral depression of background activity is more likely to coincide with the area under those electrodes than that overlying the destructive lesion, even though the polymorphic delta activity is not at highest amplitude in that area [31]. The background activity was, however, spared nonevident only at the contralateral occipital or parietal region in our patients, and it seemed difficult to localize the maximum of the EEG abnormality.

Jonkman [25] used an EEG score rating of five categories based on the visual inspect of EEG charts to correlate EEG and rCBF data in 36 patients. He found a parallel between EEG score and rCBF values in patients with either focal or diffuse EEG abnormalities, although there was no strict linear correlation. Tolonen and Ahonen [32] found a good correlation between EEG score based on the conventional EEG reading and rCBF data and pertechnetate cerebral circulation time. In the conventional EEG reading, the magnitude of the EEG abnormalities is primarily determined by the amount of slow-wave component and suppression of background activity. In our efforts to extract objective and quantitative features from EEG data, percentage alpha fraction had a positive correlation and percentage delta fraction had a negative correlation with the rCBF data. Furthermore, Tolonen and Sulg [33] reported that of four different kinds of EEG analyses, the power spectral density exhibited the best correlation with rCBF data. It seemed practical to magnify EEG abnormalities with PRI by dividing the slow-wave component by the fast-wave component calculated from EEG power data.

We believe that these metabolic and neurophysiological images bring a new dimension to the clinicopathological study of patients with neuropsychological disorders as well as those with cerebral infarction.

ACKNOWLEDGMENT

A portion of this work was generously supported by a Stroke Fellowship from the Frost Foundation.

REFERENCES

1. Gibbs, F.A., and Gibbs, E.L. Atlas of Electroencephalography. Addison-Wesley: Cambridge, 1941; 152.
2. Roseman, F., Schmidt, R.P. and Foltz, E.L. Serial electroencephalography in vascular lesions of the brain. Neurology (Minneap), 1952, 2:311–331.
3. Burchfield, R.L., Wilson, W.P., and Heyman, A. An evaluation of electroencephalography in cerebral infarction and cerebral ischemia due to arteriosclerosis. Neurology 1959; 9:859–871.
4. Ingvar, D.H. The pathophysiology of occlusive cerebrovascular disorders related

to neuroradiological findings, EEG and measurements of regional cerebral blood flow. Acta Neurol. Scand. 1967, 43(suppl 31):93–107.

5. Mosmans, P.C.M., Jonkman, E.J., Magnus, O., and Van Hullelen, A.C. Regional cerebral blood flow and EEG. Electroenceph. Clin. Neurophysiol. 1973; 33:122.

6. Lassen, N.A. Regional cerebral blood flow measurements in stroke: Necessity of a tomographic approach. J. Cereb. Blood Flow Metabol. 1981; 1:141–142.

7. Halsey, J.H. Limitation on measurement of regional cerebral blood flow in stroke. In P.L. Magistretti, ed., Functional Radionuclide Imaging of the Brain. New York: Raven Press, 1983; 73–86.

8. Metter, E.J., Wasterlain, C.G., Kuhl, D.E., Hanson, W.R., and Phelps, M.E. 18-FDG positron emission computed tomography in a study of aphasia. Ann. Neurol. 1981; 10:173–183.

9. Lenzi, G.L., Frackowiak, R.S.J., Jones, T. Cerebral oxygen metabolism and blood flow inhuman cerebral ischaemic infarction. J. Cereb. Blood Flow Metabol. 1982; 2:321–335.

10. Gibbs, J.M., Wise, R.J.S., Leenders, K., Jones, T. The relationship of regional cerebral blood flow, blood volume and oxygen metabolism in patients with carotid occlusion: Evaluation of perfusion reserve. J. Cereb. Blood Flow Metabol. 1983, 3(suppl 1):S590–591.

11. Ackerman, R.H., Alpert, N.M., Correia, J.A., et al. Positron imaging in ischemic stroke disease. Ann. Neurol. 1984; 15(suppl):S126–130.

12. Matsuoka, S., Aragaki, Y., Numaguchi, K., and Ueno, S. Effects of dexamethasone on electroencephalograms in patients with brain tumors. J. Neurosurg. 1978; 48:601–608.

13. Duffy, F.H., Burchfiel, J.L., and Lombroso, C.T. Brain electrical activity mapping (BEAM): A method for expanding the clinical utility of EEG and evoked potential data. Ann. Neurol. 1979; 5:309–321.

14. Nagata, K., Mizukami, M., Araki, G., Kawase, T., and Hirano, M. Topographic electroencephalographic study of cerebral infarction using computed mapping of the EEG (CME). J. Cereb. Blood Flow Metabol. 1982; 2:79–88.

15. Nagata, K., Yunoki, K., Araki, G., and Mizukami, M. Topographic electroencephalographic study of transient ischemic attacks. Electroenceph. Clin. Neurophysiol. 1984; 58:291–301.

16. Nagata, K., Yunoki, K., Araki, G., Mizukami, M. and Hyodo, A. Topographic electroencephalographic study of ischemic cerebrovascular disease. In G. Pfurtscheller, ed., Quantitative EEG and Imaging Techniques in Cerebral Ischemia. Amsterdam: Elsevier, 1984; 271–286.

17. Nagata, K., Gross, C.E., Kindt, G.W., Geier, J.M., and Adey, J.R. Topographic electroencephalographic study with power ratio index mapping in patients with malignant brain tumors. Neurosurgery. 1985; 17:613–619.

18. Ueno, S., and Matusoka, S. Topographic display of slow wave types of EEG abnormality in patients with brain lesions. Jpn. J. Med. Electr. Bioeng. 1976: 14:118–124.

19. Kanno, I., Uemura, K., Miura, Y., and Miura S. Design concepts and performance of HEADTOME, a multiring hybrid emission tomography for the brain. In W.D. Heiss and M.E. Phelps, eds., Positron Emission Tomography of the Brain. Berlin: Springer-Verlag, 1983; 46–50.

20. Uemura, K., Kanno, I., Miura, S., Miura, Y., Murakami, M., and Shishido, F. High resolution positron tomograph: HEADTOME III: System description and preliminary report on the performances. In T. Greitz. et al., eds., The Metabolism of the Human Brain: Studies with Positron Emission Tomography. New York: Raven Press, 1985; 47–55.

21. Lammertsma, A.A., and Jones, T. The correction for the presence of intravascular oxygen-15 in the steady state technique for measuring regional oxygen extraction in the brain. 1. Description of the method. J. Cereb. Blood Flow Metabol. 1983; 3:416–424.

22. Lenzi, G.L., Gibbs, J.M., Frackowiak, R.S.J., and Jones, T. Measurement of cerebral blood flow and oxygen metabolism by positron emission tomography and the 15-O steady-state technique: Aspects of methodology, reproducibility, and clinical application. In P.L. Magistretti, ed., Functional Radionuclide Imaging of the Brain. New York: Raven Press, 1983; 291–304.

23. Greenblatt, S.H. Alexia without agraphia or hemianopsia: Anatomical analysis of autopsied cases. Brain 1973; 96:307–316.

24. Benson, D.F., and Geschwind, N. The Alexias. In P.J. Vinken and G.W. Bruyn, eds., Handbook of Clinical Neurology, Amsterdam: North Holland, 1969; 4:112–140.

25. Soh, K., Larsen, K., Skinhoj, E., and Lassen, N.A. Regional cerebral blood flow in aphasia. Arch. Neurol. 1978; 35:625–632.

26. Tagawa, K., Sugimoto, K., Minematsu, K., et al. Type of aphasia and regional cerebral blood flow: A study with 133-Xe inhalation method. Neurol. Med. (Tokyo) 1982; 17:454–459.

27. Jonkman, E.J. Cerebral blood flow (CBF) and electrical activity (EEG). In J.H. Minderhoud, ed. Cerebral Blood Flow: Basic Knowledge and Clinical Implications. Amsterdam: Excerpta Medica, 1981; 202–222.

28. Daly, D.D. Brain tumors and other space occupying processes. In Handbook of Electroencephalography and Clinical Neurophysiology. Amsterdam: Elsevier, 1975; 14:5–10.

29. Gloor, P., Ball, G., and Schaul, N. Brain lesions that produce delta waves in the EEG. Neurology 1977; 27:326–333.

30. D'Alton, J.G., Ackerman, R.H., Chiappa, K.H., et al. Comparative study of positron emission tomography and electroencephalography in neurological disorders. Ann. Neurol. 1983; 14:144–145.

31. Goldensohn, E.S. Use of the EEG for evaluation of focal intracranial lesions. In D.W. Klass and D.D.Daly, eds., Current Practice of Clinical Electroencephalography. New York: Raven Press, 1979; 307–341.

32. Tolonen, U., and Ahonen, A. Relationship between regional pertechnetate cerebral circulation time and EEG in patients with cerebral infarction. Electroenceph. Clin. Neurophysiol. 1983; 56:125–132.

33. Tolonen, U., and Sulg, I.A. Comparison of quantitative EEG parameters from four different analysis techniques in evaluation of relationship between EEG and rCBF in brain infarction. Electroenceph. Clin. Neurophysiol. 1981; 51:177–185.

20
Focal Cortical Arousal in the Schizophrenias

John M. Morihisa and Frank H. Duffy

The association of abnormal brain electrical activity and schizophrenia is not a new discovery. However, recent advances in the application of computer technology and pattern recognition algorithms have facilitated a more detailed examination of this phenomenon. Furthermore, the development of new techniques for creating images of the anatomical, metabolic, and physiological functions of the brain have provided a new perspective from which to interpret these investigations [1].

In this chapter we focus on the evidence from brain electrical activity mapping that supports the hypothesis that schizophrenic patients have abnormalities of focal cortical arousal. These findings are examined in the context of the related body of work that uses complementary measures of brain function in the investigation of this disorder. We further explore the hypothesis that abnormalities of focal cortical arousal may be relevant to the disease processes grouped together as the schizophrenias. Indeed, the clinical heterogeneity of the schizophrenias provides the specific rationale for strategies, such as those used in the present analysis, which attempt to focus on measures of brain function that might provide the eventual basis for the biological subtyping of this group of diseases. A more extensive presentation of brain electrical activity mapping in schizophrenia has been reported [2].

METHODOLOGY

Brain electrical activity mapping, as developed by Duffy in 1979, has been used in the investigation of neurological [3–6] and psychiatric [1,2,7–9] disorders. Building on the pioneering work of others [10–17], this technique topographically maps the electroencephalogram (EEG) or evoked potentials. This approach was used to investigate schizophrenic patients from the research wards of the Neuropsychiatry Branch (formerly the Adult Psychiatry Branch) of the National Institute of Mental Health, Washington, D.C.

371

Subjects

The subjects consisted of 11 drug-free chronic schizophrenic patients who fulfilled DSM-III and Research Diagnostic Criteria. As EEG patterns are particularly susceptible to the effects of drugs, all patients had been without medication for at least four weeks prior to testing.

The control group consisted of 11 normal subjects who had negative neurological and psychiatric histories. There were no significant differences between patients and controls for age, gender, or handedness.

EEG and Evoked Potentials: Data Collection

Subject data was collected in a neurophysiological testing chamber controlled for light and sound. Data were acquired from 20 standard EEG scalp electrodes referenced to linked ears. In addition, two eye electrodes and one ground were attached to each subject. Signals were processed by an EEG amplifier that was set to pass 1 to 300 Hz. A 28-channel FM taperecorder was used to record the data for analysis on a PDP 11/60 computer that incorporated the SIGSYS biomedical software package (Braintech, Inc., Spottswood, N.J.) and the TI-CAS statistical software package [18].

For the EEG spectral data, 10 minutes or more of EEG in the eyes open alert state were recorded for each subject. Eye movements were monitored visually and electrophysiologically. Care was taken to obtain adequate muscle relaxation with monitoring of both subject and the raw EEG record. For the visual evoked potential data, subjects were stimulated by stroboscopic light flashes from a Grass PS-2 photostimulator that was set on intensity 8 and placed 16 cm in front of the subject's closed eyes. Further issues of methodological concern have been discussed elsewhere [1,2].

Data Analysis

Data were tightly bandpass-filtered from 0.5 to 50 Hz at 24 db/octave so as to minimize contamination by 60 Hz interference and muscle activity. In order to limit the contribution to error caused by aliasing we conducted clocked analog-to digital conversion at the rate of 128 samples per second. At this point raw EEG data, including eye channels, were visually inspected, and those segments containing eye blinks, eye movements, muscle potentials, movement artifacts, or 60 Hz interference were eliminated by individuals blind to diagnosis. Then a conventional fast Fourier transform algorithm was used to provide a spectrum over the range of 0 to 64 Hz with a resolution of two data points per hertz. The process of integration used in our method was performed across 1-Hz bands with the final spectral values proportional to the original data values (microvolts). Then, a mean spectrum summarizing 2–4 minutes or more of background spectral content was formed. Data was analyzed from 0 to 32 Hz and broken down into the following EEG frequency bands: delta (0 to 3.5 Hz), theta (4 to 7.5 Hz), alpha (8 to 11.5 Hz), beta-1 (12 to 15.5 Hz), beta-2 (16 to 19.5 Hz), beta-3 (20 to 23.5 Hz), beta-4 (24 to 27.5 Hz), and beta-5 (28 to 31.5 Hz).

Visual evoked potentials were averaged for data from each of the 20 electrodes with the averaging program automatically rejecting segments that contained high-voltage eye movement artifact. In each case the background polygraphic record was examined and the rejection level was individually optimized. At least 110 evoked potentials were averaged for every individual with between 200 and 350 usable trials acquired for most subjects. For each trial the stimulus occurred midway through an epoch that consisted of 256 sampled data points spaced over 1024 msec. The first 512 msec formed a prestimulus baseline that provided the basis for establishing a 0 μV reference point for the evoked potential of each channel. The adequacy of signal averaging was visually confirmed by an inspection of this evoked-potential-free epoch.

Topographic Map Formation

Topographic maps could now be formed from these sets of 20 spectra or 20 evoked potentials. For each of the 20 electrodes, a single value representing the amount of energy in a given EEG frequency range (such as alpha) and obtained by integration across that range, was acquired for the topographic mapping of spectra. For evoked potentials, a single value representing the magnitude of the evoked potential at each 4-msec poststimulus latency point for each of the 20 electrodes was obtained for topographic mapping. A 64-×-64 grid matrix was laid over the 20 individual values. This matrix defines 4096 picture elements (pixels) that were assigned a numerical value through the linear interpolation of the values of the three nearest electrodes. A colored gray scale was then fitted to the pixel values, with each color corresponding to a different voltage range. Thus, a summarized presentation was obtained of the topographic distribution of the spectral energy in the given EEG frequency bands or of the evoked potential voltage at any 4-msec epoch.

A form of exploratory data analysis, significance probability mapping [19], was applied to delineate regional between-group difference in our study of drug-free schizophrenic patients compared to normal controls. Significance probability mapping uses a parametric statistical test of the difference between group means, with set significance levels, to define areas of regional difference in our two subject groups. A more detailed explanation of topographic map formation and the process of data analysis is available elsewhere [3].

RESULTS

In this chapter we focus on findings relevant to inappropriate focal cortical arousal in unmedicated schizophrenic patients. A more extensive discussion of brain electrical activity mapping findings in schizophrenia is presented elsewhere [2], as is a specific examination of frontal lobe dysfunction [20].

In the eyes open alert resting state, a regional between-group difference in fast beta activity (28 to 31.5 Hz) was delineated that encompassed the entire postcentral cortex but was most marked over the left posterior quadrant. Plate 21 is a significance probability map that presents regional differences between patients and controls for fast beta activity. The coefficient of variation was relatively increased for this region of difference between our drug-free schizophrenic patients and normal controls. The coefficient of variation for this fast beta group comparison is displayed topographically in Plate 22.

The comparison of drug-free schizophrenic patients and controls yielded a regional difference in the left posterior quadrant late in the visual evoked potential. This regional between-group difference persisted for over 20 msec. For the delineated regional difference the patient amplitudes were augmented over the controls. Plate 23 is a significance probability map that summarizes the regional difference between these two populations from 448 to 468 msec after the visual stimulus onset (light flash).

DISCUSSION

In our investigation of the hypothesis of inappropriate focal cortical arousal in drug-free schizophrenic patients, we found increased fast beta activity and an abnormality of the visual evoked response. Both of these regional differences involved the left posterior quadrant. First the regional differences are discussed with regard to relevant studies and artifact exclusion. Then these findings are considered in the context of the hypothesis of abnormal focal cortical arousal in schizophrenic patients. Finally, this work is examined from the perspective of other complementary techniques of measuring brain function.

The finding of greater beta activity in schizophrenic patients is consistent with some previous investigations of schizophrenia [21, 22]. Moreover, a recent study employing brain electrical activity mapping of a different group of schizophrenic patients also reported increased beta activity [8].

It must be noted, however, that the beta frequency range of brain electrical activity is susceptible to contamination by muscle artifact. For this reason we subjected the data to three levels of artifact exclusion and evaluation. We first took care to acquire and maintain adequate muscle relaxation during the data acquisition with monitoring of both the subject and the EEG. Data were then tightly bandpass-filtered from 0.5 to 50 Hz at 24/db octave to minimize 60 Hz interference and muscle artifact. Then, prior to further data analysis, all raw

EEG data was visually inspected and all segments containing muscle potentials or movement artifacts were eliminated. The elimination of contaminated data was performed blind to diagnosis. Next, an evaluation of the topographic distribution of the beta activity, as well as a topographic analysis of the coefficient of variation, was performed. In this case, we found our beta regional differences to be maximal in the left parietal region and extending over the entire postcentral region, and this is not consistent with the usual topographic distribution of muscle-induced abnormalities. Finally, the topographic analysis of the coefficient of variation for this posterior region of beta difference was found to be increased in the schizophrenic patients compared to the controls. This would suggest greater beta variability in this region. It has been our experience that the most likely manifestation of undetected group-specific muscle activity occurs as a constant, low-level contaminant. Intermittent muscle activity can be easily detected visually and is eliminated during the careful inspection of raw data prior to the spectral analysis. If constant, lateralized, and group-specific low-level muscle activity were the cause of the increased beta activity, we would expect a relative reduction of overall variability in this region, not the increase that was found. Thus, our findings of increased beta in drug-free schizophrenic patients, associated with an increased coefficient of variation, are unlikely to be artifacts of undetected low-level muscle activity.

The meaning of this regional, somewhat focal, but sporadic increase in beta activity is difficult to interpret. In general, increased beta activity has been seen as indicative of increased cortical arousal or activity. Stevens [23] had found evidence of inappropriate focal cortical arousal in schizophrenia, and our findings further support the existence of this phenomenon associated with this disorder or at least with a subgroup of the schizophrenias.

Further support for the finding of focal cortical arousal in schizophrenia may be found in the body of research that uses other measures of central nervous system activity in the investigation of this disorder. One of the earliest attempts to directly measure in vivo information about possible abnormalitities of brain funcion in schizophrenia found relatively increased blood flow in postcentral cortical regions [24]. This study used regional cerebral blood flow as an indication of regional brain metabolism. Thus, these findings might provide evidence for increased cortical arousal in postcentral regions. Moreover, a positive correlation between mean EEG frequency and cerebral blood flow has been reported [25]. Thus, our findings of increased beta activity are theoretically consistent with the previous report of increased postcentral cortical blood flow. A more recent application of regional cerebral blood flow using the xenon-133 inhalation technique also delineates findings that may support our hypothesis. Gur [26] reported that unmedicated schizophrenic patients demonstrated overactivation of the left hemisphere compared to controls in resting regional cerebral blood flow. Gur's hypothesis of left hemispheric overactivation in schizophrenia is theoretically consistent with our observation of regional differences that are maximal in the left hemisphere. Finally, a recent positron emission tomography study by DeLisi et al. [27] that reports increased temporal lobe glucose use in chronic schizophrenic patients may also be consistent with these findings.

These metabolic findings in the temporal lobe provide another perspective from which we may view our present findings. The focal cortical arousal we report in schizophrenia may parallel the findings of Flor-Henry [28], Lindsay et al. [29], Sherwin [30], and Trimble and Perez [31], who reported that patients with temporal lobe epilepsy who presented with "schizophrenia-like" psychoses were more commonly associated with left-sided foci. Further, it has been reported by Trimble and Perez [31] that of 12 patients with temporal lobe epilepsy who were classified as schizophrenic, 11 met the criteria for the diagnosis for nuclear schizophrenia, based upon Schneiderian first-rank symptoms. Thus, it would appear that in at least some instances schizophreniform symptoms might be related to abnormal brain electrical activity in the left hemisphere. Further support for this relationship may be found in our findings of increased focal cortical arousal.

If we consider together the abnormality of fast activity with the finding of increased visual evoked potentials in this same left posterior region, we have a combination of focal beta increase and a regionally augmented evoked potential amplitude. Based upon empirical findings, it has been suggested [32] that this combination of phenomena is consistent with irritable if not epileptogenic cortex. Finally, when we consider the findings of a brain electrical activity mapping study [9] that found decreased P300 amplitudes in related topographic regions, we have a configuration of characteristics that has been considered [32] to be suggestive of epileptic foci. Specifically, we see in the left hemisphere of schizophrenic patients both elements of irritability (focal increases of beta activity and augmented visual evoked potential amplitudes) and hypofunction (diminished P300 amplitudes). Indeed, it has been suggested [32] that the finding of diminished and augmented activity in close proximity might suggest a region of atrophy surrounded by epileptogenic cortex.

Further evidence is suggested by Sherwin [33] that considers neurochemical findings in temporal lobe epilepsy and schizophrenia. Stevens [34] has suggested that a dysfunction of certain dopaminergic substrates may be shared by temporal lobe epilepsy and schizophrenia. Indeed, a study comparing the cerebral spinal fluid levels of homovanillic acid (a dopamine metabolite) found significant differences between subjects with left temporal lobe epilepsy who manifested schizophrenia-like symptomatology compared to those who did not [35].

Moreover, animal evidence [36] suggests that kindling of the mesolimbic dopamine system can lead to behavioral changes (rather than seizure activity) that persist beyond the cessation of kindling. Trimble [37], based on these findings, speculates that similar mechanisms may exist in humans such that chronic subictal activity might lead to the development of psychoses.

CONCLUSION

Our findings should not be interpreted as indicating that schizophrenia is a form of epilepsy. Rather we have pursued an approach that uses complementary techniques of brain function investigation to delineate parallel phenomena that may be related mainly by a similarity in their behavioral manifestations, i.e., schizophrenic symptomatology. This apparent commonality of presentation may provide the basis for useful models of the pathophysiological processes underlying neuropsychiatric disorders, and more importantly, it may provide a means of exploring an aspect of abnormal brain function that may be characteristic of subgroups within neuropsychiatric disorders. Thus, the utility of such a selectively focused examination of brain electrical phenomena lies in its attempt to recognize neurophysiological patterns of pathologic function. In this way we may be able to elucidate biological bases for the division of the heterogeneous group of schizophrenias into physiologically meaningful subtypes based on selective phenomena such as focal cortical arousal.

REFERENCES

1. Morihisa, J.M. Brain Imaging in Psychiatry. Washington, D.C.: American Psychiatric Press, 1984.
2. Morihisa, J.M., Duffy, F.H., and Wyatt, R.J. Brain electrical activity mapping (BEAM) in schizophrenic patients. Arch. Gen. Psychiatry, 1983; 40:719–728.
3. Duffy, F.H., Burchfiel, J.L., and Lombroso, C.T. Brain electrical activity mapping (BEAM): A method for extending the clinical utility of EEG and evoked potential data. Ann. Neurol. 1979; 5:309–321.
4. Duffy, F.H., Denckla, M.D., Bartels, P.H., et al. Dyslexia: Regional differences in brain electrical activity by topographic mapping. Ann. Neurol. 1980; 7:412–420.
5. Lombroso, C.T., and Duffy, F.H. Brain electrical activity mapping as an adjunct to CT scanning. In R. Canger, F. Angeleri, and JK Penry, eds., Advances in Epileptology: 11th Epilepsy International Symposium. New York: Raven Press: 1980; 83–88.
6. Duffy, F.H. Topographic display of evoked potentials: Clinical applications of brain electrical activity mapping (BEAM). Ann. N.Y. Acad. Sci. 1982; 388: 183–196.
7. Morihisa, J.M., Duffy, F.H., and Wyatt, R.J. Topographic analysis of computer processed electroencephalography in schizophrenia. In E. Usdin and I. Hanin, eds., Biological Markers in Psychiatry and Neurology. New York: Pergamon Press, 1982; 495–504.
8. Morstyn, R., Duffy, F.H., and McCarley, R. Altered P300 topography in schizophrenia. Arch. Gen. Psychiatry 1983; 40:729–734.
9. Morstyn, R., Duffy, F.H., and McCarley, R. Altered topography of EEG spectral content in schizophrenia. Electroenceph. Clin. Neurophysiol. 1983; 56:263–271.
10. Walter, W.G., and Shipton, H.W. A new toposcopic display system. Electroenceph. Clin. Neurophysiol. 1951, 3:281–292.

11. Rémond, A. Orientations et tendences des methodes topographiques dans l'etude de l'activite electrique du cerveau. Rev. Neurol. 1955; 93:399–410.
12. Bickford, R.G., Brimm, J., Berger, L., et al. Application of compressed spectral array in clinical EEG. In P. Kellaway and J. Petersen, eds., Automation of Clinical Electroencephalography. New York: Raven Press, 1973; 55–64.
13. Estrin, T., and Uzgalis, R. Computer display of spatio-temporal EEG patterns. IEEE Trans. Biomed. Eng. 1969; 16:192–196.
14. Lehmann, D. Multichannel topography of human alpha EEG fields. Electroenceph. Clin. Neurophysiol. 1971; 31:439–449.
15. Childers, D.G., Perry, N.W., Jr., Halpeny, O.S., and Bourne, J.R. Spatio-temporal measures of cortical functioning in normal and abnormal vision. Comput. Biomed. Res. 1972; 5:114–130.
16. Gotman, J., Gloor, P., and Ray, W.G. A quantitative comparison of traditional reading of the EEG and interpretation of computer extracted features in patients with supratentorial brain lesions. Electroenceph. Clin. Neurophysiol. 1975; 38:623–639.
17. Petsche, H. Topography of the EEG: Survey and prospects. Clin. Neurol. Neurosurg. 1976; 79:15–28.
18. Bartels, P.H., and Wied, G.L. Extraction and evaluation of information from cell images. Proceedings of the First Annual Life Sciences Symposium: Mammalian Cells, Probes and Problems. Los Alamos, N.M., October 1973.
19. Duffy, F.H., Bartels, P.H., and Burchfiel, J.L. Significance probability mapping: An aid in the topographic analysis of brain electrical activity. Electroenceph. Clin. Neurophysiol. 1981; 51:455–462.
20. Morihisa, J.M., and McAnulty, G.B. Structure and Function: Brain electrical activity mapping and computed tomography in schizophrenia. Biol. Psychiatry 1985; 20:3–19.
21. Itil, T.M., Saletu, B., and Davis, S. EEG findings in chronic schizophrenics based on digital computer period analysis and analog power spectra. Biol. Psychiatry 1972; 5:1–13.
22. Flor-Henry, P. Lateralized temporal-limbic dysfunction and psychopathology. Ann. N.Y. Acad. Sci. 1976; 280:777–797.
23. Stevens, J.R., Livermore, A. Telemetered EEG in schizophrenia: spectral analysis during abnormal behavior episodes. J. Neurol. Neurosurg. Psychiatry 1982; 45:385–395.
24. Ingvar, D.H., and Franzen, G. Abnormalities of cerebral blood flow distribution in patients with chronic schizophrenia. Acta Psychiatr. Scand. 1974; 50:425–462.
25. Ingvar, D.H., Sjolund, B., and Ardo, A. Correlation between dominant EEG frequency, cerebral oxygen uptake and blood flow. Electroenceph. Clin. Neurophysiol. 1976; 41:268–276.
26. Gur, R.E. Regional cerebral blood flow in psychiatry: The resting and activated brains of schizophrenic patients. In J.M. Morihisa, ed., Brain Imaging in Psychiatry. Washington, D.C.: American Psychiatric Press, 1984; 65–76.
27. DeLisi, L.E., Buchsbaum, M.S., Holcomb, H.H., et al. Increased temporal lobe glucose utilization in chronic schizophrenic patients, submitted for publication.
28. Flor-Henry, P. Schizophrenic-like reactions and affective psychoses associated with temporal lobe epilepsy: Etiologic factors. Am. J. Psychiat. 1969; 126:148–152.

29. Lindsay, J., Ounsted, C., and Richards, P. Long term outcome in children with temporal lobe seizures. III. Psychiatric aspects in childhood and adult life. Dev. Med. Child Neur. 1979; 21:630–636.

30. Sherwin, I., Peron-Magnan, P., Bancaud, J., et al. Prevalence of psychoses of epilepsy as a function of the laterality of the epileptogenic lesion. Arch. Neurol. 1982; 39:621–625.

31. Trimble, M.R., and Perez, M.M. The phenomenology of the chronic psychoses of epilepsy. In W.P. Koella and M.R. Trimble, eds., Advances in Biological Psychiatry: Temporal Lobe Epilepsy, Mania and Schizophrenia and the Limbic System. Basel: Karger, 1982; 98–105.

32. Lombroso, C.T., and Duffy, F.H. Brain electrical activity mapping in the epilepsies. In H. Akimoto, H. Kajamatsuri, M. Seino, et al., eds., Advances in Epileptology: The 13th Epilepsy International Symposium. New York: Raven Press, 1982; 173–179.

33. Sherwin, I. The effect of the location of an epileptogenic lesion on the occurrence of psychosis in epilepsy. In W.P. Koella and M.R. Trimble, eds., Advances in Biological Psychiatry: Temporal Lobe Epilepsy, Mania, and Schizophrenia and the Limbic System. Basel: Karger, 1982; 81–97.

34. Stevens, J.R. An anatomy of schizophrenia? Arch. Gen. Psychiat. 1972; 29:177–189.

35. Peters, J.G. Dopamine, noradrenaline, and serotonin spinal fluid metabolites in temporal lobe epileptic patients with schizophrenic symptomatology. Eur. Neurol. 1979; 18:15–18.

36. Stevens, J.R., and Livermore, A. Kindling in the mesolimbic dopamine system: Animal model of psychosis. Neurology 1978; 28:36–46.

37. Trimble, M.R. The Psychopathology of Epilepsy. Horsham: Geigy, 1981; 234–245.

Commentaries

21

The Use of Topographic Mapping Techniques in Clinical Studies in Psychiatry

Michael W. Torello and Robert W. McCarley

The conference on topographic mapping techniques on which this volume is based provided an excellent forum for a critical discussion of this emerging technology, with expression of both enthusiasm and caveats. This chapter deals with areas of methodological concern that surfaced at the conference by discussing ways in which our experimental procedures have addressed these issues.

Two major areas of concern emerged: (1) technical issues relating to the use of appropriate reference points, assumptions of linear interpolation, source localization, and artifact handling; and (2) general scientific issues about the generalizability of findings and the selection of representative subjects. While the use of appropriate references, the assumptions of linear interpolation models, and the questions surrounding source localization measurements are important theoretical issues, in a clinical setting such as ours it is often unnecessary to specify completely the neural generators of the scalp potentials being recorded as long as the data provide diagnostically useful information. For example, delta waves are practically useful indicators of a stage of sleep although we are not certain of their generator. For us, the especially critical areas are subject selection and artifact handling. We comment on these by using as an example the recent studies in our laboratory using the brain mapping technique (Torello et al., unpublished observations) [1, 2, 3].

RECORDING MONTAGE AND METHODOLOGY

In these studies, the international 10–20 system was used for placement of 20 scalp electrodes used in monopolar recordings with linked ears serving as reference. FPz was used as ground. Additional control electrodes were used to identify and minimize artifact from eye blinks and muscle activity. To record eye movements and blink, one set of electrodes was placed above and below one eye and another set lateral to the left and right canthus (for recording lateral eye movements). To monitor muscle artifact, a pair of electrodes was placed above the left and right nuchal strap muscles, 20% below O1 and O2, respectively, and two electrodes were placed on the left and right preauricular area to monitor temporalis muscle activity. Each subject was placed in an electrically shielded, sound-attenuated chamber and was asked to relax in a comfortable reclining chair. Each subject was instructed to sit quietly during the test and was asked to minimize body movements, eye movements, and eye blinks. The experimenter was with the subject throughout the session to check for compliance during the test.

Signals in both the 10–20 system electrodes and the control electrodes were initally amplified with standard Grass polygraphs with bandpass filters set at 0.5–70 Hz. The data were recorded on a 28-channel tape recorder for off-line analysis and upon playback there was further tight filtering from 0.5 to 50 Hz at 24 db/octave prior to computer digitization. Computer sampling was 128 samples/sec., permitting definition of the spectrum from 0 to 64 Hz. During evoked potential averaging, the computer automatically rejected any high-voltage artifacts greater than 50 μV.

ARTIFACT CONTROL

Artifacts represent a potentially serious confounding factor interfering with the assessment of brain activity, so our general strategy has been to attend to the wide variety of artifacts at each step in data acquisition and processing using strict control procedures. To this end, we have (1) used three sets of electrodes, which allow artifact recognition, to help minimize artifact from eye movements, blinks, and muscle activity; (2) minimized muscle and eye artifact at the source during the experiment; (3) monitored the effectiveness of (1) and (2) by watching the paper write-out of the electroencephalogram (EEG) during the course of the experiment; (4) eliminated segments with artifact, insofar as possible, at the time of analysis; and (5) used the control electrodes at the time of analysis to detect any possible effects of artifacts on the analysis.

Specifically, the control electrode channels showing blink, eye movements, and muscle activity were monitored on-line during the recordings and a number of maneuvers were used in the experimental sessions to reduce the frequency and amplitude of this activity. Subjects were asked to suppress blinks and time was spent during the recording session with each subject so as to obtain good relaxation and thus diminish muscle artifact. For the spectral energy topography studies done in the eyes open condition, we asked the subject to fixate on a target and we monitored eye movements on-line and after computer digitization. In the eyes closed condition, we monitored on-line and determined if additional procedures to control eye movement and blinks were necessary; we have found the use of lightly attached eye pads or gentle touching of the eyelid with the fingers makes subjects aware of eye movements and blinks and helps to diminish them. Using feature analysis techniques, as well as simple inspection, we monitor whether or not the optimum feature classifier or maximum contribution is from muscle or electro-oculogram (EOG) channels. If it is, we discard the data. If not, we examine the data even with some artifact present so as to avoid throwing away potentially useful data.

SUBJECT SELECTION

Using these control procedures with the brain mapping technique, we have tested 10 chronic male schizophrenics and 10 men with no history of psychopathology. These subjects, right-handed (save for 1 left-handed schizophrenic inadvertently included), were between 20 and 40 years of age, had no history of electroconvulsive therapy or neurological illness, no significant drug or alcohol abuse (defined by impairment of health, social relations, or job function), and no medication for medical disorders that would have deleterious EEG or cognitive functioning consequences (e.g., reserpine or barbiturates for hypertension), no hearing difficulties, IQ above 85, with English as a primary language. Also, the patients were diagnosed as schizophrenic using RDC (Research Diagnostic Criteria) and DSM-III (*Diagnostic and Statistical Manual*, 3rd edition) criteria and were matched to the normal group on education, social class, IQ, and age. These procedures of subject selection are strict but necessary to decrease within- and between-group variance.

USE OF THE P300 AS A COGNITIVE PROBE

In addition to its usefulness as a measure of the kind of information processing likely to be deficient in schizophrenia, the P300 is advantageous technically because (1) the P300 paradigm provides a greater degree of experimental control over and comparability of subjects' mental activity than simple spontaneous or resting samples of EEG; and (2) the absence of strict time-locking of any artifacts with trial onset and their easy detection in averaging of artifact channels simplifies artifact control. The spatiotemporal evolution of the P300 waveform to the auditory oddball paradigm was topographically mapped in these subjects using brain mapping technology [4]. A group average P300 waveform was constructed for the schizophrenic and control groups. The control group's P300 showed a concentric development about a maximum in the centroparietal area, slightly displaced to the left (Plate 24). In contrast, the schizophrenic group's P300 maximum was more anterior and to the right, with a deficiency in left temporal activity. Topographic mapping of the statistical between-group difference (significance probability mapping, SPM) confirmed the presence of persistently deficient activity at the left temporal electrode sites when compared to the control group. It was further found that this left temporal amplitude feature discriminated individual members of each group with 90% accuracy.

SPECTRAL DATA

EEG data was also recorded with eyes open and closed. EEG spectral energy was computed using the fast Fourier transform, and numerical matrices representing the topographic distribution of spectral energy in a specified band were constructed and displayed as color images. SPM was employed to identify regions of maximal group difference; it was found that the schizophrenic group showed increased low frequency energy (primarily delta) in the frontal regions and increased beta in the postcentral areas and the left anterior temporal area. Our data, suggesting frontal lobe dysfunction, agree with the studies of Morihisa et al. [5] and are consistent with cerebral blood flow and PET studies indicating reduced metabolism in this area. The left temporal abnormalities are consistent with our data showing a left temporal abnormality in the P300 in this group. Further studies are now under way to replicate and extend these findings and to determine if these effects were due to medication and were specific to the schizophrenia syndrome and not to other psychopathologies. We believe that we have demonstrated that through the proper use of strict control procedures of subject selection and artifact handling, diagnostically useful data can be collected using the topographic mapping technique.

However, an important limitation of this study was the lack of extensive cognitive, structural (computed tomography (CT) and magnetic resonance imaging), and clinical information on these same subjects. Consequently, it was not possible to determine, for example, which structural and neurophysiological findings are associated with which cognitive deficits and which clinical features. We are now addressing this problem by including specific, quantitative measures in each of these domains on a new group of patients. We believe that this strategy will lead to progress in understanding which symptom/sign groupings occur together so as to facilitate the discovery of natural subgroups within the schizophrenic syndrome and differentiate the schizophrenic syndrome from affective psychoses. Furthermore, we believe that electrophysiological studies of complex behavioral or psychiatric syndromes, which are probably made up of several underlying pathologies, necessitate a multidisciplinary approach that looks for converging lines of evidence about diagnostic subgroups. The ability of topographic techniques to reduce the data to a small set of meaningful features that can be more easily integrated with other information represents an important step in the use of EEG techniques in psychiatry.

ACKNOWLEDGMENTS

This work is supported in part by Scottish Rite Schizophrenia Research Program of the Northern Masonic Jurisdiction (Dr. McCarley).

REFERENCES

1. Morstyn, R., Duffy, F.H., and McCarley, R.W. Altered P300 topography in schizophrenia. Arch. Gen. Psychiatry 1983; 40:729–734.
2. Morstyn, R., Duffy, F.H., and McCarley, R.W. Altered topography of EEG spectral content in schizophrenia. Electroenceph. Clin. Neurophysiol. 1983; 56:263–271.
3. Torello, M.W., Shenton, M.E., Cassens, G.P., Duffy, F.H., and McCarley, R.W. Schizophrenia: P300 Temporal Lobe Deficit Confirmed. (Abstract) Presented at the American Psychiatric Association Convention in Dallas, Texas, May 23, 1985.
4. Duffy, F.H., Burchfiel, J.L., and Lombroso, C.T. Brain electrical activity mapping (BEAM): A method for extending the clinical utility of EEG and evoked potential data. Ann. Neurol. 1979; 5:309–321.
5. Morihisa, J.M., Duffy, F.H., Wyatt, R.J. Brain electrical activity mapping (BEAM) in schizophrenic patients. Arch. Gen. Psychiatry 1983; 40:719–728.

22

Topographic Mapping in Depressed Patients

Alan F. Schatzberg, Glen R. Elliott, Jan E. Lerbinger,
Barbara Marcel, and Frank H. Duffy

The development of computer-enhanced neurophysiological techniques represents a great stride forward in our ability to understand both neurological and psychiatric disorders. In the past few years, we have been exploring the use of brain electrical activity mapping in the assessment of chronic and refractory patients, particularly those with depression. In this chapter, we highlight our experience with brain mapping in an initial sample of 50 McLean Hospital patients; these results have recently been presented in detail. [1, 2].

Depression is one of the commonest psychiatric disorders, with a total 6-month prevalence of major depression and dysthymia of approximately 6% [3]. Although depression is highly responsive to therapy, some 10–15% of patients with depression do not respond even when traditional antidepressant treatments are aggressively prescribed. Chronic depressives probably represent a heterogeneous group of disorders. One subgroup appears to exhibit symptoms, e.g., depersonalization and perceptual distortions, suggestive of possible seizure disorders. Indeed, Himmelhoch has estimated that 10% of his depression clinic population suffered from a variant of temporal lobe epilepsy [4]. Our experience has been that many depressed patients with symptoms suggestive of seizure disorders have relatively normal routine electroencephalograms, thus posing diagnostic and treatment problems for the clinician. Our group has explored the use of mapping techniques in conjunction with global clinical assessment, neuropsychological testing, and computed tomography (CT) scanning, to assist in the evaluation and diagnosis of these patients.

We reviewed the records of the first 50 McLean Hospital patients who had brain electrical activity mapping studies. Raters, blind to the results, were employed to determine psychiatric diagnosis using Research Diagnostic Criteria (RDC) [5] and the Diagnostic Inventory for Borderline States (DIBS) [6]. Hospital records were used to determine diagnosis. Of the 50 patients, 31 met criteria for a depressive disorder. BEAM [7] reports were reviewed blind to clinical data and rated for normality or degree of abnormality using a global four-point scale. In addition, on the extended electroencephalogram (EEG) and spectral analysis/evoked response (SA/ER), quantitative data underlying these 31 patients were compared with those of 31 normal age-, handedness-, and sex-matched control subjects, using statistical methods described previously [7]. When compared to normal controls, statistically significant differences were observed in depressives in the eyes closed state: (1) increased slowing (delta and theta) on spectral analysis in the right posterior temporal region; and (2) increased frontal beta bilaterally, predominantly on the left side. On visual evoked and auditory evoked responses, significant deviations between groups were observed in the right anterior and mid-temporal regions but not in any other brain regions.

A number of statistically significant correlations were observed between degree of abnormality on SA/ER (but not extended EEG) and total borderline score or subscores of depersonalization/derealization and episodic psychosis. Spearman correlations were approximately 0.33 ($p < 0.05$) [1].

Moreover we observed differences in mapping results when we subclassified the depressed patients on the basis of specific signs and symptoms of depersonalization/derealization or paranoia. Depersonalized/derealized patients could be discriminated from nondepersonalized patients on the basis of visual and auditory evoked responses. Specifically, differences between groups were observed in the bilateral posterior quadrants and right central and right anterior temporal regions. In contrast to comparisons between the overall depressed group and normal controls, no differences were observed in spectral analysis when the depressed patients were subdivided according to the presence or absence of depersonalization/derealization.

When the paranoid and nonparanoid depressives were compared, significant differences were not observed on spectral analysis or visual evoked responses. However, differences were observed on auditory evoked responses—particularly in the left frontal-temporal area and the left posterior quadrant. Minor deviations were observed in the right central and bilateral medial frontal regions.

These data are particularly intriguing in light of the clinical phenomena studied. Depersonalization/derealization, as defined in the rating instrument used in this study, involves a sense of detachment and unreality, and odd experiences. The finding of differences in the posterior regions and right posterior regions, areas involved in nonverbal and visual phenomena, is intriguing when one considers that depersonalization could intuitively involve visual and nonverbal phenomena.

Similarly, there has long been an association among auditory hallucinosis, poor hearing, and paranoia in patients with psychotic disorders, particularly with the schizophrenias. In this study, differences between paranoid and nonparanoid depressives were observed on auditory evoked responses (but not on visual evoked responses or spectral analysis) predominantly on the left side. These data not only point to the use of mapping to separate subgroups but suggest that it may be helpful in identifying electrical phenomena that may underlie specific clinical symptomatology.

Since our patients were generally chronically depressed, it is difficult to determine whether our results are generalizable to acutely depressed patients or are limited to those with long-standing or atypical disorders. Recently, Silberman et al. [8] reported symptoms of temporal lobe epilepsy in patients with affective disorders, suggesting that dysfunction in specific brain regions (e.g., temporal lobes) may be involved in both temporal lobe epilepsy and mood disorders. Further studies are thus required to ferret out whether the relationships we observed between electrical abnormalities and depression reflect underlying processes in depression per se rather than in a specific, chronic or atypical subtype. To further examine the relationship of electrical abnormalities and symptoms of depression, depersonalization and paranoia, studies should include specific neuropsychological tests of cortical function in posterior brain regions (particularly on the right side) as well as testing of left temporal function. Such tests should include specific visual and auditory components to aid in discriminating subtypes either on clinical symptomatology or brain mapping results. We are pursuing these studies in our laboratory.

REFERENCES

1. Schatzberg, A.F., Elliott, G.R., Duffy F.H., et al. Application of brain electrical activity mapping (BEAM) in chronic depression. I: Topographic differentiation from normal control subjects and among depressive subtypes, unpublished paper.
2. Elliott, G.R., Schatzberg, A.F., Duffy, F.H., et al. Application of brain electrical activity mapping (BEAM) in chronic depression. II: Specific clinical examples, unpublished paper.
3. Myers, J.K., Weissman, M.M., Tischler, G.L., et al. Six-month prevalence of psychiatric disorders in three communities. Arch. Gen. Psychiatry 1984; 41:959–967.
4. Himmelhoch, J.M. Major disorders related to epileptic changes. In Blumer, D., (ed);, Psychiatric Aspects of Epilepsy. Washington, D.C.: American Psychiatric Press, 1984; 271–294.
5. Spitzer, R.L., Endicott, J., and Robins, E. Research diagnostic criteria: rationale and reliability. Arch. Gen. Psychiatry 1978; 35:837–844.
6. Kolb, J.E., and Gunderson, J.E. Diagnosing borderline patients with a semi-structured interview. Am. J. Psychiatry 1980; 137:37–41.
7. Morihisa, J.M., Duffy, F.H., and Wyatt, R.J. Brain electrical activity mapping (BEAM) in schizophrenic patients. Arch. Gen. Psychiatry 1983; 40:719–728.
8. Silberman, E.K., Post, R.M., Nurnberger, J., et al. Epileptic-like symptoms in affective illness. Presented at New Research Section, Annual Meeting of the American Psychiatric Association, May 1983.

23
Progress in Topographic Mapping of Neurophysiological Data: Comments

Keith H. Chiappa

In recent years there has been increased interest in the topographic mapping of electroencephalograph (EEG) and evoked potential (EP) data, and the symposium on which this volume is based provided a great service to those using these techniques by assembling many of the foremost investigators in the field. The two potential applications of these mapping techniques can be defined as research and clinical, the latter referring to the use of mapping as a means of establishing a clinical diagnosis. The chapters in this volume provide sophisticated and interesting research applications, but here I discuss only the clinical applications.

There are two clinical areas in which topographic mapping has potential clinical utility. The first is a straightforward use in which the head maps are employed as a means of viewing the potential field distribution of brain electrical activity, e.g., a spike, a slow-wave focus, or an evoked potential waveform. Here the topographic map can make a mass of data more comprehensible, give neurophysiologists new insights into the physiological process, and make it easier to explain the data to the uninitiated. The topographic map is the neurophysiologist's answer to the computed tomography (CT) scan, and it is especially attractive because it is usually in color. However, in these circumstances, topographic mapping is not providing new information. Conversely, the second area of clinical application, that in which the topographic maps are based on statistical data derived from the actual electrical data, is potentially the most useful application of mapping, and it is this area that I would like to consider in more detail.

Dr. Duffy noted at the beginning of the symposium that he has interpreted almost a thousand clinical maps and that the clinicians found them extremely useful. However, Dr. Harner, whose presentation was on "Clinical Applications of Computed EEG Topography," summarized his discussion by saying that much more research is needed before the techniques can be used clinically. Although these two opinions are diametrically opposed, very little discussion ensued on this matter. Furthermore, most of the clinical examples shown during the symposium consisted of patients with rather gross lesions which must have produced marked, focal changes on the conventional EEG and EPs, although a few cases were discussed briefly where this was not so.

I suggest that the clinical utility of statistical mapping needs to be evaluated systematically, not anecdotally. The evaluation needs to reproduce the point of view of the clinical neurophysiologist faced with the electrophysiological tests from an individual patient. Thus, not only are blinded comparisons with conventional techniques necessary, but also there must be prospective studies of patient groups in whom the diagnosis can be established with some certainty. Blumhardt [1] has reviewed an analogous situation regarding the role of EPs in multiple sclerosis, and his comments are pertinent here:

> To evaluate the role of a new, potentially diagnostic test, we need to know not only the proportion of patients with a positive result amongst those in whom the disease is established by a "gold standard," but also in equivocal cases of the disease and in patients with other commonly confused conditions. What is the role of the new test in relation to established diagnostic techniques and what are its potential advantages and disadvantages? How reliable and reproducible are the results? How does the new test stand up against the "gold standard"? As the prevalence of the disease in the population will clearly affect the "abnormality rate," we need to know the methods of selection or preliminary screening of patients in studies which evaluate the test. Finally, to determine the benefits for the patient, we need to know the positive and negative abilities of EP's and the subsequent fate of the patients who had either normal or abnormal results.

Furthermore, in evaluating clinical results, a clear distinction must be made between group-versus-group studies, and group-versus-individual studies. The latter is usual in clinical laboratories. Here, a single patient is compared to "limits of normality" obtained by studying a sample (e.g., 30 normal subjects) from the normal population. In the former case (primarily a research application) a group of patients with a disease is compared statistically with a group of matched normals. The powerful statistical techniques used in this group-versus-group analysis will usually reveal differences between the two groups, especially when the number of features evaluated is in the thousands, as it is with topographic EEG and EP studies. It is then important to test yet another group of patients with the same disease to see if they differ from the normal group in the same way. If the findings are valid, they tell us something about the group of patients, but they do not necessarily tell us anything about a single patient from that group. If the single patient's test results are evaluated using the normal group data for comparison, the single patient may well be indistinguishable from the normal individual, i.e., the patient's data may be within normal limits. This last evaluation, of course, is the one forced upon the clinical neurophysiologist who, faced with the results from a single patient, is trying to determine whether the patient's results are within normal limits. Thus, the presentation at this symposium on schizophrenia was interesting academically but gives us little information about the ability of topographic mapping to diagnose schizophrenia in individual patients. Prospective studies are needed to answer this question.

These statistical topographic mapping techniques are so powerful that artifact recognition is extremely difficult. It is not clear to me how much of the electrical activity with a frequency greater than 20 Hz recorded from the scalp of an adult with an intact skull is other than muscle artifact. None of the symposium participants were able to shed light on this question after it had been posed, despite the fact that this frequency band was often used in their analyses and often provided discriminatory data. Since muscle activity contains power at all EEG frequencies, in addition to the 20 to 120 Hz band, the differentiation of muscle from brain activity is a formidable problem and no solution was apparent at this symposium. Presently there is no known method of making this distinction when muscle activity is low voltage, recorded at a distance, or filtered. To answer the question of whether there is any recordable cerebral activity above 20 Hz, ideally one would like to study normal, awake human subjects who are fully paralzyed pharmacologically, but we have had no volunteers to date for such a study. Perhaps those of us who are being anesthetized for surgical procedures would consent to this recording. Also, studies of patients with severe idiopathic polyneuritis might supply some pertinent data.

With regard to artifact, the eyes are in almost constant motion in awake subjects; even with eyes closed, many small movements occur. This eye motion makes it difficult to differentiate frontal slow activity and know that its origin is cortical. Visual observation of conventional EEG is not sufficient to evaluate the presence or absence of eye movement artifact when powerful analytic techniques are being used. Vertical and horizontal eye movement recording channels need to be included in the topographic analysis field, and it must be shown that the eye movement electrodes do not show significant amounts of activity, i.e., that the locus of an abnormal finding is not centered on the eyes.

Dr. Buchsbaum stated that the eventual aim of topographic mapping must be anatomical localization. However, in the clinical arena, this is much less important, now that positron emission tomography (PET) and nuclear magnetic resonance (NMR) capabilities are available, and subdural or epidural and depth electrode chronic recordings are performed in epilepsy centers. EEG must continue to focus on function, not anatomy. Perhaps studies using EP data, particularly short-latency EP data, will yield useful anatomical data. However, short-latency EPs are most effectively analyzed in the time domain, and the generator sites of most long-latency EP components are not yet well defined.

Much discussion centered on the choice of recording derivations, especially reference sites (ipsilateral ears, linked ears, vertex, nose, chin, noncephalic). These are important considerations, particularly with research applications where the actual potential field distribution is desired. However, in the clinical arena such matters can be handled more empirically, so that a bipolar montage, in contrast to linked ears, might have the advantage of least artifact and least cross-pollination, since, in the final analysis, we are mapping statistics, not electrical activity.

In summary, topographic mapping is presently useful for research in potential field distribution and dipole studies. However, since its clinical application requires the use of complex statistical operations, I feel that adequate prospective trials are needed before any evaluation of its clinical utility can be made.

REFERENCE

1. Blumhardt, L.D. Do evoked potentials contribute to the early diagnosis of multiple sclerosis? In Ch. Warlow and J. Garfield, eds., Dilemmas in the Management of the Neurological Patient. Edinburgh: Churchhill Livingstone, 1984; 18–42.

24
Progress in Topographic Mapping of Neurophysiological Data: A Critique

H. Richard Tyler

The topic of the conference on which this volume is based raises the hope that we are on the verge of being able to extract and demonstrate information hidden in basic electroencephalograms (EEGs) and evoked potential (EP) recordings of significant use to researchers and clinicians. There were three recurring themes throughout the conference:

1. A comparison of data elicited by topographic mapping and other "radiological techniques"
2. What kind of "information" could be generated from potentials recorded from the skull
3. What the correct number of leads are and how long a segment of tracing should be studied for meaningful analysis

I found the most interesting and rewarding parts of the conference to be interdisciplinary communication and the approaches of nonmedical investigators (engineers, statisticians) to these problems.

I was disappointed in the clinical information. It was often narrative and not statistically or conceptually sophisticated. This reached its peak when one saw slide after slide of derived "data" from a small sample of EEGs with no meaning apparent or demonstrated by the speaker. In this instance I felt there were more meaningful data seen in the original tracing than the derived! It became clear that there is no limit to the type and kind of secondary data that can be derived and the investigator needs some conceptual idea of what to look for to avoid drowning in a sea of numbers and graphs.

There was a vast amount of potentially interesting material of correlative value not touched upon. There are many areas in which the problem of how to derive meaningful data from a large amount of noise has been approached. For example, the psychology of cognitive vision and how the brain picks stimuli out of the environment, i.e., the phenomenon of visual attention would be pertinent. How we learn about the ocean and what lies under sand dunes, and how we distinguish missile sites from satellites or the details of the surface of Jupiter from rockets—all use extraction techniques and means of information enhancement. These problems of extraction of meaningful data must have common roots with picturing information in a form that the eye can perceive and understand. The whole field of information theory and its mathematical and physical concepts would be of interest.

The problem that seemed to be always there but never verbalized was the value, appropriateness, and nature of the questions the researchers asked. We seemed to see results before questions were clearly enunciated and the questions asked were often the biggest problems. How can we determine the number of electrodes one should use unless we know the question and information sought? The discussion of whether to use 16 or 100 electrodes with intermediate stages at 32 and 48 all seemed baseless if dealt with abstractly. One could easily generate questions that could be answered by three electrodes, and others by 100. Similar discussion on the ground or reference electrode also seemed difficult for the nontechnician to understand. The nature of the information sought and the means of displaying this information should be critical to this determination. As one author capably pointed out, he could make a topographic display look as different as the number of leads he had by using different reference electrodes.

The seduction of the color graphics was impressive. If not effectively controlled, color can be misleading. It is difficult to get a clear picture of quantitative data as one is seduced by beautiful rainbow displays. One could make the reader or receiver see what one wanted by adjusting colors to the data. Clearly, conventions are needed.

I was impressed with techniques that tried to identify the dipole that generated the fields of electrical activity rather than the techniques that tried to plot the fields of electrical surface activity. It was clear that the center of fields could move over the surface of the skull even if the dipole did not traverse a similar path. Attempts to localize functions to anatomical sites using interpretation or data from surface potentials of fields might give misleading impressions of the origins of the activity. The localization of the dipole generating fields in three-dimensional space might have significant clinical utility, especially in epilepsy research.

The clinical situation in which topographic mapping techniques were shown to have utility were those with focal and particularly lateralized pathology or processes. It appeared relatively easy to program and demonstrate differences between right and left or front and back. In most clinical situations, this is also usually obvious from neurological history and examination, and the simpler techniques, i.e., basic EEG or EPs. The question, therefore, must be raised of justifying expense in terms of equipment need, complexity, and expert interpretation if topographic and computerized analysis is to be practical and clinically useful. The wide variety of techniques, the lack of any general agreement as to format, and the difficulty in relating what one laboratory is doing to another all detract from the clinical application of these procedures, except in situations that capitalize on the geographic residence of the researchers. Some general agreement on standardizations to make data comparable are necessary. The clinical areas of highest interest are those that are not easily localizable at the bedside. These include dyslexia, mental retardation, and psychiatric states. Can these procedures demonstrate focal deficits not seen otherwise? There were only hints that this might be the case.

Topographic procedures should not be developed to compete with computed tomography (CT) or nuclear magnetic resonance (NMR) scanners, or to replace EEGs. They must be used intelligently when a specific question is posed and programmed for specific answers. This raises the question: Do we need this procedure? And if so, at what cost? Since funds for medical care are limited, as we develop new procedures, we have to give up others. We cannot afford the luxury of doing positron emission tomography (PET), CT, NMR scans, and topographic mapping in routine problems.

Dr. Bartels presented a lucid and clear demonstration of the utility of statistical theories and how they can be applied to data analysis of the type under discussion at these sessions. It is clear that these statistical concepts must be accepted and used if the final outcome, i.e., the pictorial representation of data, is to have any meaning at all. This was a major weakness of many of the papers. Statistical sophistication must match the computer capability in generating graphs and numbers or we will have reams of data that will be overinterpreted.

It is clear this meeting was a beginning. As one looked around the room, one was impressed with the small number of young people. Discussion and presentation was primarily provided by established figures. The need to draw in new blood, and especially, interested investigators in fields other than medicine is obvious. Fresh approaches and imagination in applying new technical advances from ancillary fields are needed. Many in the room were electroencephalographers applying new techniques to their art. Interaction with more engineers, statisticians, physicists, theoreticians from logic, information analysts, decision analysts, etc., to help develop the field and appreciate the strengths and weaknesses of these techniques is needed.

The potential use of three-dimensional techniques and representation of the source of electrical abnormality rather than the field it creates offers potential for clinical localization. It is important to agree to some set of working rules as to what is, and what is not, acceptable. Can you portray a three-dimensional head onto a flat surface and picture it as a rectangular linear area without correction? Should the flat surface look like a map with longitude and latitude or be square boxed? Are these important or unimportant factors? Should there be standard references, placing of leads, or minimal number of leads? One would like to see the problems studied more focused so that the questions asked could be more sophisticated. Much more study should go into the questions. Most successful scientific studies are based on carefully designed questions that are then approached by techniques that can give results. It is much less productive to study techniques and figure out the questions. The latter leads to much less rigorous science. It is clear, as was demonstrated at this conference, that you can get answers with the present techniques, but they were only as good as the questions. It was neither clear that the limitation of the techniques, on the one hand, or the full potential of the methodology, on the other, was designed into studies. Statistical concepts should be part of the design, not an afterthought to see which data are significant (whatever that means). When you generate an infinite amount of data, you cannot arbitrarily pick out the 5% that are significant.

Descriptive electroencephalography has reached a plateau in development. Most findings that could be correlated with recordings of scalp fields had been done. The field of evoked potential study appears to be following the course of the development of the EEG, i.e., exploration of techniques, improvement in technique, correlation with clinical states. The promise of this conference is that it could reawaken interest in research and science in the area, and make it more than a correlative tool of the clinician. It could be the basis for meaningful research into the anatomy and physiology of the sources of both spontaneous and induced electrical fields recordable from the head. It is an area of high promise, but it will require an amplification and addition to the work reported in this conference. It will be the prime responsibilities of the participants to see that such is allowed and encouraged to occur. One will look back in five to ten years with interest to assess which were the seminal papers. I would bet on the more significant use of statistics as suggested by P.N. Bartels and the development of the dipole localization and recognition as demonstrated by D.H. Fender.

25

Brain Electrical Activity Mapping: Issues and Answers

Frank H. Duffy

Topographic mapping, as a means of enhancing the diagnostic capabilities of neurophysiologic data, has rapidly advanced in interest and activity over the past decade. The recent availability of small but powerful computers with sophisticated image graphics capability at affordable cost has facilitated new research in bioelectric cartography. This rapid growth was the germinating force for the conference from which this volume is derived. Salient details on the developmental history of cartography for electroencephalographic interpretation are provided by other authors herein. While advances in the viable application of these techniques have clearly occurred (several noted in this volume), there remains a great deal more to know and this will be the focus of much research activity for the next several years.

At international conferences which focus on newly evolved and more narrowly defined research topics, it is not unusual for more questions to be generated than answered. Our symposium "Progress in Topographic Mapping" was no exception, and this fact is underscored by several chapters in the present volume which outline critical concerns of leading experts in the field. As my contribution to this volume, I should like to address some of the issues raised.

WHY TOPOGRAPHIC MAPPING?

As our laboratory set out to develop a computerized system to extract more information from neurophysiologic data [11–21, 32–37], our goal was to mimic, through electronics, the analytic processes we believed clinicians performed in their minds during evaluation of multichannel data (e.g., electroencephalography). Such a system would allow the observer to visualize what he would otherwise have to imagine, and, in so doing, perceive underlying data structure in finer grain.

As a clinician evaluates a multichannel electroencephalogram (EEG), he must mentally address a series of questions such as:

1. Are there any epileptiform discharges, and, if so, where do they arise?
2. Is there too much slow activity, and, if so, is it constant or intermittent, generalized, lateralized or focal?
3. Is alpha activity present in normal amounts and is it symmetrical?
4. Is there evidence of medication-induced fast activity, and, if so, is it equally manifest in both right and left frontal areas?

Intrinsic to such questions are five separable analytic processes:

1. Detection of discontinuities and discrimination of those which have clinical importance as distinct from those of artifactual origin (are there any epileptiform discharges?)
2. Spectral analysis or decomposition of EEG into frequency bands (is alpha present?, slow activity?, fast activity?)
3. Topographic mapping, i.e., localization and definition of extent (where do they arise?, generalized, lateralized, or focal?, equal in both frontal areas?)
4. Temporal summation (is it constant or intermittent?)
5. Statistical analysis or comparison to some standard of normal brain wave activity (is there too much or a normal amount?)

Expressing EEG analysis in these terms emphasizes both its complexity and the crucial demands placed on the electroencephalographer in terms of skill based on training and experience. Many investigators have simultaneously appreciated this complexity and the role that recent advances in electronics, computer architecture, and analytical techniques could play in alleviating the clinician's analytical burden [5,30,31,38,40].

Detection of Discontinuities

A most thorough approach to the automated detection of discontinuities has been described by Gotman and Gloor [24,25]. In our opinion this valuable technique serves primarily as a labor saver, useful for quantifying the numbers of discharges detected in long EEG recordings. As such it has proven to be extremely helpful in the management of epilepsy. However, none of the automated methods used for spike detection are superior to human visual analysis, especially in the discrimination of true spikes from artifacts. Gotman and Gloor, for example, broaden their detection criteria so that no true discharges are missed and then rely upon visual inspection to eliminate artifact (e.g., eye blink, electrode pop, muscle activity, sharp alpha, benign paroxysms, etc.). The human eye continues to be the "gold standard" for spike detection.

In most instances the clinically important features of an epileptiform discharge are immediately apparent to the trained eye. In some instances, however, the picture may be confusing and difficult to synthesize from raw polygraphic tracings. We have found spatiotemporal mapping useful in understanding such complex discharges, especially when they are generated by horizontal dipoles or dipoles that slightly change their orientation during activation (Figure 25.1) (Duffy and Bousounis, work in progress).

Spectral Analysis and Temporal Summation

In contrast to its usefulness in recognizing discontinuities, the human eye has proved to be a less successful analyzer of EEG background activity. Many significant clinical neuropathologies fail to generate obvious and easily recognizable discontinuities, but they do alter background spectral content. Fortunately, spectral analysis has been available for many years [2], has been efficiently coded for software implementation as the fast Fourier transform of Cooley and Tukey [7], and has been extensively applied to EEG [4].

An advantage of this spectral analysis is that it may be performed on EEGs of any duration, thereby allowing one spectral value to represent the average of any desired epoch. It is customary to perform spectral analysis on brief epochs (2–16 seconds) and then average the resulting spectra from sequential epochs to estimate the spectral content of longer time periods. This is done for computational simplicity, as it is less demanding of computer memory to form spectra on multiple short segments than on single long segments. However, the creation and averaging of multiple short segments provide two additional advantages. First, segments containing artifact can be eliminated with minimal loss of accompanying real data. Second, one can obtain an estimate of the constancy or variability of spectral content with time. One need only calculate the standard deviation and related coefficient of variation (CV) [39] during the averaging of the set of short epoch spectra. This results in a direct measure of spectral stability or lack thereof.

Topographic Mapping of EEG Data

No matter what measure one takes from EEG, spatial distribution of this measure across the scalp becomes an important consideration. The value of topographic mapping has been recognized since the toposcans of Walter and Shipton [43] and the surprisingly sophisticated early computer-driven systems of Estrin and Uzgalis [22] and Harris et al. [28]. Recent efforts, including our own [11–21], have capitalized upon advances in microcomputer and minicomputer technology [23] to produce complete systems capable of fulfilling a variety of clinical and research needs. Indeed, as we write this chapter, there exist five US-based and several European and Asian companies that manufacture topographic devices specifically for neurophysiologic mapping. Uncounted are the many investigators who have constructed their own unique topographic mappers. Many EEG parameters have been mapped, such as spike frequency [27,24], spike distribution [26], raw EEG [6], frequency content [11,42], and mobility [29], among others.

Once such maps are constructed and inspected for symmetry and focality, it is natural to question whether what one sees is "normal." To address this issue directly, we have used a technique known as significance probability mapping (SPM) to render visible regions where a subject's topographic data differ from that of an appropriate control population [12]. This procedure involves calculation of the Z score between corresponding points of the matrix underlying the subject's data and corresponding points of the mean and variance matrix of the control group. Results are displayed as topographic images, known as Z-statistic SPM, which retain the spatial framework of the original data and are used to delineate regions where the subject differs from the "normal" group. This form of exploratory data analysis [41] has been useful in the clinical interpretation of topographic data especially for the localization of abnormal regions. The consistency of localization may be addressed by investigation of a second sample of a subject's data. For research purposes two or more groups may be similarly compared by student's *t*-statistic (*t*-SPM) or analysis of variance (F-SPM). Once again, data consistency is best addressed on a second data set. The general principle of SPM is to make visible via topographic mapping any one of a large number of statistical properties of the underlying data structure that are too complex to be readily grasped by simple inspection of the raw data components.

Topographic Mapping of EP Data

Many of the issues concerning interpretation of clinical EEG also apply to its cousin, the long-latency sensory evoked potential (EP). These evoked electrical transient responses vary in their morphology across both space and time. Most clinical laboratories limit themselves to a small set of EP electrodes, usually 1 to 4, placed so as to record activity over the primary cortex of the particular sensory modality being employed and over the vertex to record nonspecific late components. Few laboratories have simultaneously recorded from a full head of 10 to 20 electrodes, for the resulting set of EPs appear hopelessly complex and virtually impossible to analyze by visual inspection. It is traditional to search for and measure EP "components" such as the "N1," "P2," or "P300," waves named for their appearance at certain latencies. Normative data are usually gathered from electrodes overlying primary cortex. The complicating factor for interpretation of multichannel EP data is that although channels distant from primary cortex may show well-developed EPs, their morphology is diverse. For example, visual EPs (VEPs) recorded from anterior electrodes are not simple attenuated and prolonged analogs of the VEP recorded from the occiput. Even for occipital VEPs there may be a surprising diversity of waveform morphology. Blumhardt et al. [3] report at least six different morphologies in normal subjects to pattern-reversal stimulation. To no small degree, this complexity may explain why inspection of long-latency EP data has failed to achieve the universal application and acceptance afforded EEG. Data from psychophysiology laboratories tell us that various EP components are sensitive to stimulus intensity, stimulus type, stimulus omission, and anticipated stimulus change. However, most such laboratories select normal subjects whose baseline EPs fulfill traditional expectations, and discard normals whose EPs appear unusual. Thus, although EPs appear very sensitive to brain function, individual variability — even further modified by pathology — renders multiple channel EP data difficult to employ universally in clinical settings.

To some degree, much of this difficulty may be explained by the speculation that EP data, especially earlier components, may arise from discrete brain regions and may be adequately modeled by electrical dipole sources. What one observes on the scalp from a dipole source is a function not only of the location and magnitude of the dipole but also of its orientation. Slight anatomic variations within visual cortex may produce differing dipole orientations which would result in markedly differing spatial distributions of activity on the scalp surface. Thus the same EP component might appear at different scalp locations in different subjects. The use of multiple electrodes, assisted by topographic mapping, would be required to define the variety of spatial distributions produced by the normal variability in dipole orientation. We have observed, for example, that the flash evoked response in normal subjects universally produces an early negative component from 44 to 52 msec, usually midline and maximal between the Oz and Pz electrodes. However, the location may vary from Oz to Pz to Cz in different subjects (Plate 26). If one were only recording from O1, O2, Oz, and Cz, a maximum at Pz might escape detection.

We commonly form topographic maps of the spatial distribution of a multichannel EP every 4 msec and view the resulting images in endless-loop cinematography via a computer-controlled color graphics terminal. Such displays permit the simultaneous appreciation of both spatial and temporal data characteristics. Unique spatiotemporal patterns may be observed. For example, waves of positive or negative activity may arise in the occiput, sweep forward into the posterior and midtemporal electrodes, and then disappear. Thus, activity appearing in different electrode locations at different times may in fact reflect activity from the same generator as it progressively changes its net dipole orientation over time. As such, sequential topographic mapping of EP data permits visualization of features not readily seen by inspection of the multichannel EPs themselves. Trajectory analyses of the sweeps of such hills of potential maxima or valleys of potential minina have proven useful in the localization of both normal and abnormal function (Sandini, Chapter 15; Duffy and Sandini, submitted for publication).

So in response to the question "Why topographic mapping?", I would respond as follows. The techniques of signal averaging, spike detection, spectral decomposition, and statistical analysis have been with us for some time. In my opinion, the limiting factor has been and will remain our ability to handle the massive amounts of data produced by the application of these techniques to multichannel data. It makes no sense to struggle to visualize spatial distribution from polygraphic tracings. Indeed, Skrandries (see Chapter 2) has clearly demonstrated how we can be deceived by so doing. Computer-generated cartography is now readily available, and I vehemently propose that this process will greatly augment our collective efforts to achieve the full potential of clinical neurophysiology.

ISN'T IT ALL ARTIFACT?

It is a common observation of those who engage in topographic mapping of brain electrical activity that much more can be "seen" by inspection of such images than by inspection of the EEG or EP data from which the images were constructed. The reasons why this is so are discussed above. Unfortunately, topographic mapping does not discriminate between electrical activity of brain origin and that of extracerebral origin, i.e., artifact. Thus the appearance of focal delta at C4 in the 0–4 Hz spectral map of a patient might just as easily arise from "electrode pops" as from true focal slowing. Simply looking at the map may not provide enough information to make the crucial discrimination between "real" activity and artifact. The SPM technique is not helpful for artifact detection which may be even more deviant from normal than true cerebral abnormality. The vividness by which abnormalities may be perceived stands in contrast to the uncertainty as to their real or artifactual origin. This discrepancy may be particularly apparent when visual graphics are adjusted to emphasize unusual features through the use of color coding (e.g., white or bright red). Indeed, the discrepancy between the ease of visualizing topographic anomalies and the difficulty in excluding their artifactual origin may be the basis for Bickford's chromophobia (see Chapter 11) and the cautions rendered in this book by Harner, Chiappa, Tyler, and others. Many critics have reacted by claiming that topographic mapping is all artifact.

A common retort to this criticism emphasizes that topographic mapping creates no new information but merely displays data intrinsic to the basic recordings. Mapping does not create artifact, though it may emphasize it. Nonetheless, such arguments do not directly solve the issue, a problem which is one of poor signal-to-noise ratio (SNR) [8]. Suppose, for example, one is listening to a distant medium-wave AM radio broadcast station during a thunderstorm and experiences difficulty understanding the broadcast due to lightning-induced static. Turning up the volume fails to improve intelligibility because both signal (the broadcast) and noise (the static) become louder. By analogy, topographic mapping may be compared to "turning up the volume" of EEG. This may enhance the visibility of both real and artifactual signals, but it results in no net improvement in SNR. The solution in both cases has to be selective reduction of noise. For radio usage one may employ a "noise limiter" control, but it may be necessary to let the storm and its static pass by. For EEG, the appropriate response is one of selective reduction or elimination of artifact.

The critic may ask, "Can anything be done?" Isn't EEG usually as "clean" as possible? Our experience has been that clinical EEG records are not clear of artifact, as there is ordinarily no need to reduce artifact below a level acceptable to analysis by visual inspection. However, since the sensitivity of topographic mapping is greater than that of simple visual inspection, artifact must be reduced to a comparable degree.

Our approach to artifact reduction is fourfold: (1) reduce it at the time of data gathering, (2) monitor the adequacy of artifact reduction with special electrodes, (3) remove residual artifact at the time of data processing, and (4) detect the presence of residual artifact at the time of data inspection or statistical analysis.

The major sources of noise consist of 50 or 60 Hz mains, eye blinks, eye movements, head movements, and myographic, ECG, and electrode artifacts. In addition, poor control of the subject's state, inadequate system calibration, and improper electrode placement may confound accurate interpretation.

Prior to the commencement of data gathering, the system should be accurately calibrated. The usual bandpass-filtered 50 μV square wave pulses used for EEG are inadequate, for their peak amplitude is as much a function of the frequency characteristics of each amplifier as the gain. Ideally, a sweep frequency calibration should be performed by precision sine waves or white noise. At the least, a single sine wave at mid-EEG frequency (10 Hz) should be employed. The next step is to monitor ongoing activity during data gathering via multichannel polygraphic recordings (EEGs). Only by such means can one readily appreciate artifact and take steps to eliminate or reduce it. Those topographic mapping systems which simplify hardware by eliminating the polygraph are functioning in a blinded state.

At the time of data gathering, muscle activity should be reduced by the technologist, who must both allay anxiety and postion the patient for minimum resting muscle tone. Eye blink and movement are reduced in eyes open recording states by providing a suitable small fixation target. Subjects are instructed to view the target and avoid blinking. They are given frequent "blink holidays" when they may blink, close their eyes, and readjust their position. During eyes closed recording states, transparent or translucent eye pads serve to make the subject aware of residual (often unconscious) eye blinks. Special electrodes should be placed on or around all sources of artifact (e.g., eyes, temporal muscles, occipital muscles, heart, tongue) and monitored at the same time as the standard EEG. By careful monitoring during data intake, the examiner can assess the adequacy of the above measures while simultaneously watching for 60 Hz and electrode artifact. ECG artifact is a contaminant that must be carefully eliminated, for it produces broad band spectral noise. Because of its tendency to be lateralized to the left, it may be a source of left posterior artifact. Proper choice of reference electrode and a neck ground collar [38] are often helpful in reducing ECG artifact. Electrode, 60 Hz, and movement artifact are best handled by the accurate and secure application of low-impedance electrodes. We have found electrode attachment by collodion to specially prepared scalp areas a necessity. Naturally, accurate electrode placement by actual measurement is mandatory. During data gathering, the technologist should carefully monitor the subject's EEG for signs of state change, particularly drowsiness. Spectral content and distribution are quite different for drowsiness and sleep than for waking. The comparison of a drowsy normal subject to an awake control group will result in the appearance of abnormality just as for classic EEG.

Before data are submitted for spectral analysis, each segment should be visually inspected for residual artifact and flagged for elimination should it be found. Sampling rate for spectral analysis should be set at least twice that of the highest frequency present. Since the highest frequency is usually produced by muscle and extends to slightly above 100 Hz, sampling rates over 200 Hz are desired and 256 Hz per channel are typical. Less frequent sampling rates cause high frequencies to appear falsely as low frequencies, an effect known as aliasing. Prior to signal averaging for EP, at the very least, one should set a threshold voltage which would cause segment elimination for overvoltage artifact.

Despite the researcher's best efforts, total or even substantial elimination of artifact from the data of all subjects may be impossible. However, all is not lost, since artifact can be recognized in topographic maps by its spatial/spectral signature much as it is visually recognized and consciously ignored during standard EEG evaluation. Single channel noise on the map stands out by its severe spatial restriction to one electrode location, just as it does on EEG paper tracings. Muscle activity manifests itself by a broad band increase of beta activity, generally increasing at higher frequencies. Moreover, it is primarily seen to be maximal over the physical extent of the offending muscle, and greatest in the scalp periphery. Thus an asymmetry of beta, maximal at the scalp periphery and more for beta 5 than beta 1, would be suspect as muscle activity. Similarly, eye blink artifact is maximal in the prefrontal electrodes, primarily in the delta and theta ranges. Just as it becomes simpler to appreciate the real data structure by topographic mapping, so artifacts can be more easily recognized by their topographic signatures.

The ultimate test for artifact is to perform the same statistical comparison on the artifact channels as for the standard 10-20 channels. If apparent subject-group or between-group difference is greater in these artifact channels than in the adjacent scalp channels, the case for artifact contamination is strong indeed.

Thus, topographic mapping is not all artifact; however, great care is needed to achieve optimal artifact reduction. In our opinion, the results are worth the effort.

IS TOPOGRAPHIC MAPPING READY FOR CLINICAL APPLICATION?

Over the past four years the BEAM laboratory of the Seizure Unit at Children's Hospital Medical Center, Boston, has performed more than 1000 clinical studies involving topographic mapping. Such studies are reimbursable by Blue Cross of Massachusetts and most common insurance carriers. Brain electrical activity mapping as a "new technology" was investigated in detail by the federally funded Health Planning Council of Boston and approved. Thus it is our opinion and the opinion of a blue ribbon panel of health experts that topographic mapping of neurophysiologic data is indeed ready for general clinical use.

In our experience the typical referral is that of a patient with disturbed behavior (e.g., seizure? [32, 33], emotional dysfunction? [35–37], early encephalopathy or dementia? [18, 42]) who has a normal CT scan and often a normal neurological examination. The question posed is whether the patient's brain electrical activity is abnormal, and the findings are taken as evidence for or against organic brain disease.

How topographic mapping is used may best be illustrated by two brief clinical case presentations.

Case 1

A 21-year-old white man was employed and functioning normally until four years prior to study, when he was involved in a minor automobile accident where he struck his forehead on the vehicle's windshield as it abruptly halted. There was no loss of consciousness, and he was dismissed from the emergency room with a normal examination and skull x-ray. His subsequent work performance was inadequate; he became clinically depressed and began to hear voices. He was hospitalized in several major mental institutions where he was given a total of three CT scans, all normal, and two EEGs, which showed nondiagnostic minor abnormalities (slight theta slowing). He was originally diagnosed as a paranoid schizophrenic. Because he failed to respond to typical pharmacological therapy, he was eventually transferred to a Harvard psychiatric teaching hospital and additional tests were ordered. A CT scan and standard EEG were again normal. BEAM results, illustrated in Plate 27 and described in the accompanying legend, suggested bihemispheric abnormality of a type associated with irritable cortex [32]. The left frontal/right posterior abnormalities were taken as possible evidence of a coup/contracoup head injury. Because of the irritable nature of the electrophysiological abnormality, carbamazepine was started. The patient's response was rapid, wth cessation of hallucinations within three days. Ten days later he was discharged from a mental institution for the first time in four years.

Case 2

A 29-year-old white woman was referred for evaluation of depression and "chronic ruminative condition." Although she graduated at the top of her class in college, she was unable to hold a job. She was preoccupied with concerns over her mental state and was particularly worried that she was not as "good inside" as she may have appeared to be to others. She had seen several psychiatrists for this condition with only minor improvement. She was referred to our laboratory for a BEAM evaluation. As illustrated in Plate 28 and described in the accompanying legend, her EEG was within normal limits. However, the spectral and EP data demonstrated marked bitemporal abnormalities. As a result of the BEAM findings, she was referred for a neurological examination and CT scan. Although her neurological examination was normal, the patient was hyperverbose, kept a diary, was excessively serious, and never smiled. She denied religious conversion but was often concerned about how religion failed to appropriately address issues which she thought were critical. She reported sexual behavior that ranged from prolonged celibacy to promiscuity. She denied "seizures" or "epilepsy" but admitted "fainting" three times at ages 10, 11, and 13. Each faint involved the feeling of a hot poker up her spine and a strange feeling in her mouth and throat prevented speech, followed by loss of consciousness. These were interpreted as evidence for partial complex seizures. She was ultimately diagnosed as having the "personality of temporal lobe epilepsy" syndrome [1] and was started on long-term anticonvulsant therapy. After five months of treatment she was considered much improved. A subsequent CT scan was normal.

Case 1 (see Plate 27) is a patient who suffered a minor head injury which appeared to provoke a syndrome resembling paranoid schizophrenia with hallucinations. Only by topographic mapping was a pattern of abnormality recognized that led to more appropriate and effective pharmacotherapy. Case 2 (Plate 28) is a patient with behavioral disturbance (depression and excessive rumination) whose organic component (temporal lobe) was first recognized by topographic mapping and confirmed by neurological history and examination. These two cases represent the ways in which topographic mapping of neurophysiological data can be useful in complex diagnostic situations.

Recently we have been investigating the value of sequential studies in patients with unstable neurological conditions. In collaboration with Dr. F. Hochberg of the Massachusetts General hospital, we have been performing serial studies on patients with glioblastoma multiforme after completion of chemotherapy. These patients typically respond well to therapy and become completely symptom free for a variable period (e.g., 4–24 months). The earlier their inevitable relapse is detected, the more likely re-treatment will be effective. Unfortunately, although CT scan is the most useful technique for initial diagnosis, it has not proved to be similarly valuable in detection of tumor recurrence. This appears due to the presence of residual tumor debris obscuring signs of regrowth. Serial BEAM studies have proved significantly more useful in early detection of recurrent glioblastoma than either CT scan or clinical examination (Duffy, Hochberg, McAnulty, manuscript in preparation). The value of serial studies in the follow-up of patients in coma or after cerebral vascular accident is now under investigation.

Topographic mapping, therefore, is indeed ready for clinical application —an opinion shared by us (on the basis of extensive clinical experience), a governmental panel of experts (on the basis of extensive invited testimony), and industry (as indicated by the increasing number of companies offering mapping systems). By no means, however, are the genuine cautions put forth by several contributors to this volume invalid. Successful clinical application of neurophysiologic cartography requires a number of critical elements: (1) adequate equipment — the ability to form, visualize, and manipulate topographic images with reasonable speed, the ability to provide control groups for statistical comparison, and the availability of artifact management software; (2) a skilled technologist — the requirements for accuracy and quality of electrode placement exceed that of routine EEG, and great care must be taken to reduce artifact and monitor state; (3) a specially trained neurophysiologist — one must be skilled in the recognition of cartographic artifact in addition to possessing skills in the reading of classic EEG and EP data.

WILL TOPOGRAPHIC MAPPING OBVIATE CLASSIC EEG?

Electroencephalography is a complex specialty. Following residency in neurology, neurosurgery, or psychiatry, one must invest a minimum of one year in an approved EEG training program. Following this, one or more years of experience are required to be truly competent, even more if one specializes, for example, in neonatal EEG. Accordingly, the development of a technology which could impact upon EEG interpretation raises the possibility of rendering classic electroencephalography (and electroencephalographers) obsolete. Equipment manufacturers are quick to attempt to exploit this possibility, often without discretion. Quite naturally, a reaction—often quite overt— builds among electroencephalographers who fear for their specialty.

In our opinion such claims and fears are both quite unjustified. For although topographic mapping shows promise of becoming a major adjunct to EEG, it will never replace the technology. As of this writing, no algorithm appears capable of extracting from the EEG all the diagnostic information which the human eye can perceive. As we have discussed, spike detection algorithms use the human eye as their benchmark measure of accuracy. Thus clinical epileptology will continue to rely upon visually interpreted EEGs. In our BEAM laboratory a 28-channel EEG is collected throughout any study and separately interpreted.

For conditions where assessment of background spectral content is required, topographic mapping with SPM has proven a major adjunct. But, here also, visual inspection remains of value. Ultimately, a trained electroencephalographer must interpret the entire data set and make appropriate recommendations. In our opinion the only "diagnostic device" in clinical neurophysiology is the physician. We are a long way from *automatically* sorting and assigning significance to the massive data sets produced during clinical studies.

Furthermore, topographic mapping is a secondary process where the primary process is the decision of "what to map." One can map spikes, but someone must detect them and verify their authenticity. Spectral content can be mapped and analyzed, but the meaning of outcome must be interpreted in light of disease, state, residual artifact, etc. No doubt there exist EEG features we are sensitive to when we inspect EEG but have not yet quantified so as to facilitate mapping. Thus, far from obviating electroencephalography, topographic mapping extends the field. Moreover, only electroencephalographers with additional specialized training can appropriately employ topographic mapping in clinical settings.

One area where topographic mapping may impact upon clinical neurophysiology is that of long-latency EPs. Current clinical practice emphasizes short-latency EPs, seldom beyond 50 msec. Long-latency EPs, lasting up to 512 msec and beyond, have been largely the purview of the physiological psychologists. As shown in Case 2, topographic mapping of long-latency EPs can produce much information of clinical value.

Thus the advent of topographic mapping will increase both the complexity and utility of the practice of clinical electroencephalography (and neurophysiology), and will enlarge rather than diminish the field.

HOW MANY ELECTRODES SHOULD BE USED AND HOW SHOULD MISSING VALUES BE INTERPOLATED?

The appropriate number and placement of electrodes is a theoretical and practical issue. If it were technically feasible, 1024 scalp electrodes might be employed in a 32 by 32 grid. In such circumstances, minimal or no interpolation would be required for imaging and no scalp region would be left unexplored. However, anyone with practical experience in clinical neurophysiology appreciates how, with today's technical capabilities, this could be accomplished only as a "tour de force." Typically, laboratories performing topographic mapping employ from 12 to 45 scalp electrodes. Thus electrode placement and interpolation algorithms assume great importance.

To address the question of the optimal number of electrodes, one would wish for a scalp map of "information" plotted in x and y coordinates. A spatial frequency analysis would dictate electrode placement density on the basis of a two-dimensional extension of the Nyquist theorem. Unfortunately, no such map of information now exists. Moreover, there would theoretically be different maps for each experimental state and/or analytical objective. Creation of a fine-grained topographic map of the somatosensory EP to stimulation of individual fingers would require dense packing of electrodes [10]. In contrast, detection and assessment of a diffuse encephalopathy might be accomplished with relatively few electrodes. Any single universally applicable answer to the question of how many electrodes should be used in topographic mapping is unlikely. The first qualification must always be, "For what purpose" are we engaged in mapping?

Despite the absence of a theoretical model, empirical evidence does seem to place a minimum on the number of electrodes to be used in clinical applications. Following the model of classic EEG, the basic set of 19 scalp electrodes in the international 10-20 system montage gives equal weight to all areas, including the midline, where many activities are maximal. Schemes to reduce electrode number often call for the exclusion of electrodes where artifact is often maximal (FP1, FP2, T3, T4, Fz). In our clinical experience, midline electrodes are essential for symmetry estimates. Artifact-prone electrodes are needed to help estimate the presence of artifact in adjacent electrodes. In recent research, we have added eight additional electrodes in the center of rectangular regions such as that bounded by C4, T4, T6, and P4. We have also used one additional electrode at Oz for a total of 28. To this we add four artifact electrodes to bring our current electrode total up to 32. Various other schemes for electrode placement and number are discussed by other researchers in this book.

We noted a big improvement in clinical data visibility as we went from 16 to 20 scalp electrodes but so far we have not noted a substantial difference between 20 and 28. Until further data accumulates, we would recommend that clinical mapping systems accommodate a minimum of 32 channels, that a grid based upon the international 10-20 system be used for clinical screening, but that the system be sufficiently flexible to permit the placement of all 32 electrodes in a denser grid for special purposes (such as spike localization). Algorithms for interpolation and filling of empty areas between electrodes have employed three-point linear [11], four-point [26], polynomial approximations [9], and inverse of cubic distance [Etevenon, Chapter 6]. There seems to be little theoretical difference between the three- and four-point methods. Both assume that the best predictors of activity at an unknown locus are the values at the nearest (three or four) electrodes. Rapid computational algorithms exist for both methods. We have chosen the three point method because it is easier to break down irregularly outlined regions to be displayed into a series of triangles than squares. Other approaches weigh electrodes beyond the nearest three or four and assume some underlying topological model of brain electrical activity distribution to calculate values at unknown locations. Although all interpolation techniques appear to provide satisfactory images for purposes of visual inspection we have found empirically that multichannel approximation methods, such as polynomial approximation, are no more and are often less accurate than the simpler linear "nearest three electrode" method. This has been determined by comparing the results of each approximation with the real value obtained from an extra electrode placed at the location to be predicted. One advantage of the three point linear method is that under ordinary circumstances the underlying triangular structures used for interpolation are invisible; however, when single electrode artifact is present, triangular irregularities stand out. With the multichannel approximation methods artifact tends to be smoothed and thereby harder to identify. Until the relative merits of the various interpolation algorithms have been more thoroughly clarified, it would be wise to use them primarily for imaging purposes. If a finer grained spatial information is required the best solution would be to increase the number of electrodes rather than to refine the interpolation algorithms.

The hope is, of course, that advances in analog to digital converter technology, amplifier miniaturization, and cost will be paralleled by advances in electrode miniaturization and speed of application. Perhaps application of hundreds of electrodes will someday be simple and rapid, thereby reducing concerns about electrode placement and interpolation.

WHAT REFERENCE ELECTRODES SHOULD BE EMPLOYED?

Concern over the differential effects that result from the placement of reference electrodes has been a point of continuing interest and debate since the beginning of clinical electroencephalography. Early disagreements concerning the use of "unipolar" versus "bipolar" EEG recording techniques now see their parallel in debates concerning the use of physical reference versus "reference-free" techniques (e.g., average reference, Laplacian, field strength). Indeed, the Laplacian technique is sensitive to field curvature and may be thought of as a "two-dimensional bipolar" recording. It is unnecessary to summarize the many opinions, in this book and elsewhere, on the theoretical advantages of one technique over another. In our opinion, each has merit for specific situations but none is yet worthy of universal application. For example, the average reference technique shows merit for physiological investigations in normal subjects when electrodes are densely placed over a limited scalp region. On the other hand, when the whole scalp is studied and pathological spatial discontinuities exist, reference averaging may artifactually change nonpathological regions.

Our solution is to carry along sufficient information to reconstruct and remap data using alternative referencing techniques. We routinely record scalp electrode data referential to earlobes. However, we are able to reconstruct a midfacial or midposterior neck reference by suitable off-line recombinations.

Furthermore, we have implemented Hjorth's Laplacian approximation algorithm. So far, it is clear that no single referencing technique is adequate and that the ability to shift reference points aids in more accurately pinpointing lesions. The Laplacian techinque tends to constrict the spatial extent of topographic features yet simultaneously increases the overall image complexity. This is an interesting parallel to the role of bipolar recording in EEG, which is shown by its proponents to aid in localization but claimed by its detractors to distort waveform morphology.

In summary, we think that the ability to choose different electrode referencing algorithms will prove to be an important feature of analytic software and an important facet for the neurophysiologist as he employs cartography in clinical applications.

CONCLUSION

It is usual for a critic or expert to conclude his or her comments with a statement of cautious optimism moderated by the caveat that more carefully designed studies are needed before a final judgment can be rendered. This is a universal formula that is absolutely applicable to brain electrical activity mapping in general and to clinical cartography in particular.

On the other hand, I would like to suggest that with our sophisticated hardware and our understanding of field theory and statistics, we, as modern neurophysiologists, have come a considerable distance. It is now time to test our diverse approaches and hypotheses in the theater of clinical medicine. After all, if cartographic analysis is to make a lasting contribution, one area will be in the detection and description of neurological disease. We stand collectively on a great threshold, and the time has come to take a big step.

REFERENCES

1. Bear, D.M. Temporal lobe epilepsy: a syndrome of sensory-limbic hyperconnection. Cortex 1979; 15:357–384.
2. Bingham, C., Godfrey, M.D., and Tukey, J.W. Modern techniques of power spectrum estimation. IEEE Trans. Audio Electroacoust. 1967; AV-15:56–66.
3. Blumhardt, L.D., Barrett, G., Kriss, A., and Halliday, A.M. The pattern-evoked potential in lesions of the posterior visual pathways. Ann. N.Y. Acad. Sci. 1982; 388:264–289.
4. Bickford, R.G., Fleming, N.I., and Billinger, T.W. Compressing of EEG data by isometric power spectral plates. Electroenceph. Clin. Neurophysiol.1971; 31: 631–636.
5. Childers, D.G., ed. Modern Spectrum Analysis. New York: IEEE Press, 1978.
6. Childers, D.G., Perry, N.W., and Bourne, J.R. Spatio-temporal measures of cortical functioning in normal and abnormal vision. Comput. Biomed. Res. 1972; 5: 114–130.

7. Cooley, J.W., and Tukey, J.W. An algorithm for the machine calculation of Fourier series. Math. Comp. 1965; 19:297–301.

8. Davenport, W.B., and Root, W.L. Random Signals and Noise. New York: McGraw-Hill, 1958.

9. Dubinsky, J., and Barlow, J.S. A simple dot-density topogram for EEG. Electroenceph. Clin. Neurophysiol. 1980; 48:473–477.

10. Duff, T.A. Topography of scalp recorded potentials by stimulation of the digits. Electroenceph. Neurophysiol. 1980; 49:452–460.

11. Duffy, F.H., Burchfiel, J.L., Lombroso, C.T. Brain electrical activity mapping (BEAM): A new method for extending the clinical utility of EEG and evoked potential data. Ann. Neurol. 1979; 5:309–321.

12. Duffy, F.H., Bartels, P.H., Burchfiel, J.L. Significance probability mapping: An aid in the topographic analysis of brain electrical activity. Electroenceph. Clin. Neurophysiol. 1981; 51:455–462.

13. Duffy, F.H. Brain electrical activity mapping (BEAM): Computerized access to complex brain function. Int. J. Neurosci. 1981; 13:55–65.

14. Duffy, F.H. Topographic display of evoked potentials-clinical applications of brain electrical activity mapping (BEAM). Ann. N. Y. Acad. Sci. 1982; 388: 183–196.

15. Duffy, F.H., Als, H. Neurophysiological assessment of the neonate: An approach combining brain electrical activity mapping (BEAM) with behavioral assessment (APIB). In T.B. Brazelton, B.M. Lester, eds. New approach to developmental screening of infants. New York: Elsevier North Holland, 1983; 175–196.

16. Duffy, F.H., Jensen, F., Erba, G., Burchfiel, J.L., Lombroso, C.T. Extraction of clinical information from electroencephalographic background activity—the combined use of brain electrical activity mapping and intravenous sodium thiopental. Ann. Neurol. 1984; 15(1):22–30.

17. Duffy, F.H., Albert, M., McAnulty, G., Garvey, A.J. age-related differences in brain electrical activity in mapping of healthy subjects. Ann. Neurol. 1984; 16: 430–438.

18. Duffy, F.H., Albert, M.S., McAnulty, G. Brain electrical activity in patients with presenile and senile dementia of the Alzheimer's type. Ann. Neurol. 1984; 16: 439–448.

19. Duffy, F.H., Denckla, M.B., Bartels, P.H., Sandini, G., Keissling, L.S. Dyslexia: Automated diagnosis by computerized classification of brain electrical activity. 1980; Ann. Neurol. 7:421–428.

20. Duffy, F.H., McAnulty, G.B. Brain electrical activity in mapping (BEAM): The search for a physiological signature of dyslexia. In F.H. Duffy, N. Geschwind, eds., Dyslexia: A Neuroscientific Approach to Clinical Evaluation. Boston: Little, Brown, 1985; 105–122.

21. Duffy, F.H., Denckla, M.B., McAnulty, G., Holmes, J.M. Dyslexia: Neurophysiologic difference among language based subgroups. (submitted).

22. Estrin, T., and Uzgalis, R. Computer display of spatio-temporal EEG patterns. IEEE Trans. Biomed. Eng. 1969; BME-16:192–196.

23. Flanagan, D., ed. Computer Software. Sci. Am. September 1984; 251.

24. Gotman, J. Automatic recognition of epileptic seizures in the EEG. Electroenceph. Clin. Neurophysiol 1982; 54:53–540.

25. Gotman, J., and Gloor, P. Automatic recognition and quantification of interectal epileptic activity in the human scalp. Electroenceph. Clin. Neurophysiol. 1976; 41: 513–529.

26. Gregory, D.L., and Wong, P.K. Topographical analysis of the centrotemporal discharges in benign rolandic epilepsy of childhood. Epilepsia 1984; 25:705–711.

27. Harner, R.N. Computer analysis and clinical EEG interpretation perspective and application. In G. Dolce, ed. CEAN: Computerized EEG Analysis. Stuttgart: Gustav Fischer, 1974; 337–343.

28. Harris, J.A., Melby, G.M., Bickford, R.G. Computer-controlled multidimensional display device for investigation and modeling of physiologic systems. Comput. Biomed. Res. 1969; 2:519–538.

29. Hjorth, B. An on-line transformation of EEG scalp potentials into orthogonal source derivation. Electroenceph. Clin. Neurophysiol. 1975; 39:526–530.

30. Kellaway, P., and Petersen, A. eds. Quantitative Studies in Epilepsy. New York: Raven Press, 1976.

31. Lassen, N.A., Ingvar, D.H., Skinhoj, E. Brain function and blood flow. Sci. Am. 1978; 239:62–71.

32. Lombroso, C.T., Duffy, F.H. Brain electrical activity mapping as an adjunct to CT scanning. In R. Canger, F. Angeleri, J.K. Perry, eds., Advances in epileptology: Proceedings of XIIIth Epilepsy International Symposium. New York: Raven Press, 1980; 83–88.

33. Lombroso, C.T., Duffy, F.H. Brain electrical activity mapping in the epilepsies. In H. Akimoto, H. Kazamatsuri, M. Seino, A. Ward, eds., Advances in epileptology, Proceedings of XIIIth Epilepsy International Symposium. New York: Raven Press, 1982; 173–179.

34. McCarley R.W., Winkelman, J.W., Duffy, F.H. Human cerebral potentials associated with REM sleep rapid eye movements: links to PGO waves and waking potentials. Brain Res. 1983; 274:359–364.

35. Morihisa, J.M., Duffy, F.H., Wyatt, R.J. Brain electrical activity mapping (BEAM) in schizophrenia patients. Arch. Gen. Psychiatry 1983; 40:719–728.

36. Morstyn, R., Duffy, F.H., McCarley, R.W. Altered P300 topography in schizophrenia. Arch. Gen. Psychiatry 1983; 40:729–734.

37. Morstyn, R., Duffy, F.H., McCarley, R.W. Altered topography of EEG spectral content in schizophrenia. Electroenceph. Clin. Neurophysiol. 1983; 56:263–271.

38. Nunez, P.L. Electric Fields of the Brain. New York: Oxford University Press, 1981.

39. Pargen, E. Modern Probability Theory and Its Applications. New York: John Wiley and Sons, 1960.

40. Rémond, A., ed. EEG Informatics. A Didactic Review of Methods and Applications of EEG Data Processing. Amsterdam: Elsevier, 1977.

41. Tukey, J.W. Exploratory Data Analysis. Addison-Wesley, Reading, Massachusetts: 1977.

42. Ueno, S., Matsuoka, T., Misoguchi, T., Nagashima, M., Cheng, C.L. Topographic computer display of abnormal EEG activities in patients with CNS disease. Mem. Fac. Enging. Kyushu Univ. 1975; 24: 3:196–209.

43. Walter, W.G., Shipton, H.W. A new topographic display system. Electroenceph. Clin. Neurophysiol. 1951; 3:281–292.

Index